WEIGHT IN AMERICA

OBESITY, EATING DISORDERS, AND OTHER HEALTH RISKS

ISSN 1551-2118

WEIGHT IN AMERICA
OBESITY, EATING DISORDERS, AND OTHER HEALTH RISKS

Barbara Wexler

INFORMATION PLUS® REFERENCE SERIES
Formerly Published by Information Plus, Wylie, Texas

GALE
CENGAGE Learning·

Farmington Hills, Mich • San Francisco • New York • Waterville, Maine
Meriden, Conn • Mason, Ohio • Chicago

GALE
CENGAGE Learning®

Weight in America: Obesity, Eating Disorders, and Other Health Risks

Barbara Wexler

Kepos Media, Inc.: Steven Long and Janice Jorgensen, Series Editors

Project Editors: Laura Avery, Tracie Moy

Rights Acquisition and Management: Ashley M. Maynard, Carissa Poweleit

Composition: Evi Abou-El-Seoud, Mary Beth Trimper

Manufacturing: Rita Wimberley

Cover photograph: © Marques/Shutterstock.com.

Gale
27500 Drake Rd.
Farmington Hills, MI 48331-3535

ISBN-13: 978-0-7876-5103-9 (set)
ISBN-13: 978-1-57302-706-9

ISSN 1551-2118

This title is also available as an e-book.
ISBN-13: 978-1-57302-710-6 (set)
Contact your Gale sales representative for ordering information.

Printed in the United States of America
1 2 3 4 5   20 19 18 17 16

TABLE OF CONTENTS

PREFACE

Weight in America: Obesity, Eating Disorders, and Other Health Risks is part of the *Information Plus Reference Series*. The purpose of each volume of the series is to present the latest facts on a topic of pressing concern in modern American life. These topics include the most controversial and studied social issues of the 21st century: abortion, capital punishment, care for the elderly, crime, the environment, health care, immigration, race and ethnicity, social welfare, women, youth, and many more. Although this series is written especially for high school and undergraduate students, it is an excellent resource for anyone in need of factual information on current affairs.

By presenting the facts, it is the intention of Gale, Cengage Learning, to provide its readers with everything they need to reach an informed opinion on current issues. To that end, there is a particular emphasis in this series on the presentation of scientific studies, surveys, and statistics. These data are generally presented in the form of tables, charts, and other graphics placed within the text of each book. Every graphic is directly referred to and carefully explained in the text. The source of each graphic is presented within the graphic itself. The data used in these graphics are drawn from the most reputable and reliable sources such as from the various branches of the U.S. government and from private organizations and associations. Every effort has been made to secure the most recent information available. Readers should bear in mind that many major studies take years to conduct and that additional years often pass before the data from these studies are made available to the public. Therefore, in many cases the most recent information available in 2016 is from 2013 or 2014. Older statistics are sometimes presented as well, if they are landmark studies or of particular interest and no more-recent information exists.

Although statistics are a major focus of the *Information Plus Reference Series*, they are by no means its only content. Each book also presents the widely held positions and important ideas that shape how the book's subject is discussed in the United States. These positions are explained in detail and, where possible, in the words of their proponents. Some of the other material to be found in these books includes historical background, descriptions of major events related to the subject, relevant laws and court cases, and examples of how these issues play out in American life. Some books also feature primary documents or have pro and con debate sections that provide the words and opinions of prominent Americans on both sides of a controversial topic. All material is presented in an evenhanded and unbiased manner; readers will never be encouraged to accept one view of an issue over another.

HOW TO USE THIS BOOK

The United States has a serious weight problem. The majority of Americans weigh more than they should, and roughly one-third are considered obese. Being overweight or obese has serious health consequences, and epidemic levels in the United States have had a major impact on society. Overweight and obesity, however, are not the only problems that Americans face when it comes to food. Some suffer from eating disorders, such as anorexia nervosa and bulimia nervosa, disorders that also have a devastating effect on health. This book brings together information from academic and governmental sources on myriad aspects of overweight, obesity, and eating disorders, including their prevalence in the United States, their consequences, public opinion about them, and preventive measures.

Weight in America: Obesity, Eating Disorders, and Other Health Risks consists of 11 chapters and three appendixes. Each chapter is devoted to a particular aspect of weight in the United States. For a summary of the information that is covered in each chapter, please see the synopses that are provided in the Table of Contents. Chapters generally begin with an overview of the basic facts and background information on the chapter's topic, then proceed to examine subtopics of particular interest. For example, Chapter 5: Dietary Treatment for Overweight and Obesity begins by tracing the history of dieting and describes selected milestones in diet and nutrition. This is followed by a discussion of popular diets in the 20th century and the first decades of the 21st century. The chapter also describes the development and use of nonnutritive sweeteners. It concludes with a discussion of the development of the 2015 Dietary Guidelines for Americans and information about how diets work and how to choose a weight-loss diet. Readers can find their way through a chapter by looking for the section and subsection headings, which are clearly set off from the text. They can also refer to the book's extensive Index if they already know what they are looking for.

Statistical Information

The tables and figures featured throughout *Weight in America: Obesity, Eating Disorders, and Other Health Risks* will be of particular use to readers in learning about this issue. These tables and figures represent an extensive collection of the most recent and important statistics on weight and related issues. For example, graphics cover the percentage of obese adults by state, race, and ethnicity; the prevalence of obesity among adults; the names found on ingredient labels for added sugars; dubious diet claims; and fruit and vegetable consumption rates of adults and adolescents. Gale, Cengage Learning, believes that making this information available to readers is the most important way to fulfill the goal of this book: to help readers understand the issues and controversies surrounding overweight and obesity in the United States and reach their own conclusions about them.

Each table or figure has a unique identifier appearing above it, for ease of identification and reference. Titles for the tables and figures explain their purpose. At the end of each table or figure, the original source of the data is provided.

To help readers understand these often complicated statistics, all tables and figures are explained in the text. References in the text direct readers to the relevant statistics. Furthermore, the contents of all tables and figures are fully indexed. Please see the opening section of the Index at the back of this volume for a description of how to find tables and figures within it.

Appendixes

Besides the main body text and images, *Weight in America: Obesity, Eating Disorders, and Other Health Risks* has three appendixes. The first is the Important Names and Addresses directory. Here, readers will find contact information for a number of government and private organizations that can provide further information on aspects of overweight and obesity and weight and eating disorders. The second appendix is the Resources section, which can also assist readers in conducting their own research. In this section, the author and editors of *Weight in America: Obesity, Eating Disorders, and Other Health Risks* describe some of the sources that were most useful during the compilation of this book. The final appendix is the detailed Index. It has been greatly expanded from previous editions and should make it even easier to find specific topics in this book.

COMMENTS AND SUGGESTIONS

The editors of the *Information Plus Reference Series* welcome your feedback on *Weight in America: Obesity, Eating Disorders, and Other Health Risks*. Please direct all correspondence to:

Editors
Information Plus Reference Series
27500 Drake Rd.
Farmington Hills, MI 48331-3535

CHAPTER 1
AMERICANS WEIGH IN OVER TIME

More die in the United States of too much food than of
too little.

—John Kenneth Galbraith, *The Affluent Society* (1998)

In 2015 Americans were about the heaviest since the
U.S. government started tracking patterns of body weight
of the U.S. adult population during the first half of the 20th
century. The Centers for Disease Control and Prevention
(CDC) reports in "Adult Obesity Facts" (September 21,
2015, http://www.cdc.gov/obesity/data/adult.html) that
roughly 35% (79 million) of adults in the United States
are considered obese. Despite billions of dollars spent on
diet programs, overweight and obesity are widespread
and increasingly prevalent throughout the United States.

Although Americans' body weight had been increasing incrementally during the last century, obesity skyrock-
eted between 1976–80 and 2015, from 15% to 34.9%. The
Trust for America's Health (TFAH; a nonprofit, nonpartisan organization working to make disease prevention a
national priority) and the Robert Wood Johnson Foundation report in *The State of Obesity* (2016, http://stateof
obesity.org) that although more than two-thirds (68.6%)
of American adults are either overweight or obese, after
three decades of steady increases, obesity rates in many
states appear to have leveled off. Nonetheless, every state
reports obesity rates greater than 20%.

An analysis of data from the CDC's 2014 Behavioral
Risk Factor Surveillance System reveals that the prevalence
of self-reported obesity was greater than 30% in 22 states
and between 25% and 29% in approximately half the states.
(See Figure 1.1.) (The prevalence rate is the number of
cases of a disease or condition present during a specified
interval, usually a year, divided by the population.)

In "Prevalence of Childhood and Adult Obesity in
the United States, 2011–2012" (*Journal of the American
Medical Association*, vol. 311, no. 8, February 26, 2014),
Cynthia L. Ogden et al. compare the prevalence of youth

and adult obesity data from the 2011–12 National Health
and Nutrition Examination Survey (NHANES) with data
from the 2003–04 NHANES. Although the overall prevalence of obesity among youth and adults was unchanged
from 2003 to 2012, there was a noticeable decrease in
obesity among children aged two to five years and an
increase in obesity among women aged 60 years and
older. Ogden et al. report that non-Hispanic African
Americans had the highest rates of obesity (47.8%),
compared with Asians (10.9%), non-Hispanic whites
(33.4%), and Hispanics (42%).

In the United States many researchers believe that
obesity is the second-leading cause of preventable death
after smoking. There is conclusive scientific evidence
that mortality (death) risk increases with increasing
weight and that even slightly overweight adults—people
of average height who are 10 to 20 pounds (4.5 to 9.1 kg)
above their ideal weight—are at increased risk of premature death. The rising prevalence of overweight and obesity not only foretells increasing adverse effects on health
and longevity but also guarantees increased costs for
medical care. Overweight and obesity increase the risk
of developing a range of ailments, including heart disease, stroke, selected cancers, sleep apnea (interrupted
breathing while sleeping), respiratory problems, osteoarthritis (loss of joint bone and cartilage), gallbladder disease, fatty liver disease (the deposition of fats, such as
triglycerides in the liver, which may lead to an enlarged
liver and elevated liver enzymes), and diabetes mellitus
(abnormally high blood glucose resulting from the body's
inability to use blood glucose for energy). The TFAH and
the Robert Wood Johnson Foundation observe in "Obesity Rates & Trends" (2016, stateofobesity.org/rates/)
that 10% of annual U.S. health care spending—between
$147 billion and $210 billion—is related to obesity and
that people who are obese spend 41% more on health care
than do healthy-weight people.

FIGURE 1.1

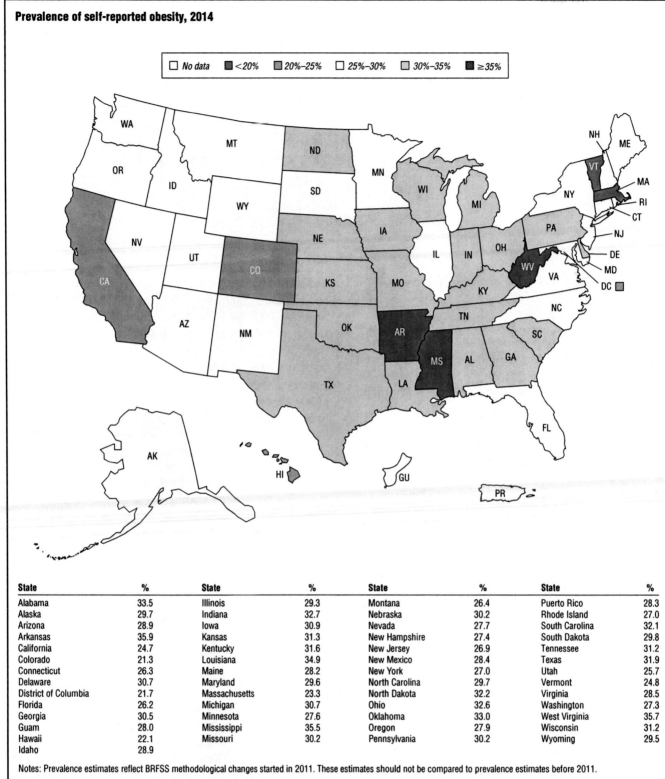

Prevalence of self-reported obesity, 2014

Legend: ☐ No data ▨ <20% ▨ 20%–25% ☐ 25%–30% ▨ 30%–35% ■ ≥35%

State	%	State	%	State	%	State	%
Alabama	33.5	Illinois	29.3	Montana	26.4	Puerto Rico	28.3
Alaska	29.7	Indiana	32.7	Nebraska	30.2	Rhode Island	27.0
Arizona	28.9	Iowa	30.9	Nevada	27.7	South Carolina	32.1
Arkansas	35.9	Kansas	31.3	New Hampshire	27.4	South Dakota	29.8
California	24.7	Kentucky	31.6	New Jersey	26.9	Tennessee	31.2
Colorado	21.3	Louisiana	34.9	New Mexico	28.4	Texas	31.9
Connecticut	26.3	Maine	28.2	New York	27.0	Utah	25.7
Delaware	30.7	Maryland	29.6	North Carolina	29.7	Vermont	24.8
District of Columbia	21.7	Massachusetts	23.3	North Dakota	32.2	Virginia	28.5
Florida	26.2	Michigan	30.7	Ohio	32.6	Washington	27.3
Georgia	30.5	Minnesota	27.6	Oklahoma	33.0	West Virginia	35.7
Guam	28.0	Mississippi	35.5	Oregon	27.9	Wisconsin	31.2
Hawaii	22.1	Missouri	30.2	Pennsylvania	30.2	Wyoming	29.5
Idaho	28.9						

Notes: Prevalence estimates reflect BRFSS methodological changes started in 2011. These estimates should not be compared to prevalence estimates before 2011.

SOURCE: "Prevalence of Self-Reported Obesity among U.S. Adults by State and Territory, BRFSS, 2014," in *Overweight and Obesity: Data, Trends, and Maps*, Centers for Disease Control and Prevention, National Center for Chronic Disease Prevention and Health Promotion, Division of Nutrition, Physical Activity, and Obesity, September 11, 2015, http://www.cdc.gov/obesity/data/prevalence-maps.html (accessed September 25, 2015)

Overweight and obesity also exact a personal toll, with affected individuals at increased risk for emotional, psychological, and social problems. Overweight children, teens, and adults suffer from depression, low self-esteem, and other mental health and emotional problems more than their normal-weight counterparts. Along with a physical inability to participate in many activities, people who are overweight or obese may encounter weight-based stigmatization, bias, and discrimination in school and at the workplace and may be excluded from social opportunities.

TRENDS IN U.S. BIRTH WEIGHTS

Although the ideal birth weight varies based on the expectant mother's ethnicity, for women in the United States the average ideal birth weight is approximately 7 pounds, 8 ounces (3,402 g). In the United States the percentage of babies born with low birth weight (LBW)—less than 5 pounds, 8 ounces (2,500 g)—rose between 1990 and 2010. (See Table 1.1.) According to Joyce A. Martin et al., in "Births: Final Data for 2013" (*National Vital Statistics Reports*, vol. 64, no. 1, January 15, 2015), the LBW rate declined slightly from 8.2% in 2010 to 8% in 2013. The percentage of infants with very low birth weight (VLBW)—less than 3 pounds, 4 ounces (1,500 g)—remained steady between 1990 (1.3%) and 2013 (1.4%). In 2013 more than twice as many non-Hispanic African American mothers gave birth to LBW and VLBW infants, 13.1% and 2.9%, respectively, than did non-Hispanic white mothers (7% LBW and 1.1% VLBW).

LBW and VLBW are major predictors of infant morbidity (illness or disease) and mortality. In "CDC Grand Rounds: Public Health Approaches to Reducing U.S. Infant Mortality" (*Morbidity and Mortality Weekly*

TABLE 1.1

Percentage of low birth weights and very low birth weights by race and Hispanic origin, selected years, 1981–2013

Year	Very low birthweight[a] All races[c]	Non-Hispanic White[d]	Non-Hispanic Black[d]	Hispanic[e]	Low birthweight[b] All races[c]	Non-Hispanic White[d]	Non-Hispanic Black[d]	Hispanic[e]
				Percent				
2013	1.41	1.11	2.90	1.21	8.02	6.98	13.08	7.09
2012	1.42	1.13	2.94	1.22	7.99	6.97	13.18	6.97
2011	1.44	1.14	2.99	1.20	8.10	7.09	13.33	7.02
2010	1.45	1.16	2.98	1.20	8.15	7.14	13.53	6.97
2009	1.45	1.16	3.06	1.19	8.16	7.19	13.61	6.94
2008	1.46	1.18	3.01	1.20	8.18	7.22	13.71	6.96
2007	1.49	1.19	3.20	1.21	8.22	7.28	13.90	6.93
2006	1.49	1.20	3.15	1.19	8.26	7.32	13.97	6.99
2005	1.49	1.21	3.27	1.20	8.19	7.29	14.02	6.88
2004	1.48	1.20	3.15	1.20	8.08	7.20	13.74	6.79
2003	1.45	1.18	3.12	1.16	7.93	7.04	13.55	6.69
2002	1.46	1.17	3.15	1.17	7.82	6.91	13.39	6.55
2001	1.44	1.17	3.08	1.14	7.68	6.76	13.07	6.47
2000	1.43	1.14	3.10	1.14	7.57	6.60	13.13	6.41
1999	1.45	1.15	3.18	1.14	7.62	6.64	13.23	6.38
1998	1.45	1.15	3.11	1.15	7.57	6.55	13.17	6.44
1997	1.42	1.12	3.05	1.13	7.51	6.47	13.11	6.42
1996	1.37	1.08	3.02	1.12	7.39	6.36	13.12	6.28
1995	1.35	1.04	2.98	1.11	7.32	6.20	13.21	6.29
1994	1.33	1.01	2.99	1.08	7.28	6.06	13.34	6.25
1993	1.33	1.00	2.99	1.06	7.22	5.92	13.43	6.24
1992[f]	1.29	0.94	2.97	1.04	7.08	5.73	13.40	6.10
1991[f]	1.29	0.94	2.97	1.02	7.12	5.72	13.62	6.15
1990[g]	1.27	0.93	2.93	1.03	6.97	5.61	13.32	6.06
1989[h]	1.28	0.93	2.97	1.05	7.05	5.62	13.61	6.18
1988	1.24	—	—	—	6.93	—	—	—
1987	1.24	—	—	—	6.90	—	—	—
1986	1.21	—	—	—	6.81	—	—	—
1985	1.21	—	—	—	6.75	—	—	—
1984	1.19	—	—	—	6.72	—	—	—
1983	1.19	—	—	—	6.82	—	—	—
1982	1.18	—	—	—	6.75	—	—	—
1981	1.16	—	—	—	6.81	—	—	—

—Data not available.
[a]Less than 1,500 grams (3 lb 4 oz).
[b]Less than 2,500 grams (5 lb 8 oz).
[c]Includes races other than white and black and origin not stated.
[d]Race and Hispanic origin are reported separately on birth certificates. Persons of Hispanic origin may be of any race. Race categories are consistent with 1977 Office of Management and Budget standards. Forty-four states and the District of Columbia reported multiple-race data for 2013 that were bridged to single-race categories for comparability with other states. Multiple-race reporting areas vary for 2003–2013.
[e]Includes all persons of Hispanic origin of any race.
[f]Data by Hispanic origin exclude New Hampshire, which did not report Hispanic origin.
[g]Data by Hispanic origin exclude New Hampshire and Oklahoma, which did not report Hispanic origin.
[h]Data by Hispanic origin exclude New Hampshire, Oklahoma, and Louisiana, which did not report Hispanic origin.

SOURCE: Adapted from Joyce A. Martin et al., "Table 24. Very Preterm and Preterm Births, and Very Low Birthweight and Low Birthweight Births, by Race and Hispanic Origin of Mother: United States, 1981–2013," in "Births: Final Data for 2013," *National Vital Statistics Reports*, vol. 64, no.1, January 15, 2015, http://www.cdc.gov/nchs/data/nvsr/nvsr64/nvsr64_01.pdf (accessed September 25, 2015)

Report, vol. 62, no. 31, August 9, 2013), the CDC reports that the decline observed in infant mortality since 1950 is largely due to fewer deaths associated with low birth weights. In 1950 an infant with VLBW had a 10% to 15% chance of survival, while by 2008 an infant with VLBW had more than a 60% chance of surviving the neonatal period (the first 27 days of life). The risk of delivering an LBW infant is greatest among the youngest and oldest mothers; however, many of the LBW births among older mothers are attributable to their higher rates of multiple births.

Birth Weight Influences Risk of Disease

Although the relationship between birth weight and development of disease in adulthood is an emerging field of research, and scientists cannot yet fully explain how and why birth weight is a predictor of health and illness in later life, mounting evidence indicates that both LBW and higher-than-average birth weight are linked to future health problems. For example, Janne Boone-Heinonen et al. note in "Overcoming Birth Weight: Can Physical Activity Mitigate Birth Weight–Related Differences in Adiposity?" (*Pediatric Obesity*, May 19, 2015) that low and high birth weights are associated with an increased risk of obesity-related disease.

Research reveals that LBW infants are more likely than normal-weight infants to develop disease in later life. Male infants with LBW who gain weight rapidly before their first birthday appear to be at the highest risk. Researchers hypothesize that LBW infants have fewer muscle cells at birth and that rapid weight gain during the first year of life may lead to disproportionate amounts of fat to muscle and above-average body mass. Infants with LBW who later develop above-average body mass have an increased risk for developing diseases such as type 2 diabetes (an inability to produce sufficient insulin, the hormone that regulates blood glucose), hypertension (high blood pressure), and cardiovascular disease (diseases of the heart and blood vessels).

Keith M. Godfrey, Hazel M. Inskip, and Mark A. Hanson find in "The Long-Term Effects of Prenatal Development on Growth and Metabolism" (*Seminars in Reproductive Medicine*, vol. 29, no. 3, May 2011) that LBW and poor rates of infant growth and development are associated with an increased risk for cardiovascular disease, type 2 diabetes, and osteoporosis (thinning of the bones that makes them more likely to fracture). The risk of developing these diseases increases when restricted early growth and development are followed by increased weight gain during childhood. The researchers also note that abnormally high birth weights are associated with an increased risk for obesity and type 2 diabetes.

LBW has also been linked to the development of asthma. In "Is the Association between Low Birth Weight and Asthma Independent of Genetic and Shared Environmental Factors?" (*American Journal of Epidemiology*, vol. 169, no. 11, June 1, 2009), a study of 21,588 twins, Eduardo Villamor, Anastasia Iliadou, and Sven Cnattingius find that LBW is associated with asthma during childhood and adult life.

High birth weight (HBW) is also associated with an increased risk for childhood cancer. Kate A. O'Neill et al. observe in "Infant Birthweight and Risk of Childhood Cancer: International Population-Based Case Control Studies of 40 000 Cases" (*International Journal of Epidemiology*, vol. 24, no. 1, 2015) that HBW is associated with about half of childhood cancers.

Some evidence indicates that birth weight is related to a risk of developing breast cancer. However, Zorana J. Andersen et al. report in "Birth Weight, Childhood Body Mass Index, and Height in Relation to Mammographic Density and Breast Cancer: A Register-Based Cohort Study" (*Breast Cancer Research*, vol. 16, no. 1, January 20, 2014) that their study of 13,572 women aged 50 to 69 years finds that birth weight is not associated with the risk of developing breast cancer in adulthood. In fact, the researchers indicate that overweight in childhood was associated with a reduced risk for breast cancer.

In "Birth Size, Infant Weight Gain, and Motor Development Influence Adult Physical Performance" (*Medicine and Science in Sports and Exercise*, vol. 41, no. 6, June 2009), Charlotte L. Ridgway et al. look at birth weight as an influence on adult physical performance measures, including muscle strength, endurance, and aerobic fitness. The researchers find that LBW is associated with impaired aerobic fitness and a higher resting pulse rate in adulthood, independent of adult body size. Higher birth weight is associated with earlier motor development, as evidenced in standing unaided and walking at younger ages. It is also associated with increased handgrip strength in adolescents, young adults, and even in older adults, which suggests that the effects of birth weight on physical performance may be lifelong. Higher birth weight, greater infant weight gain, and earlier motor development were independently associated with muscle strength and endurance, whereas higher birth weight and lower infant weight gain were associated with higher levels of aerobic fitness. Ridgway et al. explain that the link between higher birth weight and greater muscle strength and endurance may in part reflect the relationship between birth weight and lean muscle in adults—people with higher birth weights are likely to have increased muscle mass. Similarly, the relationship between lower infant weight gain and improved aerobic fitness may be attributable to the fact that rapid weight gain during infancy may preferentially produce fat rather than lean muscle tissue.

The only action that can alter the birth weight of an infant is if the mother modifies her weight gain during the pregnancy. In 2016 most health professionals concurred that for normal-weight women the optimal weight gain during pregnancy ranged between 15 and 25 pounds (6.8 and 11.3 kg) of fat and lean mass. Furthermore, the landmark study "Composition of Gestational Weight Gain Impacts Maternal Fat Retention and Infant Birth Weight" (*American Journal of Obstetrics and Gynecology*, vol. 189, no. 5, November 2003) conducted by Nancy F. Butte et al. of the Children's Nutrition Research Center in Houston, Texas, reveals that a newborn's birth weight and the mother's postpregnancy weight are influenced not only by how much weight is gained during the pregnancy but also by the source of the excess weight. The researchers conducted body scans of 63 women before, during, and after their pregnancies and recorded changes in the women's weight from water, protein, fat, and potassium—a marker for changes in muscle tissue, which is one component of lean mass. Butte et al. find that increases in lean mass, and not fat mass, appeared to influence infant size. Independent of how much fat the women gained during pregnancy, only lean body mass increased the birth weight of the infants, with women who gained more lean body mass giving birth to larger infants.

In "Birth Weight and Long-Term Overweight Risk: Systematic Review and a Meta-analysis Including 643,902 Persons from 66 Studies and 26 Countries Globally" (*PLoS One*, vol. 7, no. 10, October 17, 2012), Karen Schellong et al. reviewed 66 studies to analyze the relationship between birth weight and later risk of overweight. The researchers find that LBW is associated with lower long-term risk of overweight, while HBW predisposes for later overweight. Schellong et al. suggest that managing expectant mothers' nutrition and weight gain may be "a promising strategy to lower overweight risk for the long term, globally."

EARLY NUTRITION INCREASES RISK OF OBESITY. Research demonstrates that LBW and low weight gain during infancy are associated with coronary heart disease. Similarly, research indicates that rapid weight gain in infancy is shown to predict obesity in childhood. In 2004 a landmark study funded by the National Institutes of Health and conducted at the Children's Hospital of Philadelphia, the University of Pennsylvania School of Medicine, and the University of Iowa Fomon Infant Nutrition Unit found that among formula-fed infants, increased weight gain during the first week of life predicted adult obesity two to three decades later. This finding is important because it not only helps predict which infants are at higher risk for adult obesity but also identifies a target for obesity prevention efforts.

Lise Geisler Bjerregaard et al. review in "Effects of Body Size and Change in Body Size from Infancy through Childhood on Body Mass Index in Adulthood" (*International Journal of Obesity*, vol. 38, no. 10, October 2014) the weight for 1,633 subjects who were followed from birth through age 42 and weighed at birth, two weeks, and one, two, three, four, and six months. As they aged, the subjects' weights were obtained from school records. The researchers pinpoint the period between birth and age three months as potentially critical because weight gain during this period was associated with adulthood overweight status. The researchers' findings support the recommendation by the American Academy of Pediatrics that infants should be exclusively breast-fed for the first six months of life. Among the many health benefits associated with breast-feeding is the fact that breast-fed babies are less likely than formula-fed babies to become obese adults. This finding also suggests that monitoring and controlling weight gain shortly after birth may help prevent future obesity.

A high-calorie diet in infancy predicts not only faster early weight gain but also greater fat mass in childhood, which in turn increases the risk of obesity in adulthood. In "Nutrition in Infancy and Long-Term Risk of Obesity: Evidence from 2 Randomized Controlled Trials" (*American Journal of Nutrition*, vol. 92, no. 5, November 2010), Atul Singhal et al. report the results of a rigorous long-term study that followed infants randomly assigned to receive either a control formula or a formula containing more protein and calories than the control formula. When the children were examined at ages five and eight, those who had received the nutrient-rich formula had increased fat mass.

DEFINING AND ASSESSING IDEAL WEIGHT, OVERWEIGHT, AND OBESITY

Historically, the determination of desirable, healthy, or ideal weights have been derived from demographic and actuarial statistics (data compiled to assess insurance risk and formulate insurance premiums). The National Center for Health Statistics (NCHS) compiles and analyzes demographic data (the heights and weights of a representative sample of the U.S. population) to develop standards for desirable weight. In 1943 the Metropolitan Life Insurance Company (MetLife) introduced standard weight-for-height tables for men and women based on an analysis of actuarial data. The MetLife weight-for-height tables assisted adults in determining if their weight was within an appropriate range for height and frame size. Revised in 1959 and 1983, the tables were based on actuarial data, in which desirable or ideal weight was defined as the weight for height that was associated with the lowest mortality rate, or longest life span, among the client population of adults (policyholders) insured by MetLife.

Although the MetLife and other weight-for-height tables remained in use in 2015, many health professionals and medical researchers believe these tables have limited utility. Nearly every weight-for-height table shows different acceptable weight ranges for men and women, and there continues to be considerable debate among health professionals over which table to use. The tables also lack information about body composition, such as the ratio of fat to lean muscle mass; their data are derived primarily from white populations and do not represent the entire U.S. population; they generally do not take age into consideration; and it is often unclear how frame size is determined. Furthermore, it is now known that ideal, healthy, or low-risk weight varies for different populations and varies for the same population at different times and in relation to different causes of morbidity and mortality.

The limitations of weight-for-height tables have prompted health care practitioners and researchers to adopt other measures that allow comparison of weight independent of height and frame across populations to define desirable or healthy weight as well as overweight and obesity. For example, in *Scientific Report of the 2015 Dietary Guidelines Advisory Committee* (February 2015, http://health.gov/dietaryguidelines/2015-scientific-report/ PDFs/Scientific-Report-of-the-2015-Dietary-Guidelines-Advisory-Committee.pdf), the Dietary Guidelines Advisory Committee uses the body mass index (BMI), a measure that incorporates height and weight to categorize adult body weight as underweight, healthy weight, overweight, or obese. Table 1.2 shows BMIs for various heights and categorizes BMI ranges as "normal weight," "overweight," "obese," and "extreme obesity." Because children and adolescents are growing, their BMIs are compared with children of the same age and sex. This is called BMI-for-age percentile and indicates whether children and teens are underweight, healthy weight, overweight, or obese. (See Table 1.3.)

Overweight is generally defined as excess body weight in relation to height, when compared with a predetermined standard of acceptable, desirable, or ideal weight. One definition characterizes individuals as overweight if they are between 10 and 30 pounds (4.5 and 13.6 kg) heavier than the desirable weight for height. Overweight does not necessarily result from excessive body fat; people may become overweight as the result of an increase in lean muscle. For example, although muscular bodybuilders with minimal body fat frequently weigh more than nonathletes of the same height, they are overweight because of their increased muscle mass rather than increased fat.

Rather than viewing overweight and obesity as distinct conditions, many researchers prefer to consider weight as a curve or continuum with obesity at the far end of the curve. People who are obese constitute a subset of the overweight population. In this definition, only some overweight people are obese, but all obese people are overweight.

Similarly, there is still no uniform definition of obesity. Some health professionals describe anyone who is more than 30 pounds (13.6 kg) above his or her desirable

TABLE 1.3

Body mass index for children and teens

BMI-for-age percentile

Less than 5th percentile	Underweight
5th percentile to less than the 85th percentile	Healthy weight
85th percentile to less than the 95th percentile	Risk of overweight
95th percentile or greater	Overweight

SOURCE: "What Does the BMI-for-Age Percentile Mean?" in *How Are Overweight and Obesity Diagnosed?* National Heart, Lung and Blood Institute, July 13, 2012, http://www.nhlbi.nih.gov/health/health-topics/topics/obe/diagnosis (accessed September 25, 2015)

TABLE 1.2

Calculating and defining body mass index

Height	21	22	23	24	25	26	27	28	29	30	31
4'10"	100	105	110	115	119	124	129	134	138	143	148
5'0"	107	112	118	123	128	133	138	143	148	153	158
5'1"	111	116	122	127	132	137	143	148	153	158	164
5'3"	118	124	130	135	141	146	152	158	163	169	175
5'5"	126	132	138	144	150	156	162	168	174	180	186
5'7"	134	140	146	153	159	166	172	178	185	191	198
5'9"	142	149	155	162	169	176	182	189	196	203	209
5'11"	150	157	165	172	179	186	193	200	208	215	222
6'1"	159	166	174	182	189	197	204	212	219	227	235
6'3"	168	176	184	192	200	208	216	224	232	240	248

BMI	
18.5–24.9	Normal weight
25.0–29.9	Overweight
30.0–39.9	Obese
40.0 and above	Extreme obesity

SOURCE: "Body Mass Index for Adults," and "What Does Body Mass Index Mean?" in *How Are Overweight and Obesity Diagnosed?* National Heart, Lung and Blood Institute, July 13, 2012, http://www.nhlbi.nih.gov/health/health-topics/topics/obe/diagnosis (accessed September 25, 2015)

weight for height as obese. Others assert that body weight 20% or more above desirable or ideal body weight constitutes obesity. Extreme or clinically severe obesity is often defined as weight twice the desirable weight or 100 pounds (45.4 kg) more than the desirable weight. Obesity is also defined as an excessively high amount of adipose tissue (body fat) in relation to lean body mass such as muscle and bone. The amount of body fat (also known as adiposity), the distribution of fat throughout the body, and the size of the adipose tissue deposits are also used to assess obesity because the location and distribution of body fat are considered to be important predictors of the health risks that are associated with obesity. The location and distribution of body fat may be measured by the ratio of waist-to-hip circumference. High ratios have been associated with higher risks of morbidity and mortality.

Historically, overweight and obese body types have been characterized as apple- or pear-shaped, depending on the anatomical site where fat is more prominent. In the apple or android type of obesity, fat is mainly located in the trunk (upper body, nape of the neck, shoulder, and abdomen). Gynoid obesity, or the pear-shape, features rounded hips and more fat located in the buttocks, thighs, and lower abdomen. Fat cells around the waist, flank, and abdomen are more active metabolically than those in the thighs, hips, and buttocks. This increased metabolic activity is thought to produce the increased health risks that are associated with android obesity. In general, women are more likely to have gynoid obesity.

Research reported in the March 26, 2011, issue of the *Lancet* disputes the relationship between abdominal obesity (android obesity) and the increased risk for cardiovascular disease. In "Separate and Combined Associations of Body-Mass Index and Abdominal Adiposity with Cardiovascular Disease: Collaborative Analysis of 58 Prospective Studies" (vol. 377, no. 9771), researchers in the Emerging Risk Factors Collaboration who tracked 221,934 adults for nearly a decade find that although obesity (BMI greater than 30) significantly increases the risk for cardiovascular disease, the distribution of the excess fat does not appear to influence this risk. The researchers deemed all distributions of body fat equally harmful in terms of heart health and suggest that in addition to obesity, high blood pressure and cholesterol and a history of diabetes are important predictors of future risk of developing cardiovascular disease.

In an effort to characterize more accurately the relationship between weight, the distribution of body fat, and the risk for cardiovascular disease, Axel Carl Carlsson et al. compared a variety of measures including weight, height, waist circumference (WC), waist-hip ratio (WHR), waist-hip-height ratio (WHHR), WC-to-height ratio (WCHR), and BMI. In "Novel and Established Anthropometric Measures and the Prediction of Incident

Cardiovascular Disease: A Cohort Study" (*International Journal of Obesity*, vol. 37, no. 12, March 28, 2013), the researchers report that WHHR is the most accurate predictor of cardiovascular risk.

There are many ways to measure body fat. Weighing an individual underwater in a laboratory with specialized equipment provides a highly accurate assessment of body fat. By performing hydrostatic or underwater weighing, an examiner obtains an estimate of whole-body density and uses this to calculate the percentage of the body that is fat. First, the subject is weighed on a land scale. The subject then puts on a diver's belt with weights to prevent floating during the weighing procedure, sits on a chair that is suspended from a precision scale, and is completely submerged. When maximum expiration of breath is achieved, the subject remains in this submerged position for about 10 seconds while the investigator reads the scale. This procedure is repeated as many as 10 times to obtain reliable, consistent values. The weight of the diver's belt and chair are subtracted from this weight to obtain the true value of the subject's mass in water.

Simpler, but potentially less accurate assessments of body fat include skinfold thickness measurements, which involve measuring subcutaneous (immediately below the skin) fat deposits using an instrument called a caliper in locations such as the upper arm. Skinfold thickness measurements rely on the fact that a certain fraction of total body fat is subcutaneous and by using a representative sample of that fat, overall body fatness (density) may be predicted. Several skinfold measurements are obtained, and the values are used in equations to calculate body density. Using a caliper, the examiner grasps a fold of skin and subcutaneous fat firmly, pulling it away from the underlying muscle tissue that follows the natural contour of the skin. The caliper jaws exert a relatively constant tension at the point of contact and measure skinfold thickness in millimeters. Most obesity researchers believe there is an acceptable correlation between skinfold thickness and body fat—that it is possible to estimate body fatness from the use of skinfold calipers. However, skinfold thickness measurements are considered more subjective than underwater weights because the accuracy of measurements of skinfold thickness depends on the skill and technique of the examiner, and there may be variations in readings from one examiner to another.

Another technique used to evaluate body fat is bioelectric impedance analysis (BIA). BIA offers an indirect estimate of body fat and lean body mass. It entails passing an electrical current through the body and assessing the body's ability to conduct the current. It is based on the principle that resistance is inversely proportional to total body water when an electrical current (with a frequency of 70 megahertz) is applied through several electrodes that are placed on body extremities. Because greater conductivity occurs when there is a higher percentage of body water and because a higher percentage of body water indicates larger amounts of muscle and other lean tissue (fat cells contain less water than muscle cells), people with less fat are better able to conduct electrical current. BIA has been shown to correlate well with total body fat that has been assessed by other methods.

Other means of estimating the location and distribution of body fat include waist-to-hip circumference ratios and imaging techniques such as ultrasound, computed tomography, or magnetic resonance imaging.

Waist Circumference and Waist-to-Hip Ratio

Along with height and weight, waist circumference is a common measure used to assess abdominal fat content. An excess of body fat in the abdomen or upper body is considered to increase the risk of developing heart disease, high blood pressure, diabetes, stroke, and certain cancers. Like body fat, health risks increase as the waist circumference increases. For men, a waist circumference greater than 40 inches (101.6 cm) is considered to confer increased health risks. Women are considered at increased risk when a waist measurement is 35 inches (88.9 cm) or greater. Waist-circumference measures lose their incremental predictive value in people with a BMI greater than or equal to 35 because these individuals generally exceed the cutoff points for increased risk. Table 1.4 shows the relationship between BMI, waist circumference, and disease risk for people who are underweight, normal weight, overweight, obese, and extremely obese.

In fact, research demonstrates that clothing size, which serves as a surrogate for waist circumference, can help predict disease risk. Laura A. E. Hughes et al. find that skirt and trouser sizes correlate well with waist-circumference measurements and that bigger skirt and trouser sizes are associated with a greater risk of developing selected cancers.

In "Self-Reported Clothing Size as a Proxy Measure for Body Size" (*Epidemiology*, vol. 20, no. 5, September 2009), Hughes et al. indicate that skirt size predicts the risk for endometrial cancer (cancer of the lining of the uterus) and trouser size predicts the risk for renal cell carcinoma (kidney cancer).

However, the utility of clothing size as a surrogate for weight has been called into question by studies that find great variability in sizing, especially in women's clothing. Vanity sizing, in which clothing manufacturers scale down clothing sizes such that a women's size 12 becomes a size 8 or 10, has been found to increase weight misperception because despite size variations, many people still monitor their weight using clothing sizes. For this reason, Dustin T. Duncan et al. call in "Does Perception Equal Reality? Weight Misperception in Relation to Weight-Related Attitudes and Behaviors among Overweight and Obese U.S. Adults" (*International Journal of Behavioral Nutrition and Physical Activity*, vol. 8, no. 20, March 22, 2011) for an end to vanity sizing.

The waist-to-hip ratio is the ratio of waist circumference to hip circumference, which is calculated by dividing waist circumference by hip circumference. For men and women, a waist-to-hip ratio of one or more is considered to place them at greater risk. Most people store body fat at the waist and abdomen (android body fat distribution) or at the hips (gynoid body fat distribution).

Body Mass Index

BMI is a single number that evaluates an individual's weight status in relation to height. It does not directly measure the percentage of body fat; however, it offers a more accurate assessment of overweight and obesity than weight alone. It is a direct calculation based on height and weight, and it is not gender specific. BMI is the preferred measurement of health care professionals and obesity researchers to assess body fat and is the most

TABLE 1.4

Classification of overweight and obesity by body mass index, waist circumference, and associated disease risk

	BMI (kg/m²)	Obesity class	Disease risk[a] relative to normal weight and waist circumference	
			Men ≤ 102 cm (≤ 40 in) Women ≤ 88 cm (≤ 35 in)	> 102 cm (> 40 in) > 88 cm (> 35 in)
Underweight	<18.5		—	—
Normal[b]	18.5–24.9		—	—
Overweight	25.0–29.9		Increased	High
Obesity	30.0–34.9	I	High	Very high
	35.0–39.9	II	Very high	Very high
Extreme obesity	≥40	III	Extremely high	Extremely high

[a]Disease risk for type 2 diabetes, hypertension, and cardiovascular disease.
[b]Increased waist circumference can also be a marker for increased risk even in persons of normal weight.

SOURCE: "Classification of Overweight and Obesity by BMI, Waist Circumference, and Associated Disease Risk," in *Aim for a Healthy Weight*, National Institutes of Health, National Heart, Lung, and Blood Institute, https://www.nhlbi.nih.gov/health/educational/lose_wt/BMI/bmi_dis.htm (accessed September 25, 2015) common method of tracking overweight and obesity among adults. BMI, which is calculated by dividing weight in kilograms by the square of height in meters, classifies people as underweight, normal weight, overweight, or obese. Table 1.5 shows the formula used to calculate BMI when height is measured in either inches or centimeters and weight is measured in either pounds or kilograms.

The World Health Organization and the National Institutes of Health consider individuals overweight when their BMI is between 25 and 29.9, and they are classified as obese when their BMI exceeds 30. Table 1.2 shows the relationship between height, weight, and BMI. It also shows the classification of overweight and obesity by BMI and distinguishes between obesity and extreme obesity. Table 1.6 shows weights in pounds and kilograms that represent the three levels of obesity at two different heights: 5 feet, 4 inches (162.6 cm) and 5 feet, 9 inches (175.3 cm).

BMI is a simple, inexpensive tool for assessing weight, but it has several limitations. BMI may deem muscular athletes overweight when they are extremely fit and excess weight is the result of a larger amount of lean muscle. It may similarly misrepresent the health of older adults who as the result of muscle wasting (loss of muscle mass) may be considered to have a normal or healthy weight when they may actually be nutritionally depleted or overweight in terms of body fat composition. Although it is an imperfect method for assessing individuals, BMI is useful for tracking weight trends in the population.

Definitions and Estimates of Prevalence Vary

Historically, varying definitions of, and criteria for, overweight and obesity have affected prevalence statistics and made it difficult to compare data. Some overweight- and obesity-related prevalence rates are crude or unadjusted estimates; others are age-adjusted estimates that offer different values. Early efforts to track overweight and obesity in the U.S. population relied on the 1943, 1959, and 1983 MetLife tables of desirable weight-for-height as the reference standard for overweight. During the last four decades, most government agencies and public health organizations have estimated overweight using data from a series of surveys conducted by the NCHS. These surveys include the National Health Examination Surveys, NHANES, and the Behavioral Risk Factor Surveillance System.

Despite changing definitions of overweight and obesity and various methods to track changes in the U.S. population, there is irrefutable evidence that the prevalence of overweight and obesity has steadily increased among people of both sexes, all ages, all racial and ethnic groups, and all educational levels. The prevalence of obesity in the United States was first reported in the 1960 National Health Examination Survey. Most obesity data referenced in the medical literature in 2015 were drawn from the 2011–12 NHANES study and the 2015

TABLE 1.5

How to calculate body mass index (BMI)

You can calculate BMI as follows

$$BMI = \frac{Weight\ (kg)}{Height\ squared\ (m^2)}$$

If pounds and inches are used

$$BMI = \frac{Weight\ (pounds) \times 703}{Height\ squared\ (inches^2)}$$

Calculation directions and sample

Here is a shortcut method for calculating BMI. (Example: for a person who is 5 feet 5 inches tall weighing 180 lbs.)

1. Multiply weight (in pounds) by 703

$$180 \times 703 = 126{,}540$$

2. Multiply height (in inches) by height (in inches)

$$65 \times 65 = 4{,}225$$

3. Divide the answer in step 1 by the answer in step 2 to get the BMI.

$$126{,}540/4{,}225 = 29.9$$

$$BMI = 29.9$$

SOURCE: "You Can Calculate BMI As Follows," in *The Practical Guide: Identification, Evaluation, and Treatment of Overweight and Obesity in Adults*, National Institutes of Health, National Heart, Lung, and Blood Institute, North American Association for the Study of Obesity, October 2000, http://www.nhlbi.nih.gov/files/docs/guidelines/prctgd_c.pdf (accessed September 25, 2015)

TABLE 1.6

Obesity cut points for adults 5'4" and 5'9"

Height	Obesity class I	Obesity class II	Obesity class III
5'4"	174 pounds	204 pounds	232 pounds
5'4"	79 kilograms	93 kilograms	105 kilograms
5'9"	203 pounds	236 pounds	270 pounds
5'9"	92 kilograms	107 kilograms	123 kilograms

SOURCE: Margot Shields, Margaret D. Carroll, and Cynthia L. Ogden, "Table. Obesity Cut Points for Adults 5'4" and 5'9"," in "Adult Obesity Prevalence in Canada and the United States," *NCHS Data Brief*, no. 56, National Center for Health Statistics, March 2011, http://www.cdc.gov/nchs/data/databriefs/db56.pdf (accessed September 25, 2015)

National Health Interview Studies, along with several other national studies. Data from the 1960 National Health Examination Survey and prior NHANES studies indicated that the prevalence of obesity was relatively constant between 1960 and 1980 and sharply increased between the late 1980s and 2010.

Overweight and obesity have steadily progressed at an alarming rate since the 1980s. Cheryl D. Fryar, Margaret D. Carroll, and Cynthia L. Ogden observe in "Prevalence of Overweight, Obesity, and Extreme Obesity among Adults: United States, Trends 1960–1962 through 2011–2012" (September 2014, http://www.cdc.gov/nchs/data/hestat/obesity_adult_11_12/obesity_adult_11_12.pdf) that the prevalence of obesity in the United States doubled between 1976–80 and 2011–12. During the same period the prevalence of overweight remained relatively stable until an uptick in 2009–10. Figure 1.2 shows trends in overweight, obesity, and extreme obesity among men and women aged 20 to 74 years from 1960 to 2012.

Data from the National Health Interview Study reveal that the prevalence of obesity among adults aged 20 years and older has increased over time, from 19.4% in 1997 to 30.2% in March 2015. (See Figure 1.3.) The prevalence of overweight and obesity generally increases with advancing age, then starts to decline among people over the age of 60 years. In January through March 2015

for men and women combined, the prevalence of obesity was highest among adults aged 40 to 59 years (34.1%) and lowest among adults aged 20 to 39 years (26.5%). (See Figure 1.4.) There was no significant difference in the prevalence of obesity between men and women in all four age groups.

The age-adjusted prevalence of obesity in racial and ethnic minorities, especially minority women, is generally higher than in whites in the United States. According to Tainya C. Clarke et al. of the NCHS, in *Early Release of Selected Estimates Based on Data from the January–March 2015 National Health Interview Survey* (September 2015, http://www.cdc.gov/nchs/data/nhis/earlyrelease/early release201509_06.pdf), in 2015 for both sexes, non-Hispanic African Americans were more likely than Hispanics and non-Hispanic whites to be obese. The age-adjusted prevalence of obesity was highest among non-Hispanic African American women (47.7%) and lowest among non-Hispanic white women (26.7%). (See Figure 1.5.)

WHY ARE SO MANY AMERICANS OVERWEIGHT?

Historically, overweight and obesity were largely attributed to gluttony (excess in eating). The scientific study of obesity has identified genetic, biochemical, viral,

FIGURE 1.2

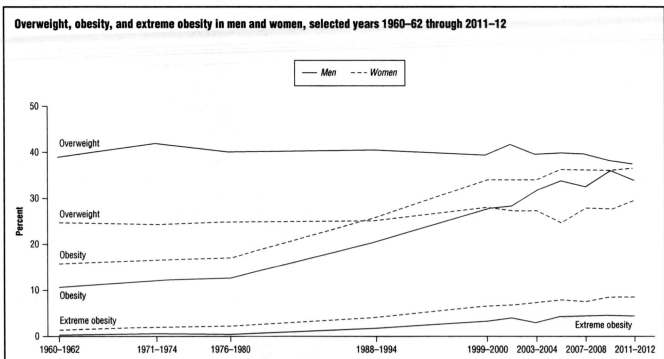

Overweight, obesity, and extreme obesity in men and women, selected years 1960–62 through 2011–12

Notes: Age-adjusted by the direct method to the year 2000 U.S. Census Bureau estimates using age groups 20–39, 40–59, and 60–74. Pregnant females were excluded. Overweight is body mass index (BMI) of 25 or greater but less 30; obesity is BMI greater than or equal to 30; and extreme obesity is BMI greater than or equal to 40.

SOURCE: Cheryl D. Fryar, Margaret D. Carroll, and Cynthia L. Ogden, "Figure. Trends in Adult Overweight, Obesity, and Extreme Obesity among Men and Women Aged 20–74 Years: United States, Selected Years 1960–1962 through 2011–2012," in "Prevalence of Overweight, Obesity, and Extreme Obesity among Adults: United States, 1960–1962 through 2011–2012," *NCHS Health E-Stats*, Centers for Disease Control and Prevention, National Center for Health Statistics, September 2014, http://www.cdc.gov/nchs/data/hestat/obesity_adult_11_12/obesity_adult_11_12.pdf (accessed September 25, 2015)

FIGURE 1.3

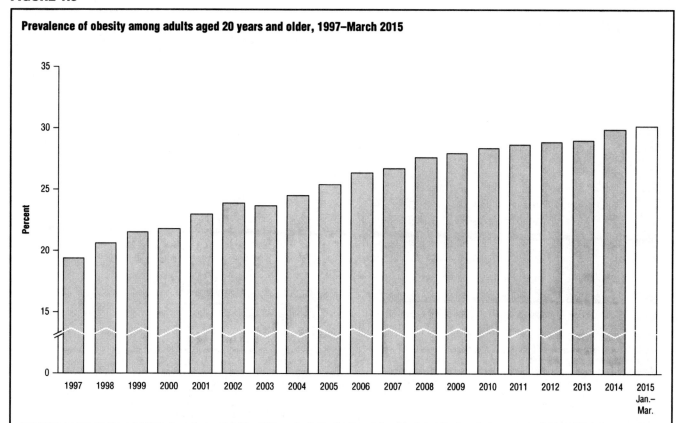

Prevalence of obesity among adults aged 20 years and older, 1997–March 2015

Notes: Data are based on household interviews of a sample of the civilian noninstitutionalized population. Obesity is defined as a body mass index (BMI) of 30 kg/m² or more. The measure is based on self-reported height (m) and weight (kg). Estimates of obesity are restricted to adults aged 20 and over for consistency with the Healthy People 2020 (3) initiative. The analyses excluded people with unknown height or weight (about 6% of respondents each year).

SOURCE: Tainya C. Clarke et al., "Figure 6.1. Prevalence of Obesity among Adults Aged 20 Years and over: United States, 1997–March 2015," in *Early Release of Selected Estimates Based on Data from the January–March 2015 National Health Interview Survey*, Centers for Disease Control and Prevention, National Center for Health Statistics, September 2015, http://www.cdc.gov/nchs/data/nhis/earlyrelease/earlyrelease201509_06.pdf (accessed September 25, 2015)

and metabolic alterations in humans and experimental animals, as well as the complex interactions of psychosocial and cultural factors that create susceptibility to overweight and obesity. Although overweight and obesity are thought to result from multiple causes, for the overwhelming majority of Americans overweight and obesity result from excessive consumption of calories and inadequate physical activity—eating too much and exercising too little.

Some observers maintain that Americans were destined to become overweight when their diets remained unchanged even as the inventions of the industrial revolution such as cars, automation, and a variety of laborsaving devices sharply reduced levels of physical activity. The widespread availability of high-calorie foods and less physically demanding jobs conspired to make Americans fatter. Others contend that the rise in overweight and obesity began during the 1970s, when Americans came to rely on processed, convenient, and calorie-dense, saturated-fat-laden fast foods.

Research also implicates a viral cause of obesity. Eleonora Ponterio and Lucio Gnessi note in "Adenovirus

36 and Obesity: An Overview" (*Viruses*, vol. 7, no. 7, July 8, 2015) that the human adenovirus-36 (Ad-36) is capable of inducing adiposity in experimentally infected animals and that in humans it is associated with obesity in adults and children. (Adenoviruses typically produce respiratory infections.) In the United States antibodies to Ad-36 are more prevalent in obese people (about 30% are infected) than in people who are not obese (11% are infected).

Research confirms genetic origins of obesity. In "Current Review of Genetics of Human Obesity: From Molecular Mechanisms to an Evolutionary Perspective" (*Molecular Genetics and Genomics*, vol. 290, no. 4, August 2015), David Albuquerque et al. describe the complexity of the genetics underlying obesity and susceptibility or risk of developing obesity. The researchers note that although obesity due to single-gene disorders has been well described and genome-wide searches have identified specific sites, called loci, where genetic variants associated with polygenic (caused by more than one gene) obesity are located, the genes within these many loci have not yet been identified. Albuquerque et al. also

FIGURE 1.4

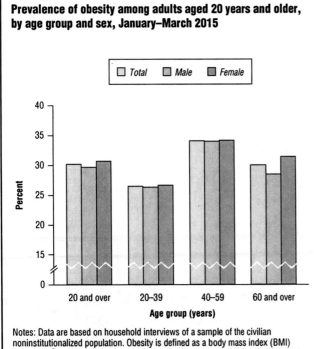

Prevalence of obesity among adults aged 20 years and older, by age group and sex, January–March 2015

☐ Total   ☐ Male   ☐ Female

Percent / Age group (years)

Notes: Data are based on household interviews of a sample of the civilian noninstitutionalized population. Obesity is defined as a body mass index (BMI) of 30 kg/m² or more. The measure is based on self-reported height (m) and weight (kg). Estimates of obesity are restricted to adults aged 20 and over for consistency with the Healthy People 2020 (3) initiative. The analyses excluded the 4.0% of persons with unknown height or weight.

SOURCE: Tainya C. Clarke et al., "Figure 6.2. Prevalence of Obesity among Adults Aged 20 Years and over, by Age Group and Sex: United States, January–March 2015," in *Early Release of Selected Estimates Based on Data from the January–March 2015 National Health Interview Survey*, Centers for Disease Control and Prevention, National Center for Health Statistics, September 2015, http://www.cdc.gov/nchs/data/nhis/earlyrelease/earlyrelease201509_06.pdf (accessed September 25, 2015)

FIGURE 1.5

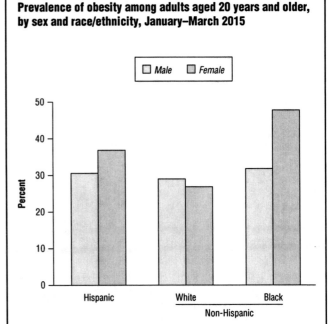

Prevalence of obesity among adults aged 20 years and older, by sex and race/ethnicity, January–March 2015

☐ Male   ☐ Female

Percent

Notes: Data are based on household interviews of a sample of the civilian noninstitutionalized population. Obesity is defined as a body mass index (BMI) of 30 kg/m² or more. The measure is based on self-reported height (m) and weight (kg). Estimates of obesity are restricted to adults aged 20 and over for consistency with the Healthy People 2020 (3) initiative. The analyses excluded the 4.0% of persons with unknown height or weight. Estimates are age adjusted using the projected 2000 U.S. population as the standard population and using five age groups: 20–24, 25–34, 35–44, 45–64, and 65 and over.

SOURCE: Tainya C. Clarke et al., "Figure 6.3. Age-Adjusted Prevalence of Obesity among Adults Aged 20 Years and over, by Sex and Race/Ethnicity: United States, January–March 2015," in *Early Release of Selected Estimates Based on Data from the January–March 2015 National Health Interview Survey*, Centers for Disease Control and Prevention, National Center for Health Statistics, September 2015, http://www.cdc.gov/nchs/data/nhis/earlyrelease/earlyrelease201509_06.pdf (accessed September 25, 2015)

indicate that there are different obesity-linked loci in children and among ethnic groups.

The American Diet Has Changed

The American diet has changed dramatically since the mid-20th century. According to the U.S. Department of Agriculture (USDA), in *Agriculture Fact Book, 2001–2002* (March 2003, http://www.usda.gov/factbook/2002factbook.pdf), during the 1950s food production in the United States provided about 800 fewer calories per person per day than in 2000. Of the 3,800 calories produced per person per day in 2000, the USDA estimates that about 1,100 calories were wasted, either through spoilage, plate waste, or cooking, leaving an average of about 2,700 calories per person per day. The USDA data reveal that between 1970 and 2000 the average number of calories consumed daily rose by 530 calories, an increase of 24.5%. This 24.5% increase consisted of 9.5 percentage points of grains (primarily refined grain products), 9 percentage points of added fats and oils, 4.7 percentage points of added sugars, 1.5 percentage points of fruits and vegetables, and 1 percentage point of meats and nuts.

There was a 1.5 percentage point decline in dairy product and egg consumption.

The USDA states that Americans consumed an average of 4 pounds (1.8 kg) more fish and shellfish, 7 pounds (3.2 kg) more red meat, and 46 pounds (20.9 kg) more poultry per person per year in 2000 than they did during the 1950s. Americans consumed more meat—57 pounds (25.9 kg) more per year in 2000 than they did during the 1950s. Despite record-high per capita (per person) consumption of meat in 2000, the proportion of fat in the U.S. food supply from meat, poultry, and fish declined from one-third (33%) during the 1950s to a quarter (24%) in 2000. This decline resulted from the marketing of lower-fat ground and processed meat products, a shift away from red meat to poultry, and closer trimming of outside fat on meat, which commenced in 1986.

According to the USDA, the consumption of milk dropped from an annual average of 36.4 gallons (137.8 L) per person during the 1950s to 22.6 gallons (85.6 L) in 2000, a decrease of 38%. The USDA posits a link between the trend toward dining out and the reduction in beverage milk consumption. According to the USDA, soft drinks, fruit drinks, and flavored teas appear to be displacing milk as the beverages of choice for Americans. By contrast, Americans ate more cheese, from 7.7 pounds (3.5 kg) during the 1950s to 29.8 pounds (13.5 kg) in 2000.

The average use of added fats and oils increased 67%, from 44.6 pounds (20.2 kg) during the 1950s to 74.5 pounds (33.8 kg) in 2000. Added fats include butter, shortenings, and oils used in commercially prepared foods. All fats that naturally occur in foods, such as those in milk and meat, were excluded from the USDA analysis. Americans consumed an average of 23% more salad and cooking oil in 2000 than they did during the 1950s, and more than twice as much shortening. During the same period the consumption of butter and margarine declined by about the same proportion—25%. During the 1950s added fats and oils accounted for the largest proportion of fat in the food supply (41%), followed by animal proteins—meat, poultry, and fish (32%). By 2000 added fats and oils accounted for 53% of total fat consumption, most likely because Americans' appetites for fried foods in fast-food outlets and high-fat snack foods grew, as did the use of salad dressings. USDA food consumption surveys, which assess the prevalence of discretionary fats in the American diet, continue to find that margarine, salad dressing, and mayonnaise, along with cakes and other sweet baked goods, are among the top-10 food sources of fat in the American diet.

The USDA indicates that the consumption of fruit and vegetables increased 20%, from 587.5 pounds (266.5 kg) during the 1970s to 707.7 pounds (321 kg) in 2000. The USDA attributes some of the increase to the introduction of convenient, ready-to-eat, precut, and packaged fruit and vegetables and to increasing consumer health awareness. Despite these gains, the CDC explains in *State Indicator Report on Fruits and Vegetables, 2013* (May 2013, http://www.cdc.gov/nutrition/downloads/State-Indicator-Report-Fruits-Vegetables-2013.pdf), a state-by-state study of fruit and vegetable consumption, that 37.7% of adults report consuming fruit less than one time daily and 22.6% consumed less than one serving of vegetables in 2013. (See Table 1.7.) Vegetable consumption by adolescents was even worse—37.7% said they ate vegetables less than once a day and 36% said they ate less than one serving of fruit per day. Among adults the median (half are higher and half are lower) vegetable intake was higher in California, Oregon, and New Hampshire and lower in North Dakota, South Dakota, Iowa, Louisiana, and Mississippi. (See Table 1.7 and Figure 1.6.) In "Adults Meeting Fruit and Vegetable Intake Recommendations—United States, 2013" (*Morbidity and Mortality Weekly Report*, vol. 64, no. 26, July 10, 2015), Latetia V. Moore and Frances

E. Thompson compare these data to the Dietary Guidelines for Americans, which contain federal intake recommendations, and find that less than 18% of adults consumed the recommended amount of fruit and less than 14% consumed the recommended amount of vegetables.

According to the USDA, the per capita use of flour and cereal products reached 199.9 pounds (90.7 kg) in 2000, up from an annual average of 155.4 pounds (70.5 kg) during the 1950s and 138.2 pounds (62.7 kg) during the 1970s, when grain consumption was at a record low. This increase reflects plentiful grain stocks, robust consumer demand for store-bought bakery items and grain-based snack foods, and increased consumption of fast-food products such as buns, pizza dough, and tortillas. However, in *USDA Wheat Baseline, 2015–24* (June 22, 2015, http://www.ers.usda.gov/topics/crops/wheat/usda-wheat-baseline,-2015-24.aspx), the Economic Research Service indicates that the 2013 annual average of 134.7 pounds (61.1 kg) of flour was down 11.6 pounds (5.3 kg) from the 2000 peak and 3.6 pounds (1.6 kg) lower than the most recent peak in 2007. Despite the overall increase in grain consumption, the average American's diet contained mostly refined grain products and fell short of the recommended minimum three daily servings of whole-grain products.

Although NHANES (August 29, 2013, http:www.ars.usda.gov/ba/bhnrc/fsrg) reports that Americans' consumption of whole grains increased 23.4% between 2008 and 2010, American adults still consumed far less than the recommended three to five servings per day. Likewise, the USDA notes in *Scientific Report of the 2015 Dietary Guidelines Advisory Committee* that Americans' diets still do not meet recommendations for vegetables, fruit, dairy, or whole grains

The USDA cites a variety of factors that have contributed to the changes in the American diet over the past 50 years, including fluctuations in food prices and availability, increases in real (adjusted for inflation) disposable income, and more food assistance for the poor. New products, particularly the expanding array of convenience foods, also alter patterns of consumption, as do more imports, growth in the away-from-home food market, intensified advertising campaigns, and increases in nutrient-enrichment standards and food fortification. Social and demographic trends driving changes in food choices include smaller households, more two-wage earner households, more single-parent households, an aging population, and increased ethnic diversity.

Americans Enjoy Eating Out

A variety of societal trends are thought to contribute to Americans' propensity to overeat, including eating outside the home, as well as ready access to, and preference for, sugar- and fat-laden foods. Table 1.8 shows how

TABLE 1.7

Fruit and vegetable consumption by adults and adolescents, by state, 2013

	Adults				Adolescents			
	Percentage who report consuming fruits and vegetables less than one time daily		Median intake of fruits and vegetables (times per day)		Percentage who report consuming fruits and vegetables less than one time daily		Median intake of fruits and vegetables (times per day)	
State	Fruits	Vegetables	Fruits	Vegetables	Fruits	Vegetables	Fruits	Vegetables
U.S. national	37.7	22.6	1.1	1.6	36.0	37.7	1.0	1.3
Alabama	43.8	24.3	1.0	1.6	44.4	45.7	1.0	1.0
Alaska	38.7	19.7	1.1	1.7	39.1	34.1	1.0	1.3
Arizona	38.0	20.6	1.1	1.7				
Arkansas	47.5	28.6	1.0	1.5	49.4	43.2	1.0	1.0
California	30.4	16.5	1.3	1.8				
Colorado	35.7	19.1	1.1	1.7				
Connecticut	32.0	20.6	1.3	1.7	34.6	35.3	1.3	1.3
Delaware	39.2	23.8	1.0	1.6	46.0		1.0	
Dist of Columbia	31.7	20.1	1.3	1.8				
Florida	37.7	22.6	1.1	1.6	37.2	42.1	1.0	1.1
Georgia	41.9	23.2	1.0	1.6	42.9	43.1	1.0	1.0
Hawaii	39.5	22.6	1.0	1.7	45.1	40.8	1.0	1.1
Idaho	38.1	20.1	1.1	1.6	33.9	32.2	1.0	1.3
Illinois	36.0	25.2	1.1	1.6	38.7	42.3	1.0	1.1
Indiana	41.6	27.3	1.0	1.5	44.7	42.0	1.0	1.1
Iowa	39.8	26.9	1.0	1.4	36.1	35.1	1.0	1.3
Kansas	41.4	22.2	1.0	1.6	40.4	35.7	1.0	1.3
Kentucky	45.9	25.2	1.0	1.5	49.7	43.2	1.0	1.1
Louisiana	46.7	32.5	1.0	1.4	47.8	50.1	1.0	0.9
Maine	33.2	18.9	1.2	1.7	37.5		1.0	
Maryland	36.4	22.8	1.1	1.6	38.7	38.9	1.0	1.3
Massachusetts	31.6	20.7	1.2	1.7				
Michigan	37.3	23.2	1.1	1.6	37.8	36.8	1.0	1.3
Minnesota	36.2	23.6	1.1	1.5				
Mississippi	50.8	32.3	0.9	1.4	39.8	42.4	1.0	1.1
Missouri	43.9	25.2	1.0	1.5				
Montana	39.2	21.7	1.0	1.6	38.4	33.5	1.0	1.3
Nebraska	40.1	26.2	1.0	1.5	41.0	38.0	1.0	1.3
Nevada	36.9	24.4	1.1	1.6				
New Hampshire	30.3	17.6	1.3	1.8	36.8	31.8	1.0	1.3
New Jersey	33.9	22.2	1.1	1.6	39.1	34.9	1.0	1.3
New Mexico	38.0	21.9	1.1	1.7	40.8	37.1	1.0	1.3
New York	33.9	23.0	1.2	1.6	34.7		1.3	
North Carolina	40.8	21.9	1.0	1.6	44.5	39.6	1.0	1.1
North Dakota	39.1	27.1	1.1	1.4	36.4	39.4	1.0	1.1
Ohio	40.5	26.0	1.0	1.5	42.4	42.2	1.0	1.1
Oklahoma	50.2	26.8	0.9	1.5	44.3	40.4	1.0	1.1
Oregon	32.0	15.3	1.1	1.9				
Pennsylvania	36.1	23.9	1.1	1.5				
Rhode Island	32.9	20.7	1.2	1.6	36.5	35.3	1.0	1.3
South Carolina	44.4	27.3	1.0	1.5	50.6	47.8	0.7	1.0
South Dakota	39.6	26.3	1.0	1.4	41.2	38.8	1.0	1.1
Tennessee	46.3	25.4	1.0	1.6	44.9	41.4	1.0	1.1
Texas	40.3	21.8	1.0	1.6	42.1	47.5	1.0	1.0
Utah	34.9	19.8	1.1	1.7	32.5	31.8	1.0	1.3
Vermont	31.4	18.1	1.3	1.7	30.7	26.4	1.3	1.6
Virginia	38.4	22.2	1.1	1.7	39.8	41.7	1.0	1.1
Washington	35.0	18.8	1.1	1.7				
West Virginia	47.2	26.2	1.0	1.5	37.8	34.9	1.0	1.3
Wisconsin	35.6	26.0	1.1	1.5	34.1	35.7	1.0	1.3
Wyoming	38.2	22.4	1.1	1.6	37.9	31.4	1.0	1.3

Note: Some states may not have estimates for F&V intake among adolescents which may be due to either not collecting survey data, not achieving a high enough overall response rate to receive weighted results, or omitting 1 or more questionnaire items during administration of the survey.

SOURCE: "Table 1. State Indicator Report on Fruits and Vegetables, 2013: Behavioral Indicators," in *State Indicator Report on Fruits and Vegetables 2013*, Centers for Disease Control and Prevention, National Center for Chronic Disease Prevention and Health Promotion, Division of Nutrition, Physical Activity, and Obesity, May 2013, http://www.cdc.gov/nutrition/downloads/State-Indicator-Report-Fruits-Vegetables-2013.pdf (accessed October 2, 2015)

expenditures for eating away from home have steadily increased and more than doubled from $307.6 billion in 1995 to $705.9 billion in 2013. Purchases of food away from home rose between 2003 and 2008; however, the Great Recession, which lasted from late 2007 to mid-2009, prompted Americans to limit their eating out. Aylin

Kumcu and Phil Kaufman of the Economic Research Service note in "Food Spending Adjustments during Recessionary Times" (*Amber Waves*, September 2011) that there was a 5% decline in inflation-adjusted food spending during the recession—the largest decrease in 25 years. They indicate that this decline was largely

FIGURE 1.6

Median daily vegetable intake among adults, 2013

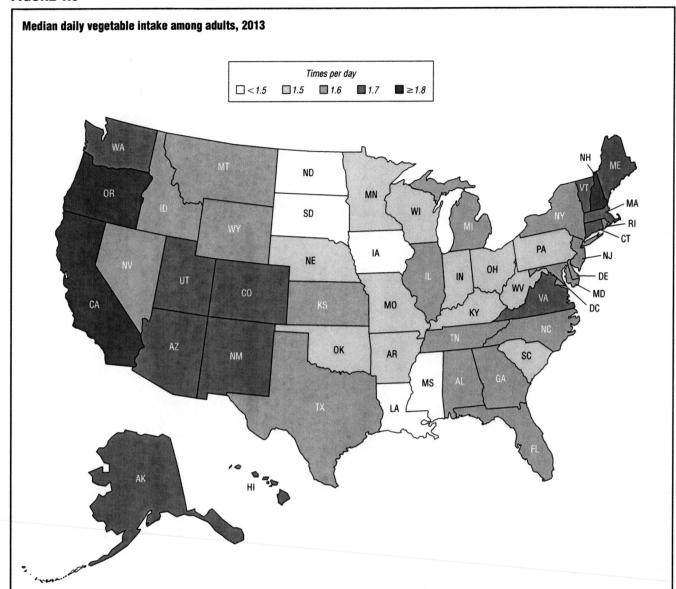

SOURCE: "Median Daily Vegetable Intake among Adults in the United States," in *State Indicator Report on Fruits and Vegetables 2013*, Centers for Disease Control and Prevention, National Center for Chronic Disease Prevention and Health Promotion, Division of Nutrition, Physical Activity, and Obesity, 2013, http://www.cdc.gov/nutrition/downloads/State-Indicator-Report-Fruits-Vegetables-2013.pdf (accessed October 2, 2015)

attributable to reductions in food-away-from-home spending, such as at fast-food and sit-down restaurants. Table 1.8 shows that after a drop in 2009, expenditures at eating and drinking places rose between 2010 and 2013.

Many nutritionists and obesity researchers assert that controlling portion size, which is key to controlling calorie consumption, is more difficult in restaurants, where portions are frequently quite large. Increasingly, restaurants have translated consumer demand for value into more food for less money. Because humans are genetically programmed to eat when food is abundant, larger portions trigger the natural impulse to eat more.

Besides portion size, large containers also appear to increase intake. In "Container Size Influences Snack

Food Intake Independently of Portion Size" (*Appetite*, vol. 58, 2012), David Marchiori, Olivier Corneille, and Olivier Klein report that larger containers stimulate food intake independent of portion size. They gave study participants a medium portion of M&M's in a small container, a medium portion in a large container, or a large portion in a large container. Marchiori, Corneille, and Klein explain that the larger container increased intake by 129% despite the portion size remaining constant.

BIGGER PORTIONS IN RESTAURANTS. Samara Joy Nielsen and Barry M. Popkin of the University of North Carolina, Chapel Hill, looked at portion sizes consumed in the United States to determine whether average portion sizes had increased over time and reported their findings in "Patterns and Trends in Food Portion Sizes, 1977–1998"

TABLE 1.8

Food away from home, total expenditures, selected years 1929–2013

Year	Eating and drinking places[a]	Hotels and motels[a]	Retail stores, direct selling[b]	Recreational places[c]	Schools and colleges[d]	All other[e]	Total[f]
			Million dollars				
1929	2,101	362	—	—	175	1,483	4,121
1933	1,235	250	—	—	105	869	2,459
1935	1,257	271	—	—	161	1,145	2,834
1936	1,430	320	—	—	175	1,236	3,161
1937	1,696	351	—	—	194	1,375	3,616
1938	1,626	312	—	—	191	1,260	3,389
1939	1,782	321	—	—	203	1,307	3,613
1940	1,938	353	—	—	219	1,385	3,895
1941	2,369	386	—	—	263	1,781	4,799
1942	2,992	453	—	—	310	2,539	6,294
1943	3,837	604	—	—	332	3,572	8,345
1944	4,471	681	—	—	326	4,415	9,893
1945	5,218	736	—	—	373	4,908	11,235
1946	5,859	846	—	—	525	3,802	11,032
1947	6,243	854	—	—	842	3,864	11,803
1948	6,338	846	—	—	983	4,069	12,236
1949	6,294	786	—	—	979	3,943	12,002
1950	6,472	774	—	—	1,051	4,172	12,469
1951	7,172	783	—	—	1,124	5,167	14,246
1952	7,549	805	—	—	1,138	5,435	14,927
1953	7,834	790	—	—	1,215	5,392	15,231
1954	8,008	752	1,416	274	1,311	3,676	15,437
1955	8,490	809	1,468	313	1,390	3,539	16,009
1956	8,992	875	1,534	354	1,530	3,506	16,791
1957	9,409	932	1,592	342	1,661	3,609	17,545
1958	9,447	922	1,599	356	1,809	3,756	17,889
1959	10,102	982	1,677	385	1,949	3,739	18,834
1960	10,505	1,028	1,716	421	2,082	3,855	19,607
1961	10,907	1,061	1,740	452	2,264	3,961	20,385
1962	11,624	1,134	1,812	472	2,463	4,090	21,595
1963	12,247	1,200	1,854	484	2,624	4,148	22,557
1964	13,156	1,289	1,988	496	2,814	4,279	24,022
1965	14,444	1,409	2,162	522	3,062	4,598	26,197
1966	15,768	1,541	2,346	544	3,329	5,173	28,701
1967	16,595	1,623	2,436	563	3,632	5,570	30,419
1968	18,695	1,703	2,713	616	3,903	5,830	33,460
1969	20,207	1,716	2,984	661	4,256	6,291	36,115
1970	22,617	1,894	3,325	721	4,475	6,551	39,583
1971	24,166	2,086	3,626	762	4,990	6,621	42,251
1972	27,167	2,390	3,811	832	5,370	7,017	46,587
1973	31,265	2,639	4,218	963	5,605	7,960	52,650
1974	34,029	2,864	4,520	1,167	6,287	9,178	58,045
1975	41,384	3,199	4,952	1,369	7,060	10,145	68,109
1976	47,536	3,769	5,341	1,511	7,854	10,822	76,833
1977	52,491	4,115	5,663	2,606	8,413	11,547	84,835
1978	60,042	4,863	6,323	2,810	9,034	13,012	96,084
1979	68,872	5,551	7,157	2,921	9,914	14,756	109,171
1980	75,883	5,906	8,158	3,040	11,115	16,194	120,296
1981	83,358	6,639	8,830	2,979	11,357	17,751	130,914
1982	90,390	6,888	9,256	2,887	11,692	18,663	139,776
1983	98,710	7,660	9,827	3,271	12,338	19,077	150,883
1984	105,836	8,409	10,315	3,489	12,950	20,047	161,046
1985	111,760	9,168	10,499	3,737	13,534	20,133	168,831
1986	121,699	9,665	11,116	4,059	14,401	20,755	181,695
1987	137,190	11,117	9,302	4,396	13,470	21,119	196,594
1988	150,724	11,905	10,359	5,082	13,889	22,474	214,433
1989	160,226	12,179	11,369	6,089	14,609	24,016	228,488
1990	171,616	12,508	12,786	7,206	15,299	25,605	245,020
1991	180,062	12,460	13,515	7,936	16,186	26,226	256,385
1992	184,697	13,204	11,817	8,509	17,666	27,596	263,489
1993	197,865	13,362	11,790	9,361	18,330	27,864	278,572
1994	207,464	13,880	12,015	10,103	19,271	28,460	291,193
1995	221,205	14,211	11,848	11,110	20,064	29,158	307,596
1996	223,406	14,553	11,959	11,512	20,867	29,696	311,993
1997	242,362	15,381	10,680	12,126	21,901	32,022	334,472
1998	255,376	16,069	11,335	12,790	23,053	32,528	351,151
1999	266,451	16,710	12,463	13,493	23,920	34,148	367,185
2000	287,332	18,003	13,608	14,224	24,468	34,997	392,631
2001	293,911	20,813	14,597	14,780	25,394	35,422	404,917
2002	295,341	21,513	17,319	15,873	26,735	36,017	412,799

TABLE 1.8

Food away from home, total expenditures, selected years 1929–2013 [CONTINUED]

Year	Eating and drinking places[a]	Hotels and motels[a]	Retail stores, direct selling[b]	Recreational places[c]	Schools and colleges[d]	All other[e]	Total[f]
			Million dollars				
2003	324,995	21,914	18,272	17,327	28,077	37,516	448,102
2004	338,105	23,462	19,430	18,265	30,184	38,491	467,938
2005	372,094	24,570	20,677	20,225	31,521	40,556	509,643
2006	397,682	25,328	21,616	22,665	33,769	43,098	544,158
2007	419,891	25,588	22,297	24,288	36,379	45,042	573,485
2008	431,391	26,085	22,990	24,639	38,524	46,028	589,656
2009	427,222	25,257	22,110	24,107	40,736	46,887	586,319
2010	441,739	25,541	22,803	24,612	43,149	46,908	604,752
2011	469,812	25,828	24,134	25,239	45,108	48,555	638,676
2012	499,929	26,411	25,033	26,372	46,618	50,426	674,789
2013	526,176	26,501	25,420	27,559	48,076	52,196	705,927

—Not available.

[a]Includes tips.

[b]Includes vending machine operators but not vending machines operated by organizations.

[c]Motion picture theaters, bowling alleys, pool parlors, sports arenas, camps, amusement parks, golf and country clubs (includes concessions beginning in 1977).

[d]Includes school food subsidies.

[e]Military exchanges and clubs; railroad dining cars; airlines; food service in manufacturing plants, institutions, hospitals, boarding houses, fraternities and sororities, and civic and social organizations; and food supplied to military forces, civilian employees and child day care centers.

[f]Computed from unrounded data.

SOURCE: "Table 3. Food away from Home: Total Expenditures," in *Food Expenditures*, U.S. Department of Agriculture, Economic Research Service, October 2015, http://www.ers.usda.gov/datafiles/Food_Expenditures/Food_Expenditures/table3.xls (accessed October 2, 2015)

(*Journal of the American Medical Association*, vol. 289, no. 4, January 22, 2003). In this landmark study, Nielsen and Popkin analyze data collected by national nutrition surveys (the Nationwide Food Consumption Survey and the Continuing Survey of Food Intakes by Individuals) that were conducted in the United States in 1977–78, 1989–91, 1994–96, and 1998, detailing the consumption habits of more than 63,000 people. For each survey year, the researchers analyze the average portion sizes that were consumed of specific food items (salty snacks, desserts, soft drinks, fruit drinks, french fries, hamburgers, cheese-burgers, pizza, and Mexican food) by eating location (home, restaurant, and fast-food outlet). Nielsen and Popkin report that between 1977 and 1996 the average portions of salty snacks such as chips increased by 60% and soft drinks grew by 50%. The average bag of chips grew from 1 ounce (28.4 g) in 1977 to 1.6 ounces (45.4 g) in 1996. During this same period an average dispensed soft drink increased from 13.1 ounces (387.4 mL) to 19.9 ounces (588.5 mL). As a result, the average chips-and-soda snack in 1996 contained 150 more calories than it did in 1977.

Portion-size increases were also observed with many fast-food offerings. During the 20 years studied, the size of the average hamburger grew by 23%, to 7 ounces (198.4 g), and the servings of fries grew by 16%, to 3.5 ounces (99.2 g). In 1996 a regular-sized burger-and-fries meal contained 155 more calories than it did in 1977. Worse still, Nielsen and Popkin find that portion size had also expanded in Americans' homes, indicating wide-spread ignorance about appropriate portion size. Interest-ingly, portion sizes were smallest in restaurants, although

they, too, had increased during the study period. For example, the average restaurant portion of spaghetti with tomato sauce and meatballs doubled in size from 500 to 1,025 calories.

In "Reducing Portion Sizes to Prevent Obesity: A Call to Action" (*American Journal of Preventive Medicine*, vol. 43, no. 5, November 2012), Lisa R. Young and Marion Nestle observe that portion sizes of many foods continued to increase throughout the first decade of the 21st century. Furthermore, nearly 150 new large-size portions, including burgers, pizza, candy bars, and bev-erages, were introduced during the same period. For example, Hardee's Monster Thickburger contains a whopping 1,420 calories. Young and Nestle observe that although European portion sizes have also grown, they are not as big as U.S. portions. For example, the largest portion of french fries offered by British Burger King has 200 fewer calories than the largest U.S. portion.

Deborah A. Cohen and Mary Story observe in "Mit-igating the Health Risks of Dining Out: The Need for Standardized Portion Sizes in Restaurants" (*American Journal of Public Health*, vol. 104, no. 4, April 2014) that restaurant portion sizes continue to grow and call for standardized portion sizes to help Americans eat appro-priate servings of food. Cohen and Story reviewed the calorie count of 30,923 menu items offered by 245 res-taurant chains and find that most restaurant meals contain considerably more calories than the 640 recommended by the Institute of Medicine for people who should be con-suming 2,000 calories per day.

DOES THE ECONOMY AFFECT FOOD CONSUMPTION AND WEIGHT? In *The Effects of the Financial Crisis on Actual and Anticipated Consumption* (October 2011, http://www.mrrc.isr.umich.edu/publications/papers/pdf/wp255.pdf), Michael D. Hurd and Susann Rohwedder compare consumption changes during the Great Recession with consumption changes during previous years. They posit that spending on necessities such as food consumed at home is likely to be reduced less than spending on dining out, which is optional. As anticipated, purchases of food to be consumed at home showed a much smaller decline than did meals eaten away from home.

Daniel J. Hruschka observes in "Do Economic Constraints on Food Choice Make People Fat? A Critical Review of Two Hypotheses for the Poverty-Obesity Paradox" (*American Journal of Human Biology*, vol. 24, no. 3, May–June 2012) that in wealthy countries, poorer and less educated people are more likely to be overweight than their more prosperous countrymen. Hruschka questions the conventional thinking that "economic deprivation leads people to choose cheaper foods which in turn fosters overconsumption of energy" and notes that during the Great Recession obesity among women slowed across income groups.

Shu Wen Ng, Meghan M. Slining, and Barry M. Popkin indicate that some researchers assert that people exhibit better health behaviors during economic downturns, whereas other researchers suggest that dietary and health behaviors worsen. Ng, Slining, and Popkin analyzed food and beverage intakes and purchasing trends in the context of major economic and sociodemographic changes, examined trends by age, race, and ethnic groups, and reported their findings in "Turning Point for US Diets? Recessionary Effects or Behavioral Shifts in Foods Purchased and Consumed" (*American Journal of Clinical Nutrition*, vol. 99, no. 3, March 2014). They find that although overall caloric intake and purchases declined between 2003 and 2013, this decline was not associated with economic conditions such as the Great Recession or food prices. Instead, Ng, Slining, and Popkin posit that public health efforts may have contributed to the decreased intake.

BIGGER PORTIONS AT HOME. Increased portion sizes at home are reflected in recipes and cookbooks. Lisa R. Young notes in *The Portion Teller: Smartsize Your Way to Permanent Weight Loss* (2005) that recipes call for bigger portions using the same ingredients than they did in past decades. For example, a brownie recipe from Irma S. Rombauer and Marion Rombauer Becker's *Joy of Cooking* (1964) recommended dividing it into 30 servings, whereas the same recipe in the 1997 edition of the book was divided into only 16 servings. Similarly, a 1987 recipe for Toll House cookies yielded 60 servings, whereas in earlier decades the same recipe yielded 100 servings. Other popular food items have increased in size and caloric content. In "Portion Distortion" (June 24, 2015, http://www.nhlbi.nih.gov/health/public/heart/obesity/wecan/portion/index.htm), the National Heart, Lung, and Blood Institute compares portion sizes and the corresponding calories of several popular foods between 1984 and 2004. For example, in 1984 a 16-ounce coffee with whole milk and sugar contained 45 calories, while in 2004 a 16-ounce mocha coffee contained 350 calories. Similarly, in 1984 a 1.5-inch-diameter chocolate chip cookie contained 55 calories, while in 2004 its 3.5-inch counterpart contained 275 calories.

Nielsen and Popkin also note other changes in eating behavior. For example, they find that in 1996 Americans obtained 19% of their total calories from snacks—double the amount of 1977—and 81% from meals. They conclude that "control of portion size must be systematically addressed both in general and as it relates to fast food pricing and marketing. The best way to encourage people to eat smaller portions is if food portions served inside and outside the home are smaller."

There is no evidence that portion sizes have returned to their previous sizes or have even decreased in size. In a review of research about portion size, Ingrid H. M. Steenhuis and Willemijn M. Vermeer of Vrije Universiteit Amsterdam observe in "Portion Size: Review and Framework for Interventions" (*International Journal of Behavioral Nutrition and Physical Activity*, vol. 6, no. 58, August 21, 2009) that since the 1970s portion sizes, especially of high energy-dense (high-calorie) foods eaten at home and in restaurants, have increased. The researchers confirm that "portion distortion," a term that is used to describe the phenomenon of people becoming acclimated to larger portions so that they not only do not view them as excessive but also have more difficulty selecting appropriate amounts of food, definitely increases consumption by at least 30%.

The contribution of increased portion size to increased daily intake of energy from food and drink was confirmed by research conducted by Kiyah J. Duffey and Barry M. Popkin and reported in "Energy Density, Portion Size, and Eating Occasions: Contributions to Increased Energy Intake in the United States, 1977–2006" (*PLoS Medicine*, vol. 8, no. 6, June 2011). The researchers analyze data from the Nationwide Food Consumption Survey (1977–78), the Continuing Survey of Food Intakes by Individuals (1989–91), and NHANES (1994–98 and 2003–06) to determine the contribution of changes in the energy density of foods consumed, the portion size, and the number of meals and snacks per day. They find that the daily total energy intake increased by 570 calories between 1977 and 2006. Duffey and Popkin indicate that although all three factors contributed to changes in the average daily total energy intake over the past 30 years, increases in the number of eating occasions and portion size accounted for most of the change. In fact, the consumption of food and beverage portions increased across all eating and drinking occasions (meals and snacks).

Is the Food Industry the Culprit?

In "The Perils of Ignoring History: Big Tobacco Played Dirty and Millions Died. How Similar Is Big Food?" (*Milbank Quarterly*, vol. 87, no. 1, March 2009), Kelly D. Brownell and Kenneth E. Warner implicate marketing strategies employed by the food industry as a significant factor in the rise of obesity. Furthermore, they liken food industry practices to those of the tobacco industry, concluding that:

> The tobacco industry had a playbook, a script, that emphasized personal responsibility, paying scientists who delivered research that instilled doubt, criticizing the "junk" science that found harms associated with smoking, making self-regulatory pledges, lobbying with massive resources to stifle government action, introducing "safer" products, and simultaneously manipulating and denying both the addictive nature of their products and their marketing to children. The script of the food industry is both similar to and different from the tobacco industry script.... Because obesity is now a major global problem, the world cannot afford a repeat of the tobacco history, in which industry talks about the moral high ground but does not occupy it.

Kelly D. Brownell et al. explain in "Personal Responsibility and Obesity: A Constructive Approach to a Controversial Issue" (*Health Affairs*, vol. 29, no. 3, March–April 2010) that people gain weight when their environment promotes highly palatable food and cite research suggesting that some foods can trigger symptoms of addiction. The researchers aver that the traditional approach to diet and obesity has been one of rugged individualism—educating individuals and exhorting them to alter their behavior, often without regard to environmental influences. Instead of focusing solely on personal responsibility, Brownell et al. propose efforts on the part of government and the food industry to create conditions that encourage responsible choices. Furthermore, they call on the food industry to limit its "relentless" and often "stealth" marketing techniques such as food marketing that is incorporated into video games.

David A. Kessler also implicates the food industry in *The End of Overeating: Taking Control of the Insatiable American Appetite* (2009). He asserts that conditioned overeating is not a personal character flaw; rather, it is a biological response to the widespread availability of foods that are high in salt, fat, and sugar. Kessler blames the food industry for engineering highly processed industrial foods that use salt, fat, and added sugar to trigger cravings in some people and addiction in other people who are susceptible.

Some industry observers believe that one ingredient in particular triggers cravings: high-fructose corn syrup (HFCS). In "Brain Functional Magnetic Resonance Imaging Response to Glucose and Fructose Infusions in Humans" (*Diabetes, Obesity, and Metabolism*, vol. 13, no. 3, March 2011), Jonathan Q. Purnell et al. explain that the brain responds differently to glucose (sugar) than it does to fructose. Consuming glucose increases responses in the reward- and executive-function parts of the brain, whereas fructose inhibits these responses. This action may explain why fructose consumption appears to promote obesity—it actually stimulates hunger, which in turn increases consumption and weight gain.

Fructose also appears to trigger fat storage more efficiently than other sugars do. Although all sugars are stored in the body as fat, some researchers think that fructose is more readily converted into fat than other sugars. Fructose encourages the liver to promote fat by activating enzymes that create higher levels of cholesterol and triglycerides (fatty substances that are normally present in the bloodstream and all the cells of the body) and make muscles more insulin resistant. Elevated levels of cholesterol and triglycerides increase the risk of coronary heart disease, and insulin resistance can lead to diabetes.

HFCS does more than sweeten; it also acts as a preservative, giving sweet foods a longer shelf life. Since the 1970s HFCS has been used to sweeten nearly every product on supermarket shelves. Some researchers feel that because it is so ubiquitous, many Americans are unknowingly consuming excessive amounts of fructose. Table 1.9 shows the per capita consumption of HFCS, which peaked in 1999 and has since slowly declined.

During the first decade of the 21st century HFCS received negative publicity, and as a result consumption continued to decline. In response, the Corn Refiners Association launched a controversial advertising campaign in 2009 that was intended to rebrand HFCS as "corn sugar." In a letter dated May 30, 2012 (http://www.fda.gov/about FDA/CentersOffices/OfficeofFoods/CFSAN/CFSANFOIA ElectronicReadingRoom/ucm305226.htm), the Food and Drug Administration (FDA) rejected the Corn Refiners Association's request to rename its sweetener. The FDA explained that the use of the term *corn sugar* for HFCS would suggest that HFCS is a solid, dried, and crystallized sweetener obtained from corn rather than a syrup. The agency also stated that because the term *corn sugar* is commonly used to describe dextrose, a different sugar, using it to describe HCFS could cause needless confusion.

In *The Fattening of America: How the Economy Makes Us Fat, If It Matters, and What to Do about It* (2008), Eric A. Finkelstein and Laurie Zuckerman observe that Americans consumed 1,000 calories more per week in 2008 than they did in 1985. Finkelstein and Zuckerman describe how declining food costs, especially for high-calorie, low-nutrient foods, and modern technology combined to reduce the cost of producing higher-calorie processed food products. They note that when the staples used to produce fast foods became cheaper, the food industry intensified marketing efforts to induce consumers to buy and eat more. Table 1.10 shows that food expenditures decreased as a percentage of disposable personal income from 10.5% in 1996 to 9.8% in 2013.

TABLE 1.9

Estimated number of per capita calories of high-fructose corn syrup consumed daily, 1970–2014

Year	Primary weight (market level)[a] lb/yr	Loss from primary to retail weight percent	Weight at retail level lb/yr	Loss from retail/institutional to consumer level percent	Weight at consumer level lb/yr	Loss at consumer level		Per capita consumption (adjusted for loss)			Calories per serving number	Serving weight grams	Calories consumed daily[b] number	Servings (teaspoons) consumed daily[c] teaspoons
						Nonedible share percent	Other (uneaten food, spoilage, etc.) percent	lbs/yr	oz/daily	g/daily				
1970	0.5	0.0	0.5	11.0	0.5	0.0	34.0	0.3	0.0	0.4	16.0	4.2	2	0.1
1971	0.8	0.0	0.8	11.0	0.7	0.0	34.0	0.5	0.0	0.6	16.0	4.2	2	0.1
1972	1.2	0.0	1.2	11.0	1.0	0.0	34.0	0.7	0.0	0.8	16.0	4.2	3	0.2
1973	2.1	0.0	2.1	11.0	1.8	0.0	34.0	1.2	0.1	1.5	16.0	4.2	6	0.4
1974	2.8	0.0	2.8	11.0	2.5	0.0	34.0	1.6	0.1	2.0	16.0	4.2	8	0.5
1975	4.9	0.0	4.9	11.0	4.3	0.0	34.0	2.9	0.1	3.6	16.0	4.2	14	0.8
1976	7.2	0.0	7.2	11.0	6.4	0.0	34.0	4.2	0.2	5.2	16.0	4.2	20	1.2
1977	9.6	0.0	9.6	11.0	8.5	0.0	34.0	5.6	0.2	7.0	16.0	4.2	27	1.7
1978	10.8	0.0	10.8	11.0	9.6	0.0	34.0	6.3	0.3	7.9	16.0	4.2	30	1.9
1979	14.8	0.0	14.8	11.0	13.1	0.0	34.0	8.7	0.4	10.8	16.0	4.2	41	2.6
1980	19.0	0.0	19.0	11.0	16.9	0.0	34.0	11.1	0.5	13.8	16.0	4.2	53	3.3
1981	22.8	0.0	22.8	11.0	20.3	0.0	34.0	13.4	0.6	16.7	16.0	4.2	63	4.0
1982	26.6	0.0	26.6	11.0	23.7	0.0	34.0	15.6	0.7	19.4	16.0	4.2	74	4.6
1983	31.2	0.0	31.2	11.0	27.8	0.0	34.0	18.3	0.8	22.8	16.0	4.2	87	5.4
1984	37.2	0.0	37.2	11.0	33.1	0.0	34.0	21.9	1.0	27.2	16.0	4.2	104	6.5
1985	45.2	0.0	45.2	11.0	40.2	0.0	34.0	26.5	1.2	33.0	16.0	4.2	126	7.9
1986	45.7	0.0	45.7	11.0	40.7	0.0	34.0	26.8	1.2	33.4	16.0	4.2	127	7.9
1987	47.7	0.0	47.7	11.0	42.5	0.0	34.0	28.0	1.2	34.8	16.0	4.2	133	8.3
1988	49.0	0.0	49.0	11.0	43.6	0.0	34.0	28.8	1.3	35.7	16.0	4.2	136	8.5
1989	48.2	0.0	48.2	11.0	42.9	0.0	34.0	28.3	1.2	35.2	16.0	4.2	134	8.4
1990	49.6	0.0	49.6	11.0	44.1	0.0	34.0	29.1	1.3	36.2	16.0	4.2	138	8.6
1991	50.3	0.0	50.3	11.0	44.8	0.0	34.0	29.5	1.3	36.7	16.0	4.2	140	8.7
1992	52.5	0.0	52.5	11.0	46.7	0.0	34.0	30.8	1.4	38.3	16.0	4.2	146	9.1
1993	55.2	0.0	55.2	11.0	49.1	0.0	34.0	32.4	1.4	40.3	16.0	4.2	153	9.6
1994	56.9	0.0	56.9	11.0	50.6	0.0	34.0	33.4	1.5	41.5	16.0	4.2	158	9.9
1995	58.0	0.0	58.0	11.0	51.6	0.0	34.0	34.1	1.5	42.3	16.0	4.2	161	10.1
1996	59.3	0.0	59.3	11.0	52.8	0.0	34.0	34.8	1.5	43.3	16.0	4.2	165	10.3
1997	62.0	0.0	62.0	11.0	55.2	0.0	34.0	36.4	1.6	45.3	16.0	4.2	173	10.8
1998	64.0	0.0	64.0	11.0	56.9	0.0	34.0	37.6	1.6	46.7	16.0	4.2	178	11.1
1999	65.4	0.0	65.4	11.0	58.2	0.0	34.0	38.4	1.7	47.8	16.0	4.2	182	11.4
2000	64.2	0.0	64.2	11.0	57.1	0.0	34.0	37.7	1.7	46.9	16.0	4.2	179	11.2
2001	63.7	0.0	63.7	11.0	56.7	0.0	34.0	37.4	1.6	46.5	16.0	4.2	177	11.1
2002	64.1	0.0	64.1	11.0	57.1	0.0	34.0	37.7	1.7	46.8	16.0	4.2	178	11.1
2003	62.5	0.0	62.5	11.0	55.6	0.0	34.0	36.7	1.6	45.6	16.0	4.2	174	10.9
2004	61.4	0.0	61.4	11.0	54.6	0.0	34.0	36.1	1.6	44.8	16.0	4.2	171	10.7
2005	60.8	0.0	60.8	11.0	54.1	0.0	34.0	35.7	1.6	44.4	16.0	4.2	169	10.6
2006	60.1	0.0	60.1	11.0	53.5	0.0	34.0	35.3	1.5	43.9	16.0	4.2	167	10.4
2007	57.7	0.0	57.7	11.0	51.3	0.0	34.0	33.9	1.5	42.1	16.0	4.2	160	10.0
2008	54.5	0.0	54.5	11.0	48.5	0.0	34.0	32.0	1.4	39.8	16.0	4.2	151	9.5
2009	51.8	0.0	51.8	11.0	46.1	0.0	34.0	30.5	1.3	37.8	16.0	4.2	144	9.0
2010	50.6	0.0	50.6	11.0	45.0	0.0	34.0	29.7	1.3	36.9	16.0	4.2	141	8.8
2011	48.6	0.0	48.6	11.0	43.2	0.0	34.0	28.5	1.3	35.5	16.0	4.2	135	8.4
2012	47.6	0.0	47.6	11.0	42.4	0.0	34.0	28.0	1.2	34.8	16.0	4.2	132	8.3
2013	45.8	0.0	45.8	11.0	40.7	0.0	34.0	26.9	1.2	33.4	16.0	4.2	127	8.0
2014	45.6	0.0	45.6	11.0	40.6	0.0	34.0	26.8	1.2	33.3	16.0	4.2	127	7.9

TABLE 1.9

Estimated number of per capita calories of high-fructose corn syrup consumed daily, 1970–2014 [CONTINUED]

[a]U.S. per capita HFCS estimated deliveries for domestic food and beverage use, calendar year.
[b]Number of daily teaspoons multiplied by calories per serving.
[c]Grams per day divided by serving weight.
Note: Estimated number of daily per capita calories calculated by adjusting HFCS deliveries for domestic food and beverage use for food losses.

SOURCE: "Table 52. High Fructose Corn Syrup: Estimated Number of per Capita Calories Consumed Daily, by Calendar Year," in *Sugar and Sweeteners Yearbook Tables*, U.S. Department of Agriculture, Economic Research Service, May 21, 2015, http://www.ers.usda.gov/data-products/sugar-and-sweeteners-yearbook-tables.aspx#.UseHQrS4reo (accessed October 2, 2015)

TABLE 1.10

Food expenditures by families and individuals as a share of disposable personal income, 1929–2013

| Year | Disposable personal income | Expenditures for food | | | | | |
| | | At home[a] | | Away from home[b] | | Total[c] | |
	Billion dollars	Billion dollars	Percent	Billion dollars	Percent	Billion dollars	Percent
1929	83.4	16.9	20.3	2.6	3.1	19.5	23.4
1930	74.7	15.8	21.2	2.3	3.1	18.1	24.2
1931	64.3	12.7	19.8	2.1	3.3	14.8	23.0
1932	49.2	9.6	19.5	1.7	3.5	11.3	23.0
1933	46.1	10.1	21.9	1.5	3.3	11.6	25.2
1934	52.8	11.1	21.0	1.7	3.2	12.8	24.2
1935	59.3	12.1	20.4	1.8	3.0	13.9	23.4
1936	67.4	12.7	18.8	2.0	3.0	14.7	21.8
1937	72.2	13.3	18.4	2.2	3.0	15.5	21.5
1938	66.6	12.6	18.9	2.1	3.2	14.7	22.1
1939	71.4	13.0	18.1	2.3	3.2	15.2	21.3
1940	76.8	13.5	17.6	2.4	3.1	15.9	20.7
1941	93.8	15.3	16.3	2.9	3.1	18.2	19.4
1942	118.6	18.5	15.6	3.6	3.0	22.1	18.6
1943	135.4	20.7	15.3	4.5	3.3	25.2	18.6
1944	148.3	22.1	14.9	5.1	3.4	27.2	18.4
1945	152.2	23.6	15.5	5.7	3.7	29.3	19.2
1946	161.4	28.4	17.6	6.5	4.0	34.9	21.6
1947	171.2	32.8	19.2	7.4	4.3	40.2	23.5
1948	190.6	34.9	18.3	7.5	3.9	42.4	22.3
1949	190.4	34.3	18.0	7.8	4.1	42.0	22.1
1950	210.1	35.7	17.0	7.6	3.6	43.3	20.6
1951	231.0	40.0	17.3	8.4	3.6	48.4	20.9
1952	243.4	41.8	17.2	8.8	3.6	50.6	20.8
1953	258.6	42.3	16.4	9.0	3.5	51.3	19.9
1954	264.3	42.4	16.0	9.3	3.5	51.7	19.6
1955	283.3	42.9	15.1	9.8	3.5	52.7	18.6
1956	303.0	44.4	14.7	10.4	3.4	54.8	18.1
1957	319.8	48.1	15.0	10.9	3.4	59.0	18.4
1958	330.5	49.8	15.1	11.1	3.4	60.9	18.4
1959	350.5	50.1	14.3	12.1	3.5	62.3	17.8
1960	365.4	51.5	14.1	12.6	3.4	64.0	17.5
1961	381.8	52.0	13.6	13.1	3.4	65.1	17.1
1962	405.1	52.9	13.1	13.9	3.4	66.8	16.5
1963	425.1	53.3	12.5	14.5	3.4	67.9	16.0
1964	462.5	55.5	12.0	15.7	3.4	71.2	15.4
1965	498.1	58.4	11.7	16.9	3.4	75.4	15.1
1966	537.5	61.0	11.3	18.6	3.5	79.6	14.8
1967	575.3	61.4	10.7	19.8	3.4	81.1	14.1
1968	625.0	64.5	10.3	21.7	3.5	86.2	13.8
1969	674.0	69.0	10.2	23.4	3.5	92.3	13.7
1970	735.7	75.5	10.3	26.4	3.6	102.0	13.9
1971	801.8	79.5	9.9	28.1	3.5	107.6	13.4
1972	869.1	86.0	9.9	31.3	3.6	117.3	13.5
1973	978.3	94.9	9.7	34.9	3.6	129.8	13.3
1974	1,071.6	107.3	10.0	38.5	3.6	145.8	13.6
1975	1,187.4	117.4	9.9	45.9	3.9	163.3	13.8
1976	1,302.5	125.1	9.6	52.6	4.0	177.7	13.6
1977	1,435.7	133.8	9.3	58.5	4.1	192.3	13.4
1978	1,608.3	147.3	9.2	67.5	4.2	214.8	13.4
1979	1,793.5	164.0	9.1	76.9	4.3	240.9	13.4
1980	2,009.0	180.8	9.0	85.2	4.2	266.0	13.2
1981	2,246.1	195.5	8.7	95.8	4.3	291.3	13.0
1982	2,421.2	201.0	8.3	104.5	4.3	305.5	12.6
1983	2,608.4	211.4	8.1	113.7	4.4	325.1	12.5
1984	2,912.0	224.0	7.7	121.9	4.2	345.8	11.9
1985	3,109.3	234.0	7.5	128.6	4.1	362.6	11.7
1986	3,285.1	242.7	7.4	137.9	4.2	380.6	11.6
1987	3,435.3	252.7	7.4	144.4	4.2	397.1	11.6
1988	3,726.3	271.7	7.3	155.5	4.2	427.2	11.5
1989	3,991.4	290.1	7.3	163.3	4.1	453.4	11.4
1990	4,254.0	314.5	7.4	175.2	4.1	489.6	11.5
1991	4,444.8	328.6	7.4	184.0	4.1	512.6	11.5
1992	4,736.7	332.1	7.0	190.8	4.0	522.9	11.0
1993	4,921.6	340.0	6.9	204.8	4.2	544.8	11.1
1994	5,184.3	352.9	6.8	215.4	4.2	568.2	11.0
1995	5,457.0	359.4	6.6	229.2	4.2	588.6	10.8
1996	5,759.6	374.2	6.5	232.1	4.0	606.3	10.5
1997	6,074.6	387.4	6.4	248.3	4.1	635.6	10.5
1998	6,498.9	396.1	6.1	260.9	4.0	657.0	10.1

TABLE 1.10

Food expenditures by families and individuals as a share of disposable personal income, 1929–2013 [CONTINUED]

| Year | Disposable personal income | Expenditures for food | | | | | |
| | | At home[a] | | Away from home[b] | | Total[c] | |
	Billion dollars	Billion dollars	Percent	Billion dollars	Percent	Billion dollars	Percent
1999	6,803.3	413.9	6.1	272.9	4.0	686.7	10.1
2000	7,400.5	431.6	5.9	292.9	4.0	724.4	9.8
2001	7,752.3	453.6	5.9	302.0	3.9	755.6	9.7
2002	8,099.2	474.7	5.9	307.7	3.8	782.4	9.7
2003	8,485.8	489.9	5.8	335.3	4.0	825.2	9.7
2004	9,002.3	509.1	5.7	350.4	3.9	859.4	9.5
2005	9,400.8	533.7	5.7	383.0	4.1	916.7	9.8
2006	10,036.9	552.0	5.5	410.2	4.1	962.2	9.6
2007	10,507.0	579.1	5.5	432.6	4.1	1,011.8	9.6
2008	10,994.4	607.7	5.5	444.5	4.0	1,052.1	9.6
2009	10,942.5	605.9	5.5	441.3	4.0	1,047.1	9.6
2010	11,237.9	622.3	5.5	454.7	4.0	1,076.9	9.6
2011	11,801.4	655.1	5.6	480.2	4.1	1,135.3	9.6
2012	12,384.0	679.7	5.5	508.0	4.1	1,187.6	9.6
2013	12,505.1	699.5	5.6	531.7	4.3	1,231.3	9.8

[a]Food-at-home includes cash purchases from grocery stores and other retail outlets, including purchases with food stamps and WIC vouchers and food produced and consumed on farms (valued at farm prices), but excludes government-donated foods.
[b]Food-away-from-home includes meals and snacks purchased by families and individuals and food furnished to employees, but excludes food paid for by government and business, such as donated foods to schools, meals in prisons and other institutions, and expense-account meals.
[c]Total may not add due to rounding.

SOURCE: "Table 7. Food Expenditures by Families and Individuals As a Share of Disposable Personal Income," in *Food Expenditures*, U.S. Department of Agriculture, Economic Research Service, December 1, 2014, http://www.ers.usda.gov/data-products/food-expenditures.aspx (accessed October 2, 2015)

CHAPTER 2
WEIGHT AND PHYSICAL HEALTH

If we could give every individual the right amount of nourishment and exercise, not too little and not too much, we would have found the safest way to health.

—Hippocrates

During the 20th century and the first two decades of the 21st century, advances in public health and medical care helped Americans lead longer, healthier lives. Two important measures of the health of the population are infant mortality (death) rates and life expectancy at birth rates. By the end of the 20th century, infant mortality rates had significantly decreased and life expectancy had increased by 29.5 years. Table 2.1 shows the long-term upward trend in life expectancy as well as recent gains. In 2013 life expectancy at birth for the total population reached a record high of 78.8 years, up from 75.4 years in 1990.

As deaths from infectious diseases declined during the second half of the 20th century, mortality from chronic diseases, such as heart disease and cancer, increased. Table 2.2 displays the 10 leading causes of death in the United States in 1980 and 2013. Overweight and obesity are considered contributing factors to at least four of the 10 leading causes of death in 2013: diseases of the heart, malignant neoplasms (cancers), cerebrovascular diseases (diseases affecting the supply of blood to the brain), and diabetes mellitus. Obesity may also be implicated in some deaths attributable to another leading cause of death: nephritis, nephrotic syndrome, and nephrosis (kidney disease or chronic renal failure). Table 2.2 also reveals the rise of diabetes as a cause of death. In 1980 it was the seventh-leading cause of death, claiming 34,851 lives. By 2013 it was the underlying cause of 75,578 deaths. Epidemiologists (scientists who study the occurrence and distribution of diseases and the factors that govern their spread) and medical researchers believe the increasing prevalence of diabetes in the U.S. population and the resultant rise

in deaths attributable to diabetes are direct consequences of the obesity epidemic in the United States.

Overweight and obesity increase not only the risk of morbidity (illness or disease) and mortality but also the severity of diseases such as hypertension (high blood pressure), arthritis, and other musculoskeletal problems. Table 2.3 lists the health consequences that may result from overweight and obesity among adults and children. It also estimates the likelihood of these health consequences. For example, adults who are obese are twice as likely to suffer from high blood pressure than adults who have a healthy weight.

In "Association between Class III Obesity (BMI of 40–59 kg/m^2) and Mortality: A Pooled Analysis of 20 Prospective Studies" (*PLoS Medicine*, vol. 11, no. 7, July 8, 2014), Cari M. Kitahara et al. examine the relationship between body mass index (BMI) and life expectancy in the United States. The researchers find that people with class III obesity (BMI 40 or higher) had a dramatic reduction in life expectancy compared with people of normal weight. Years of life lost ranged from 6.5 years for people with a BMI of between 40 and 44.9 to 13.7 years with a BMI of between 55 to 59.9. Kitahara et al. observe that the prevalence of class III obesity has grown to 6% of Americans and that the number of years of life lost for this group is comparable to or higher than that of current smokers.

IS OBESITY A DISEASE?

Researchers now recognize that obesity does not simply result from willful overeating and laziness, but from a complex combination of genetic, metabolic, behavioral, and environmental factors. Rather than viewing it as a lifestyle choice or personal failing, several groups favor declaring obesity a disease. Proponents assert that many public health benefits

TABLE 2.1

Life expectancy at birth, at 65 years of age, and at 75 years of age, according to race and sex, selected years 1900–2013

[Data are based on death certificates]

Specified age and year	All races			White			Black or African American[a]		
	Both sexes	Male	Female	Both sexes	Male	Female	Both sexes	Male	Female
At birth				Life expectancy, in years					
1900[b, c]	47.3	46.3	48.3	47.6	46.6	48.7	33.0	32.5	33.5
1950[c]	68.2	65.6	71.1	69.1	66.5	72.2	60.8	59.1	62.9
1960[c]	69.7	66.6	73.1	70.6	67.4	74.1	63.6	61.1	66.3
1970	70.8	67.1	74.7	71.7	68.0	75.6	64.1	60.0	68.3
1980	73.7	70.0	77.4	74.4	70.7	78.1	68.1	63.8	72.5
1990	75.4	71.8	78.8	76.1	72.7	79.4	69.1	64.5	73.6
1995	75.8	72.5	78.9	76.5	73.4	79.6	69.6	65.2	73.9
2000	76.8	74.1	79.3	77.3	74.7	79.9	71.8	68.2	75.1
2001	77.0	74.3	79.5	77.5	74.9	80.0	72.0	68.5	75.3
2002	77.0	74.4	79.6	77.5	74.9	80.1	72.2	68.7	75.4
2005	77.6	75.0	80.1	78.0	75.5	80.5	73.0	69.5	76.2
2006	77.8	75.2	80.3	78.3	75.8	80.7	73.4	69.9	76.7
2007	78.1	75.5	80.6	78.5	76.0	80.9	73.8	70.3	77.0
2008	78.2	75.6	80.6	78.5	76.1	80.9	74.3	70.9	77.3
2009	78.5	76.0	80.9	78.8	76.4	81.2	74.7	71.4	77.7
2010	78.7	76.2	81.0	78.9	76.5	81.3	75.1	71.8	78.0
2011	78.7	76.3	81.1	79.0	76.6	81.3	75.3	72.2	78.2
2012	78.8	76.4	81.2	79.1	76.7	81.4	75.5	72.3	78.4
2013	78.8	76.4	81.2	79.1	76.7	81.4	75.5	72.3	78.4
At 65 years									
1950[c]	13.9	12.8	15.0	14.1	12.8	15.1	13.9	12.9	14.9
1960[c]	14.3	12.8	15.8	14.4	12.9	15.9	13.9	12.7	15.1
1970	15.2	13.1	17.0	15.2	13.1	17.1	14.2	12.5	15.7
1980	16.4	14.1	18.3	16.5	14.2	18.4	15.1	13.0	16.8
1990	17.2	15.1	18.9	17.3	15.2	19.1	15.4	13.2	17.2
1995	17.4	15.6	18.9	17.6	15.7	19.1	15.6	13.6	17.1
2000	17.6	16.0	19.0	17.7	16.1	19.1	16.1	14.1	17.5
2001	17.9	16.2	19.2	18.0	16.3	19.3	16.2	14.2	17.7
2002	17.9	16.3	19.2	18.0	16.4	19.3	16.3	14.4	17.8
2005	18.4	16.9	19.6	18.5	17.0	19.7	16.9	15.0	18.3
2006	18.7	17.2	19.9	18.7	17.3	19.9	17.2	15.2	18.6
2007	18.8	17.4	20.0	18.9	17.4	20.1	17.3	15.4	18.8
2008	18.8	17.4	20.0	18.9	17.5	20.0	17.5	15.5	18.9
2009	19.1	17.7	20.3	19.2	17.7	20.3	17.8	15.9	19.2
2010	19.1	17.7	20.3	19.2	17.8	20.3	17.8	15.9	19.3
2011	19.2	17.8	20.3	19.2	17.8	20.4	18.0	16.2	19.4
2012	19.3	17.9	20.5	19.3	18.0	20.4	18.1	16.2	19.5
2013	19.3	17.9	20.5	19.3	18.0	20.5	18.1	16.3	19.5
At 75 years									
1980	10.4	8.8	11.5	10.4	8.8	11.5	9.7	8.3	10.7
1990	10.9	9.4	12.0	11.0	9.4	12.0	10.2	8.6	11.2
1995	11.0	9.7	11.9	11.1	9.7	12.0	10.2	8.8	11.1
2000	11.0	9.8	11.8	11.0	9.8	11.9	10.4	9.0	11.3
2001	11.2	9.9	12.0	11.2	10.0	12.1	10.5	9.0	11.5
2002	11.2	10.0	12.0	11.2	10.0	12.1	10.5	9.1	11.5
2005	11.5	10.4	12.3	11.5	10.4	12.3	10.9	9.4	11.2
2006	11.7	10.6	12.5	11.1	10.6	12.5	11.1	9.1	12.0
2007	11.9	10.7	12.6	11.9	10.8	12.6	11.2	9.8	12.1
2008	11.8	10.7	12.6	11.8	10.7	12.6	11.3	9.8	12.2
2009	12.1	11.0	12.9	12.1	10.4	12.9	11.6	10.2	12.5
2010	12.1	11.0	12.9	12.1	11.0	12.8	11.6	10.2	12.5
2011	12.1	11.1	12.9	12.1	11.0	12.8	11.7	10.4	12.5
2012	12.2	11.2	12.9	12.1	11.1	12.9	11.8	10.4	12.7
2013	12.2	11.2	12.9	12.1	11.1	12.9	11.8	10.4	12.7

would result from designating obesity as a disease, including:

- Reducing the social stigma and prejudice that are associated with obesity, and promoting attitudinal changes to reduce weight-based discrimination

- Enabling more people to seek treatment for obesity by providing health insurance coverage for treatment

- Increasing public awareness of the severity of obesity as a threat to health and longevity

- Stimulating scientific and medical research on the prevention and treatment of the condition and speeding approval of new antiobesity drugs

Groups that view obesity as a disease, including the World Health Organization, the National Institutes of Health (NIH), the National Academy of Sciences, the

TABLE 2.1

Life expectancy at birth, at 65 years of age, and at 75 years of age, according to race and sex, selected years 1900–2013 [CONTINUED]

[Data are based on death certificates]

Specified age and year	White, not Hispanic			Black, not Hispanic			Hispanic[d]		
	Both sexes	Male	Female	Both sexes	Male	Female	Both sexes	Male	Female
At birth				Life expectancy, in years					
2006	78.2	75.7	80.6	73.1	69.5	76.4	80.3	77.5	82.9
2007	78.4	75.9	80.8	73.5	69.9	76.7	80.7	77.8	83.2
2008	78.4	76.0	80.7	73.9	70.5	77.0	80.8	78.0	83.3
2009	78.7	76.3	81.1	74.3	70.9	77.4	81.1	78.4	83.5
2010	78.8	76.4	81.1	74.7	71.4	77.7	81.2	78.5	83.8
2011	78.8	76.4	81.1	74.9	71.7	77.8	81.4	78.8	83.7
2012	78.9	76.6	81.2	75.1	71.8	78.1	81.6	79.1	83.9
2013	78.9	76.5	81.2	75.1	71.8	78.1	81.6	79.1	83.8
At 65 years									
2006	18.7	17.2	19.9	17.1	15.1	18.5	20.2	18.5	21.5
2007	18.8	17.4	20.0	17.2	15.3	18.7	20.5	18.7	21.7
2008	18.8	17.4	20.0	17.4	15.4	18.8	20.4	18.7	21.6
2009	19.1	17.7	19.5	17.7	15.8	19.1	20.7	19.0	21.9
2010	19.1	17.7	20.3	17.7	15.8	19.1	20.6	18.8	22.0
2011	19.1	17.8	20.3	17.9	16.1	19.2	20.7	19.1	21.8
2012	19.3	17.9	20.4	18.0	16.1	19.4	21.0	19.5	22.1
2013	19.3	17.9	20.4	18.0	16.1	19.4	20.9	19.3	22.0
At 75 years									
2006	11.7	10.6	12.5	11.1	9.6	12.0	13.0	11.7	13.7
2007	11.8	10.7	12.6	11.2	9.7	12.1	13.1	11.8	13.8
2008	11.8	10.7	12.6	11.3	9.8	12.2	13.0	11.7	13.8
2009	12.0	11.0	12.9	11.6	10.1	12.4	13.3	12.0	13.8
2010	12.0	11.0	12.8	11.6	10.1	12.5	13.2	11.7	14.1
2011	12.0	11.0	12.8	11.7	10.4	12.5	13.2	12.0	13.9
2012	12.1	11.1	12.9	11.7	10.4	12.6	13.5	12.3	14.2
2013	12.1	11.1	12.9	11.7	10.4	12.6	13.4	12.3	14.1

[a]Data shown for 1900–1960 are for the nonwhite population.
[b]Death registration area only. The death registration area increased from 10 states and the District of Columbia (D.C.) in 1900 to the coterminous United States in 1933.
[c]Includes deaths of persons who were not residents of the 50 states and D.C.
[d]Hispanic origin was added to the U.S. standard death certificate in 1989 and was adopted by every state in 1997. To estimate life expectancy, age-specific death rates were corrected to address racial and ethnic misclassification, which underestimates deaths in the Hispanic population. Life expectancies for the Hispanic population are adjusted for underreporting on the death certificate of Hispanic ethnicity, but are not adjusted to account for the potential effects of return migration. To address the effects of age misstatement at the oldest ages, the probability of death for Hispanic persons older than 80 years is estimated as a function of non-Hispanic white mortality with the use of the Brass relational logit model.
Notes: Populations for computing life expectancy for 1991–1999 are 1990-based postcensal estimates of the U.S. resident population. Starting with *Health, United States, 2012*, populations for computing life expectancy for 2001–2009 were based on intercensal population estimates of the U.S. resident population. Populations for computing life expectancy for 2010 were based on 2010 census counts. Life expectancy for 2011 and beyond was computed using 2010-based postcensal estimates. In 1997, life table methodology was revised to construct complete life tables by single years of age that extend to age 100. (Anderson RN. Method for constructing complete annual U.S. life tables. NCHS. Vital Health Stat 2(129). 1999.) Previously, abridged life tables were constructed for 5-year age groups ending with 85 years and over. In 2000, the life table methodology was revised. The revised methodology is similar to that developed for the 1999–2001 decennial life tables. In 2008, the life table methodology was further refined. Starting with 2003 data, some states allowed the reporting of more than one race on the death certificate. The multiple-race data for these states were bridged to the single-race categories of the 1977 Office of Management and Budget standards, for comparability with other states. The race groups, white and black include persons of Hispanic and non-Hispanic origin. Persons of Hispanic origin may be of any race.

SOURCE: "Table 16. Life Expectancy at Birth, at Age 65, and at Age 75, by Sex, Race, and Hispanic Origin: United States, Selected Years 1900–2013," in *Health, United States, 2014: With Special Feature on Adults Aged 55–64*, Centers for Disease Control and Prevention, National Center for Health Statistics, May 2015, http://www.cdc.gov/nchs/data/hus/hus14.pdf (accessed October 5, 2015)

Federal Trade Commission, the Maternal and Child Health Bureau, the American Medical Association (AMA), the American Heart Association, the American Academy of Family Physicians, the American Society for Bariatric Surgery, the Obesity Medicine Association, and the American Obesity Association (AOA), observe that in the past, alcoholism was viewed as a personal choice or moral weakness, whereas in the 21st century it is considered a disease. They also note that eating disorders such as anorexia nervosa (intense fear of becoming fat even when dangerously underweight) and bulimia nervosa (recurrent episodes of binge eating followed by purging to prevent weight gain) are classified as diseases. In view of the size and scope of the obesity epidemic, proponents argue that the social and financial costs of allowing the problem of obesity to go unchecked will far exceed the costs associated with extending health care coverage for weight-reduction programs.

The AOA contends that obesity meets the criteria for disease because according to *Stedman's Medical Dictionary* (2005) a disease should have at least two of the following three features:

- Recognized etiologic (causative) agents

- Identifiable signs and symptoms

- Consistent anatomical alterations

The AOA describes etiologic agents for obesity as social, behavioral, cultural, physiological, metabolic, and

TABLE 2.2

Leading causes of death and numbers of deaths, according to sex and race, 1980 and 2013

[Data are based on death certificates]

Sex, race, Hispanic origin, and rank order	1980		2013*	
	Cause of death	Deaths	Cause of death	Deaths
All persons				
Rank	All causes	1,989,841	All causes	2,596,993
1	Diseases of heart	761,085	Diseases of heart	611,105
2	Malignant neoplasms	416,509	Malignant neoplasms	584,881
3	Cerebrovascular diseases	170,225	Chronic lower respiratory diseases	149,205
4	Unintentional injuries	105,718	Unintentional injuries	130,557
5	Chronic obstructive pulmonary diseases	56,050	Cerebrovascular diseases	128,978
6	Pneumonia and influenza	54,619	Alzheimer's disease	84,767
7	Diabetes mellitus	34,851	Diabetes mellitus*	75,578
8	Chronic liver disease and cirrhosis	30,583	Influenza and pneumonia	56,979
9	Atherosclerosis	29,449	Nephritis, nephrotic syndrome and nephrosis*	47,112
10	Suicide	26,869	Suicide	41,149
Male				
Rank	All causes	1,075,078	All causes	1,306,034
1	Diseases of heart	405,661	Diseases of heart	321,347
2	Malignant neoplasms	225,948	Malignant neoplasms	307,559
3	Unintentional injuries	74,180	Unintentional injuries	81,916
4	Cerebrovascular diseases	69,973	Chronic lower respiratory diseases	70,317
5	Chronic obstructive pulmonary diseases	38,625	Cerebrovascular diseases	53,691
6	Pneumonia and influenza	27,574	Diabetes mellitus*	39,841
7	Suicide	20,505	Suicide	32,055
8	Chronic liver disease and cirrhosis	19,768	Influenza and pneumonia	26,804
9	Homicide	18,779	Alzheimer's disease	25,836
10	Diabetes mellitus	14,325	Chronic liver disease and cirrhosis	23,709
Female				
Rank	All causes	914,763	All causes	1,290,959
1	Diseases of heart	355,424	Diseases of heart	289,758
2	Malignant neoplasms	190,561	Malignant neoplasms	277,322
3	Cerebrovascular diseases	100,252	Chronic lower respiratory diseases	78,888
4	Unintentional injuries	31,538	Cerebrovascular diseases	75,287
5	Pneumonia and influenza	27,045	Alzheimer's disease	58,931
6	Diabetes mellitus	20,526	Unintentional injuries	48,641
7	Atherosclerosis	17,848	Diabetes mellitus*	35,737
8	Chronic obstructive pulmonary diseases	17,425	Influenza and pneumonia	30,175
9	Chronic liver disease and cirrhosis	10,815	Nephritis, nephrotic syndrome and nephrosis*	23,619
10	Certain conditions originating in the perinatal period	9,815	Septicemia	20,162
White				
Rank	All causes	1,738,607	All causes	2,217,103
1	Diseases of heart	683,347	Diseases of heart	522,645
2	Malignant neoplasms	368,162	Malignant neoplasms	498,116
3	Cerebrovascular diseases	148,734	Chronic lower respiratory diseases	136,682
4	Unintentional injuries	90,122	Unintentional injuries	112,803
5	Chronic obstructive pulmonary diseases	52,375	Cerebrovascular diseases	107,909
6	Pneumonia and influenza	48,369	Alzheimer's disease	77,387
7	Diabetes mellitus	28,868	Diabetes mellitus*	58,925
8	Atherosclerosis	27,069	Influenza and pneumonia	49,013
9	Chronic liver disease and cirrhosis	25,240	Nephritis, nephrotic syndrome and nephrosis*	37,270
10	Suicide	24,829	Suicide	37,154
Black or African American				
Rank	All causes	233,135	All causes	302,969
1	Diseases of heart	72,956	Diseases of heart	72,010
2	Malignant neoplasms	45,037	Malignant neoplasms	67,953
3	Cerebrovascular diseases	20,135	Cerebrovascular diseases	16,269
4	Unintentional injuries	13,480	Unintentional injuries	13,413
5	Homicide	10,172	Diabetes mellitus*	13,385
6	Certain conditions originating in the perinatal period	6,961	Chronic lower respiratory diseases	9,918
7	Pneumonia and influenza	5,648	Nephritis, nephrotic syndrome and nephrosis*	8,393
8	Diabetes mellitus	5,544	Homicide	8,059
9	Chronic liver disease and cirrhosis	4,790	Septicemia	6,250
10	Nephritis, nephrotic syndrome and nephrosis	3,416	Alzheimer's disease	5,714

genetic factors. The identifiable signs and symptoms of obesity include an excess accumulation of adipose tissue (fat); an increase in the size or number of fat cells; insulin resistance; decreased levels of high-density lipoprotein and norepinephrine; alterations in the activity of the sympathetic and parasympathetic nervous system; and

TABLE 2.2

Leading causes of death and numbers of deaths, according to sex and race, 1980 and 2013 [CONTINUED]

[Data are based on death certificates]

*Starting with 2011 data, the rules for selecting renal failure as the underlying cause of death were changed, affecting the number of deaths in the nephritis, nephrotic syndrome and nephrosis and diabetes categories. These changes directly affect deaths with mention of renal failure and other associated conditions, such as diabetes mellitus with renal complications. The result is a decrease in the number of deaths for nephritis, nephrotic syndrome and nephrosis and an increase in the number of deaths for diabetes mellitus. Therefore, trend data for these two causes of death should be interpreted with caution.

Notes: Starting with 2003 data, some states allowed the reporting of more than one race on the death certificate. The multiple-race data for these states were bridged to the single-race categories of the 1977 Office of Management and Budget standards, for comparability with other states. The race groups, white, black, Asian or Pacific Islander, and American Indian or Alaska Native, include persons of Hispanic and non-Hispanic origin. Persons of Hispanic origin may be of any race.

SOURCE: Adapted from "Table 20. Leading Causes of Death and Numbers of Deaths, by Sex, Race, and Hispanic Origin: United States, 1980 and 2014," in *Health, United States, 2014: With Special Feature on Adults Aged 55–64*, Centers for Disease Control and Prevention, National Center for Health Statistics, May 2015, http://www.cdc.gov/nchs/data/hus/hus14.pdf (accessed October 5, 2015)

TABLE 2.3

Health consequences of overweight and obesity

Premature death

- An estimated 300,000 deaths per year may be attributable to obesity.
- The risk of death rises with increasing weight.
- Even moderate weight excess (10 to 20 pounds for a person of average height) increases the risk of death, particularly among adults aged 30 to 64 years.
- Individuals who are obese (body mass index (BMI) > 30) have a 50 to 100% increased risk of premature death from all causes, compared to individuals with a healthy weight.

Heart disease

- The incidence of heart disease (heart attack, congestive heart failure, sudden cardiac death, angina or chest pain, and abnormal heart rhythm) is increased in persons who are overweight or obese (BMI > 25).
- High blood pressure is twice as common in adults who are obese than in those who are at a healthy weight.
- Obesity is associated with elevated triglycerides (blood fat) and decreased high density lipoprotein (HDL) cholesterol ("good cholesterol").

Diabetes

- A weight gain of 11 to 18 pounds increases a person's risk of developing type 2 diabetes to twice that of individuals who have not gained weight.
- Over 80% of people with diabetes are overweight or obese.

Cancer

- Overweight and obesity are associated with an increased risk for some types of cancer including endometrial (cancer of the lining of the uterus), colon, gall bladder, prostate, kidney, and postmenopausal breast cancer.
- Women gaining more than 20 pounds from age 18 to midlife double their risk of postmenopausal breast cancer, compared to women whose weight remains stable.

Breathing problems

- Sleep apnea (interrupted breathing while sleeping) is more common in obese persons.
- Obesity is associated with a higher prevalence of asthma.

Arthritis

- For every 2-pound increase in weight, the risk of developing arthritis is increased by 9 to 13%.
- Symptoms of arthritis can improve with weight loss.

Reproductive complications

Complications of pregnancy
- Obesity during pregnancy is associated with increased risk of death in both the baby and the mother and increases the risk of maternal high blood pressure by 10 times.
- In addition to many other complications, women who are obese during pregnancy are more likely to have gestational diabetes and problems with labor and delivery.
- Infants born to women who are obese during pregnancy are more likely to be high birthweight and, therefore, may face a higher rate of Cesarean section delivery and low blood sugar (which can be associated with brain damage and seizures).
- Obesity during pregnancy is associated with an increased risk of birth defects, particularly neural tube defects, such as spina bifida.
- Obesity in premenopausal women is associated with irregular menstrual cycles and infertility.

Additional health consequences

- Overweight and obesity are associated with increased risks of gall bladder disease, incontinence, increased surgical risk, and depression.
- Obesity can affect the quality of life through limited mobility and decreased physical endurance as well as through social, academic, and job discrimination.

Children and adolescents

- Risk factors for heart disease, such as high cholesterol and high blood pressure, occur with increased frequency in overweight children and adolescents compared to those with a healthy weight.
- Type 2 diabetes, previously considered an adult disease, has increased dramatically in children and adolescents. Overweight and obesity are closely linked to type 2 diabetes.
- Overweight adolescents have a 70% chance of becoming overweight or obese adults. This increases to 80% if one or more parent is overweight or obese.
- The most immediate consequence of overweight, as perceived by children themselves, is social discrimination.

SOURCE: "Overweight and Obesity: Health Consequences," in *The Surgeon General's Call to Action to Prevent and Decrease Overweight and Obesity*, U.S. Department of Health and Human Services, Office of the Surgeon General, 2001, http://www.surgeongeneral.gov/topics/obesity/calltoaction/fact_consequences.htm (accessed October 5, 2015)

elevated blood pressure, blood glucose, cholesterol, and triglyceride levels. The consistent anatomical alteration of obesity is the increase in body mass.

Opponents contend that although obesity increases the risk of developing many diseases, it is not an ailment in itself but an unhealthy consequence of poor lifestyle choices. They liken it to cigarette smoking, a risk factor that predisposes people to disease, and they dispute the notion that labeling obesity as a disease will have a beneficial effect on the ability of public health organizations to alter the course of the obesity epidemic. They maintain the public tends to view diseases as conditions that are contracted or contagious; and with disease comes a victim mentality, rather than an assumption of personal responsibility. Because many health professionals consider the assumption of personal responsibility as being crucial for the long-term success of obesity treatment, any action that releases people from assuming personal responsibility is counterproductive.

For example, in "Obesity 'Disease' Discourages Prevention, Katz Argues" (YaleDailyNews.com, April 22, 2014), Elizabeth Himwich interviews David L. Katz, the director of the Yale Prevention Research Center at the Yale University School of Medicine and editor-in-chief of *Childhood Obesity*. Katz compares obesity to drowning, asserting that both result from "an interaction between a perfectly healthy body and the challenge of an environment in which they are maladapted." In both instances, people are exposed to substances that are initially beneficial, but excessive exposure is problematic. Water is necessary but too much of it for too long results in drowning. Similarly, excessive food consumption for too long results in overweight and obesity.

Furthermore, because people who are obese often function normally and can perform all the activities of daily living, opponents assert that their lives are not impaired or compromised as they might be by other chronic diseases. Some researchers, such as Silvia Migliaccio et al. of the Università Sapienza di Roma in "Is Obesity in Women Protective against Osteoporosis?" (*Diabetes, Metabolic Syndrome, and Obesity*, vol. 4, July 2011), also point to the fact that in a few instances obesity may even be protective by reducing the risk of osteoporosis.

Another concern is the lack of universally accepted, effective treatment for obesity. If obesity is classified as a disease, which treatment or therapies should be covered? For example, if exercise is deemed beneficial, then health insurers might be required to pay for gym memberships. Furthermore, some opponents believe it is not necessary to designate obesity as a disease to encourage Americans to seek treatment. They cite the more than $50 billion that is spent annually on weight-loss programs and services as evidence that Americans are not reluctant to seek treatment for obesity.

Although the debate has not been fully resolved, obesity is rapidly acquiring recognition as a disease. In 2002 the Internal Revenue Service ruled that for tax purposes obesity is a disease, allowing Americans for the first time to claim a deduction for some health care expenses that are related to obesity, just as they can for expenditures that are related to cancer, diabetes, heart disease, and other illnesses.

In 2004 the federal Medicare program discarded its long-standing position that obesity is not a disease, which effectively removed a major roadblock for people seeking coverage for treatment of obesity. After years of review, the Centers for Medicare and Medicaid Services, which administers the health program for older adults and people who are disabled, announced in *CMS Manual System: Pub. 100-03 Medicare National Coverage Determinations* (October 1, 2004, http://www.cms.hhs.gov/transmittals/downloads/R23NCD.pdf) that it eliminated the phrase "obesity itself cannot be considered an illness" from its policy that had been used to deny coverage for weight-loss treatment. Although the decision stopped short of declaring obesity a disease and did not automatically imply coverage for any specific treatment, it enabled individuals, physicians, and companies to apply to Medicare for reimbursement for a variety of weight-loss therapies. Medicare coverage for selected weight-loss procedures took effect in February 2006.

In June 2013 the AMA officially recognized obesity as a disease in an effort to increase attention to combating it and to encourage reimbursement for obesity treatment—drugs, surgery, and counseling. Andrew Pollack reports in "A.M.A. Recognizes Obesity as a Disease" (NYTimes.com, June 18, 2013) that the AMA statement characterizes obesity as a "multimetabolic and hormonal disease state" that leads to unfavorable consequences, including type 2 diabetes and cardiovascular disease.

Because private insurance companies often use Medicare as a model for their coverage and benefits, the Medicare decision prompted them to expand coverage for weight-loss procedures. As of February 2016, private health insurance coverage for weight-loss therapies and surgical procedures varied widely. The National Obesity Foundation reports in "Health Insurance Will Cover Obesity Treatment in 2015" (December 10, 2014, http://nofusa.org/news/health-insurance-cover-obesity-treatment/) that the Patient Protection and Affordable Care Act (which is more commonly known as the Affordable Care Act [ACA]), requires most insurance plans to provide some form of treatment to help obese patients lose weight. Screening and counseling for obesity as well as U.S. Food and Drug Administration–approved drug treatment must be covered by the plans; however, coverage for ongoing treatment and weight-loss surgery varies. Twenty-three states require plans to cover weight-loss surgery and 25 cover nutrition counseling. Some insurance plans provide counseling or coaching by telephone or in-person, whereas others refer patients to weight-loss programs such as Weight Watchers.

THE GENETICS OF BODY WEIGHT AND OBESITY

Genetics, the study of single genes and their effects, explains how and why traits such as hair color and blood types run in families. In the early 21st century the scientific community agreed that body shape and body weight are also regulated traits, that genes govern much of this regulation, and that altering genetically predetermined set points for body weight is often difficult. Genomics, a discipline that emerged during the 1980s, is the study of more than single genes; it considers the functions and interactions of all the genes in the genome. In terms of understanding genetics as a risk factor for obesity, genomics has broader applicability than does genetics because it is likely that humans carry dozens of genes that are directly related to body size and that most obesity is multifactorial—resulting from the complex interactions of multiple genes and environmental factors.

Because genomics is a relatively new discipline, many questions are still unanswered about how genes influence the ability to balance energy input and energy expenditure, and why individuals vary in their abilities to perform this critical body function. Table 2.4 summarizes what is known and what remains to be learned about variations in body weight, energy metabolism, and inherited obesity syndromes.

Single Mutant Genes Cause Obesity

Although most obesity in humans is not due to mutations (alterations or changes) in single genes, there are obesity syndromes caused by variations in single genes. According to Alexandra I. F. Blakemore and Philippe Froguel of the Imperial College of London, in "Investigation of Mendelian Forms of Obesity Holds Out the Prospect of Personalized Medicine" (*Annals of the New York Academy of Sciences*, vol. 1214, no. 1, December 2010), these mutations occur in genes that encode proteins that are related to the regulation of food intake and account for approximately 5% of all obesity.

The Centers for Disease Control and Prevention (CDC) reports in "Genes and Obesity" (May 17, 2013, http://www.cdc.gov/genomics/resources/diseases/obesity/obesedit.htm) that since 2006 genome-wide association studies have found more than 50 genes associated with obesity, but most exert small effects. Table 2.5 shows some of the gene variants that are associated with obesity. One example is a mutation of the leptin gene (on chromosome 7) and its receptor. The circulating hormone leptin (leptos means thin) sends the brain a satiety signal to decrease appetite. Obese mice of the ob/ob strain (obese mice that are specially bred for research) produce no leptin and tend to overeat; when given leptin, the mice stop eating and lose weight. Experiments, however, have failed to replicate these findings in humans. Blood concentrations of leptin are usually elevated in obese people,

TABLE 2.4

Obesity and genetics

What we know:	What we don't know:
Biological relatives tend to resemble each other in many ways, including body weight. Individuals with a family history of obesity may be predisposed to gain weight and interventions that prevent obesity are especially important.	Why are biological relatives more similar in body weight? What genes are associated with this observation? Are the same genetic associations seen in every family? How do these genes affect energy metabolism and regulation?
In an environment made constant for food intake and physical activity, individuals respond differently. Some people store more energy as fat in an environment of excess; others lose less fat in an environment of scarcity. The different responses are largely due to genetic variation between individuals.	Why are interventions based on diet and exercise more effective for some people than others? What are the biological differences between these high and low responders? How do we use these insights to tailor interventions to specific needs?
Fat stores are regulated over long periods of time by complex systems that involve input and feedback from fatty tissues, the brain, and endocrine glands like the pancreas and the thyroid. Overweight and obesity can result from only a very small positive energy input imbalance over a long period of time.	What elements of energy regulation feedback systems are different in individuals? How do these differences affect energy metabolism and regulation?
Rarely, people have mutations in single genes that result in severe obesity that starts in infancy. Studying these individuals is providing insight into the complex biological pathways that regulate the balance between energy input and energy expenditure.	Do additional obesity syndromes exist that are caused by mutations in single genes? If so, what are they? What are the natural history, management strategy, and outcome for affected individuals?
Obese individuals have genetic similarities that may shed light on the biological differences that predispose to gain weight. This knowledge may be useful in preventing or treating obesity in predisposed people.	How do genetic variations that are shared by obese people affect gene expression and function? How do genetic variation and environmental factors interact to produce obesity? What are the biological features associated with the tendency to gain weight? What environmental factors are helpful in countering these tendencies?
Pharmaceutical companies are using genetic approaches (pharmacogenomics) to develop new drug strategies to treat obesity.	Will pharmacologic approaches benefit most people affected with obesity? Will these drugs be accessible to most people?
The tendency to store energy in the form of fat is believed to result from thousands of years of evolution in an environment characterized by tenuous food supplies. In other words, those who could store energy in times of plenty were more likely to survive periods of famine and to pass this tendency to their offspring.	How can thousands of years of evolutionary pressure be countered? Can specific factors in the modern environment (other than the obvious) be identified and controlled to more effectively counter these tendencies?

SOURCE: "Obesity and Genetics: What We Know, What We Don't Know and What It Means," in *Genomics and Health*, Centers for Disease Control and Prevention, Office of Surveillance, Epidemiology, and Laboratory Services, Public Health Genomics, January 20, 2011, http://www.cdc.gov/genomics/resources/diseases/obesity/obesknow.htm (accessed October 5, 2015)

TABLE 2.5

Selected gene variants associated with obesity

Gene symbol	Gene name	Gene product's role in energy balance
ADIPOQ	Adipocyte-, C1q-, and collagen domain-containing	Produced by fat cells, adiponectin promotes energy expenditure
FTO	Fat mass- and obesity-associated gene	Promotes food intake
LEP	Leptin	Produced by fat cells
LEPR	Leptin receptor	When bound by leptin, inhibits appetite
INSIG2	Insulin-induced gene 2	Regulation of cholesterol and fatty acid synthesis
MC4R	Melanocortin 4 receptor	When bound by alpha-melanocyte stimulating hormone, stimulates appetite
PCSK1	Proproteinconvertasesubtilisin/kexin type 1	Regulates insulin biosynthesis
PPARG	Peroxisome proliferator-activated receptor gamma	Stimulates lipid uptake and development of fat tissue

SOURCE: "Table. Selected Genes with Variants That Have Been Associated with Obesity," in *Genomics and Health*, Centers for Disease Control and Prevention, Office of Surveillance, Epidemiology, and Laboratory Services, Public Health Genomics, May 17, 2013, http://www.cdc.gov/genomics/resources/diseases/obesity/obesedit.htm#table (accessed October 5, 2015)

suggesting that they may be insensitive or resistant to leptin, rather than leptin deficient. Most obese individuals appear to have normal genetic sequences for leptin and its receptor, although people with a demonstrable genetic leptin deficiency suffer from extreme obesity.

Melanocortin 4 receptor (MC4R) deficiency is the most commonly occurring monogenic (single gene) form of obesity. Inheriting one copy of certain variants of the gene causes obesity in some families. In "Melanocortin-4 Receptor Mutations in Obesity" (*Advances in Clinical Chemistry*, vol. 48, 2009), Ferruccio Santini et al. report that mutations in MC4R produce a distinct obesity syndrome that is inherited. The researchers observe that these mutant receptors play a pivotal role in the control of eating behavior—that the regulation of body weight in humans is sensitive to variations in the amount of functional MC4R and are present in about 6% of people who are obese.

Blakemore and Froguel observe that research on genome-wide single nucleotide polymorphisms (SNPs) associated with obesity, particularly the role of the FTO (fat mass and obesity-associated) gene, has outpaced research concentrating on a single gene that determines the occurrence of obesity. The focus on the FTO gene may be warranted because common variants of the FTO gene, which are located on chromosome 16, may be implicated in as much as 22% of obesity, according to the CDC. The FTO gene is also associated with an increased risk for diabetes.

In "Pediatric Obesity: Etiology and Treatment" (*Endocrinology and Metabolism Clinics*, vol. 58, no. 5, October 2011), Melissa K. Crocker and Jack A. Yanovski of the NIH summarize what is known about the genetic underpinnings of obesity. The researchers observe that "virtually all of the known genetic causes of obesity primarily increase energy intake. Genes regulating the leptin signaling pathway are particularly important for human energy homeostasis." They report that SNPs of many genes and chromosomal regions have been found

to be associated with body weight or body composition; however, mechanisms explaining how such SNPs exert an influence on energy balance are not fully understood. Crocker and Yanovski reiterate one of the challenges of clinical genetic research: "Even in studies including thousands of genotyped people, such SNPs can be linked to body weight only when they are relatively common in the population."

Multiple Gene Variants Involved in Body Weight and Obesity

Heritability studies seek to determine the proportion of variance of a particular trait that is attributable to genetic factors and the proportion that is attributable to environmental factors. Such studies indicate that genetic factors may account for as much as 75% of the variability in human body weight and approximately 33% of the variation in the overall BMI (body weight in kilograms divided by height in meters squared). Genetic factors affect variations in the resting metabolic rate, body fat distribution, and weight gain related to overfeeding, which explains in part why some individuals are more susceptible than others to weight gain or weight loss. To ensure survival in times of scarce food supplies, the human body has evolved to resist any loss of body fat. This biological drive to maintain weight is coordinated through central nervous system pathways, with the involvement of many neuropeptides. (Neuropeptides are released by neurons as intercellular messengers. Many neuropeptides are also hormones outside of the nervous system.) Evidence from twin, adoption, and family studies reveals that biological relatives exhibit similarities in the maintenance of body weight. First-degree relatives of moderately obese people are at three to four times the risk of obesity relative to the general population. First-degree relatives of severely obese people are at five times greater risk. Genetic predisposition to obesity does not mean that developing the condition is inevitable; however, research indicates that inherited genetic variation is an important risk factor for obesity.

Genetic factors have been implicated in the development of eating disorders such as anorexia and bulimia and appear to be involved in the extent to which diet and exercise are effective strategies for weight reduction. Furthermore, genetic variations among individuals may promote different food preferences and eating patterns that interact with environmental conditions to maintain healthy body weight or promote obesity.

These genetic risk factors tend to be familial but are not inherited in a simple manner; they may reflect many genetic variations, and each variation may contribute a small amount of risk and may interact with environmental elements to produce obesity. Tuomo Rankinen et al. present in "The Human Obesity Gene Map: The 2005 Update" (*Obesity*, vol. 14, no. 4, April 2006) the 12th update of the human obesity gene map, which was completed in October 2005. This map contains over 600 genes, markers, and chromosomal regions that are associated with or linked to human obesity. Besides offering direction for future efforts to prevent and treat obesity, mounting genetic evidence offers a compelling argument that obesity is not a personal failing and that in most cases obesity involves multiple genetic and environmental components that affect endocrine, metabolic, and regulatory mechanisms.

In "Obesity Gene Atlas in Mammals" (*Journal of Genomics*, vol. 1, 2013), Tanja Kunej et al. describe the creation of an obesity database that contains 1,736 obesity-associated loci (specific sites where genetic variants associated with polygenic obesity are located) from humans, cattle, rats, and mice. The researchers note that genes involved in polygenic (caused by more than one gene) obesity govern or play a role in a variety of biological functions, including regulation of food intake, energy expenditure, lipid and glucose metabolism, and adipose tissue development.

Extra Genes Point to a Genetic Cause of Thinness

Unlike obesity, few genetic variants associated with underweight have been identified. Sébastien Jacquemont et al. report in "Mirror Extreme BMI Phenotypes Associated with Gene Dosage at the Chromosome 16p11.2 Locus" (*Nature*, vol. 478, no. 7367, August 31, 2011) that duplication of a portion of chromosome 16 is associated with being very thin (BMI less than 18.5). The researchers analyzed the deoxyribonucleic acid of more than 95,000 people and find that more than half of children with this duplication had significantly lower than normal weight gain. Jacquemont et al. also note that people missing this gene have an increased risk for obesity.

Genetic Susceptibility and Environmental Influences

Although genetics may largely predetermine adult body weight absent specific environmental triggers or influences, genetic destiny in terms of body weight may not necessarily be realized. For example, an individual with a strong genetic predisposition for obesity will not become obese in the absence of sufficient food (caloric) intake. Similarly, when people who are genetically predisposed to normal body weight consume a largely high-fat diet, they may become overweight or obese because they may be more inclined to overeat. This is in part because the brain has difficulty conveying the satiety signal (the message to stop eating) when fatty foods are being consumed.

Besides caloric intake and physical activity, both of which are able to modify body weight, environmental influences before birth also significantly affect adult health and body weight. Research demonstrates that the pregnant mother's nutritional status affects the metabolism of her unborn child. Women who are severely malnourished during pregnancy stimulate the fetus to modify its metabolism to conserve and store energy, a survival practice that can promote overweight when the food supply is ample.

Societal and cultural norms can also cause environmental influences such as lifestyle and behavior to override genetic programming. For example, in the United States many young women with genetic predisposition to normal body weight or even overweight sharply limit their caloric intake and exercise vigorously to achieve "model thin" bodies. Similarly, in cultures where overweight is perceived as an indication of prosperity and is admired and coveted, people may override genetic tendencies to be normal weight by increasing caloric intake in an effort to achieve the culturally established ideal.

HEALTH RISKS AND CONSEQUENCES OF OVERWEIGHT AND OBESITY

People who are overweight or obese are at higher risk of developing one or more serious medical conditions, and obesity is associated with increases in deaths from all causes. Overweight and obesity significantly increase the risk for hypercholesterolemia (high cholesterol), hypertension, heart disease, and stroke; type 2 diabetes; osteoarthritis and chronic joint pain; gallbladder disease; fatty liver disease; several types of cancers; and sleep apnea (interrupted breathing while sleeping) and sleep disorders.

Hypercholesterolemia, Hypertension, Heart Disease, and Stroke

Overweight, obesity, and excess abdominal fat are directly related to cardiovascular risk factors, including high levels of total serum cholesterol, low-density lipoprotein (LDL) cholesterol (a fatlike substance often called bad cholesterol because high levels increase the risk for heart disease), triglycerides, blood pressure, fibrinogen, and insulin, and low levels of high-density lipoprotein (HDL) cholesterol (often called good cholesterol because high levels appear to protect against heart disease). The association between total serum cholesterol and coronary heart disease is largely due to LDL. A high-risk LDL cholesterol is greater than or equal to 160 milligrams per deciliter (mg/dL) with a 10 mg/dL rise in LDL cholesterol corresponding to approximately a 10% increase in risk. High-risk total serum cholesterol is greater than or equal to 240 mg/dL. The age-adjusted percentage of the population aged 20 years and older suffering from high serum cholesterol levels decreased from 20.8% in 1988–94 to 12.7% in 2011–12. (See Table 2.6.) The overall decline in high total serum cholesterol occurred in response to the increasing use of effective cholesterol-lowering statin drugs.

The percentage of the population suffering from hypertension (people with elevated blood pressure and those taking antihypertensive medication) increased between 1988–94 and 2011–12, from 25.5% to 30% of the population. (See Table 2.6.) The highest rates for those aged 20 years and older during the 2009–12 period were reported among African American females (44.5%). (See Table 2.7.) Men and women were increasingly likely to have hypertension as they aged. Hypertension is approximately three times more common in obese people than in healthy-weight people, and the relationship between weight and blood pressure is clearly one of cause and effect, because when weight increases, so does blood pressure, and when weight decreases, blood pressure falls.

The physiological processes that produce the hypertension associated with obesity include sodium retention and increases in vascular resistance, blood volume, and cardiac output (the volume of blood pumped, measured in liters per minute). Although it is not known precisely how weight loss results in a decrease in blood pressure, it is known that weight loss is associated with a reduction in vascular resistance and total blood volume and cardiac output. Weight loss also results in an improvement in insulin resistance, a reduction in sympathetic nervous system activity, and the suppression of the renin-angiotensin-aldosterone system (a group of hormones that are responsible for the opening and narrowing of blood vessels and the retention of fluids).

TABLE 2.6

Selected health conditions and risk factors by selected characteristics, selected years 1988–2012

[Data are based on interviews and physical examinations of a sample of the civilian noninstitutionalized population]

Health condition	1988–1994	1999–2000	2001–2002	2003–2004	2005–2006	2007–2008	2009–2010	2011–2012
Diabetes[a]				Percent of adults aged 20 and over				
Total, age-adjusted[b]	8.8	9.0	10.6	10.9	10.4	11.4	11.5	11.9
Total, crude	8.3	8.6	10.3	10.9	10.9	11.9	12.1	12.5
Hypercholesterolemia[c]								
Total, age-adjusted[d]	22.8	25.5	24.6	27.9	27.4	27.6	27.2	28.2
Total, crude	21.5	24.5	24.2	27.9	28.1	28.8	28.6	30.4
High cholesterol[e]								
Total, age-adjusted[d]	20.8	18.3	16.5	16.9	15.6	14.2	13.2	12.7
Total, crude	19.6	17.7	16.4	17.0	15.9	14.6	13.6	13.1
Hypertension[f]								
Total, age-adjusted[d]	25.5	30.0	29.7	32.1	30.5	31.2	30.0	30.0
Total, crude	24.1	28.9	28.9	32.5	31.7	32.6	31.9	32.5
Uncontrolled high blood pressure among persons with hypertension[g]								
Total, age-adjusted[d]	77.2	71.9	68.3	63.8	63.0	56.2	55.7	54.6
Total, crude	73.9	69.1	65.4	60.8	56.6	51.8	46.7	48.0
Overweight (includes obesity)[h]								
Total, age-adjusted[d]	56.0	64.5	65.6	66.4	66.9	68.1	68.8	68.6
Total, crude	54.9	64.1	65.6	66.5	67.3	68.3	69.2	69.0
Obesity[i]								
Total, age-adjusted[d]	22.9	30.5	30.5	32.3	34.4	33.7	35.7	34.9
Total, crude	22.3	30.3	30.6	32.3	34.7	33.9	35.9	35.1
Untreated dental caries[j]								
Total, age-adjusted[d]	27.7	24.4	21.3	29.8	24.4	21.7	—	25.5
Total, crude	28.2	25.0	21.7	30.2	24.5	21.8	—	25.5
Obesity[k]				Percent of persons under age 20				
2–5 years	7.2	10.3	10.6	14.0	11.0	10.1	12.1	8.4
6–11 years	11.3	15.1	16.3	18.8	15.1	19.6	18.0	17.7
12–19 years	10.5	14.8	16.7	17.4	17.8	18.1	18.4	20.5
Untreated dental caries[j]								
5–19 years	24.3	23.6	21.2	25.6	16.2	16.9	14.6	17.5

TABLE 2.6

Selected health conditions and risk factors by selected characteristics, selected years 1988–2012 [CONTINUED]

[Data are based on interviews and physical examinations of a sample of the civilian noninstitutionalized population]

—Data not available.

[a]Includes physician-diagnosed and undiagnosed diabetes. Estimates were obtained using fasting weights. Physician-diagnosed diabetes was obtained by self-report and excludes women who reported having diabetes only during pregnancy. Undiagnosed diabetes is defined as a fasting plasma glucose (FPG) of at least 126 mg/dL or a hemoglobin A1c of at least 6.5% and no reported physician diagnosis. Pregnant women were excluded. Adjustments to FPG recommended by NHANES for trend analysis were incorporated into the data presented here. Prior to Health, United States, 2010, the definition of undiagnosed diabetes did not consider hemoglobin A1c. The revised definition of undiagnosed diabetes was based on recommendations from the American Diabetes Association. To ensure data comparability, the revised definition of undiagnosed diabetes was applied to all data in this table.

[b]Estimates are age-adjusted to the year 2000 standard population using three age groups: 20–44 years, 45–64 years, and 65 years and over. Age-adjusted estimates in this table may differ from other age-adjusted estimates based on the same data presented elsewhere if different age groups are used in the adjustment procedure.

[c]Hypercholesterolemia is defined as measured serum total cholesterol greater than or equal to 240 mg/dL or reporting taking cholesterol-lowering medication. Respondents were asked, "Are you now following this advice [from a doctor or health professional] to take prescribed medicine [to lower your cholesterol]?" Risk levels for serum total cholesterol have been defined by the Third Report of the National Cholesterol Education Program Expert Panel on Detection, Evaluation, and Treatment of High Blood Cholesterol in Adults. National Heart, Lung, and Blood Institute, National Institutes of Health. September 2002.

[d]Estimates are age-adjusted to the year 2000 standard population using five age groups: 20–34 years, 35–44 years, 45–54 years, 55–64 years, and 65 years and over. Age-adjusted estimates in this table may differ from other age-adjusted estimates based on the same data and presented elsewhere if different age groups are used in the adjustment procedure.

[e]High cholesterol is defined as greater than or equal to 240 mg/dL (6.20 mmol/L). This second measure of cholesterol presented in Health, United States is based solely on measured high serum total cholesterol.

[f]Hypertension is defined as having measured high blood pressure and/or taking antihypertensive medication. High blood pressure is defined as having measured systolic pressure of at least 140 mm Hg or diastolic pressure of at least 90 mm Hg. Those with high blood pressure also may be taking prescribed medicine for high blood pressure. For antihypertensive medication use, respondents were asked, "Are you now taking prescribed medicine for your high blood pressure?"

[g]Uncontrolled high blood pressure among persons with hypertension is defined as measured systolic pressure of at least 140 mm Hg or diastolic pressure of at least 90 mm Hg, among those with measured high blood pressure or reporting taking antihypertensive medication.

[h]Overweight is defined as body mass index (BMI) greater than or equal to 25, based on the NHANES variable, Body Mass Index. Excludes pregnant women.

[i]Obesity is defined as body mass index (BMI) greater than or equal to 30, based on the NHANES variable, Body Mass Index. Excludes pregnant women.

[j]Untreated dental caries refers to decay on the crown or enamel surface of a tooth (i.e., coronal caries) that has not been treated or filled. The presence of caries was evaluated in primary and permanent teeth for persons aged 5 and older. The third molars were not included. Persons without at least one natural tooth (primary or permanent) were excluded. Over time, there have been changes in the NHANES oral health examination process, ages examined, and methodology.

[k]Obesity is defined as body mass index (BMI) at or above the sex- and age-specific 95th percentile BMI (based on the variable BMXBMI) using cutoff points from the 2000 CDC growth charts for the United States: Methods and development. NCHS. Vital Health Stat 11(246). 2002. Starting with Health, United States, 2010, the terminology describing height for weight among children changed from previous editions. The term obesity now refers to children who were formerly labeled as overweight. This is a change in terminology only and not measurement; the previous definition of overweight is now the definition of obesity. Changes in terminology for childhood overweight and obesity. National health statistics report; no. 25. Hyattsville, MD: NCHS; 2010. Excludes pregnant girls.

Notes: Some data have been revised and differ from previous editions of Health, United States.

SOURCE: Adapted from "Table 59. Selected Health Conditions and Risk Factors, by Age: United States, Selected Years 1988–1994 through 2011–2012," in *Health, United States, 2014: With Special Feature on Adults Aged 55–64*, Centers for Disease Control and Prevention, National Center for Health Statistics, May 2015, http://www.cdc.gov/nchs/data/hus/hus14.pdf (accessed October 5, 2015)

Obesity increases the risk for coronary artery disease, which in turn increases the risk for future heart failure. Congestive heart failure is not a disease but a condition that occurs when the heart is unable to pump enough blood to meet the needs of the body's tissues. When the heart fails, it is unable to pump out all the blood that enters its chambers. Congestive heart failure is a frequent complication of severe obesity and a major cause of death. The duration of obesity is a strong predictor of congestive heart failure because over time elevated total blood volume and high cardiac output cause the left ventricle of the heart to increase in size (known as left ventricular hypertrophy) beyond that expected from normal growth. Left ventricular hypertrophy is frequently identified in cardiac patients with obesity and in part results from hypertension, but abnormalities in left ventricular mass and function also occur in the absence of hypertension and may be related to the severity of obesity.

Inflammation in blood vessels and throughout the body is thought to increase the risk for heart disease and stroke (sudden injury to the brain due to a compromised blood and oxygen supply). People with more body fat have higher blood levels of substances such as plasminogen activator inhibitor-1, an enzyme produced in the kidneys that inhibits the conversion of plasminogen to plasmin and initiates fibrinolysis. Fibrinolysis leads to the breakdown of fibrin, which is responsible for the semisolid character of a blood clot that can occlude (block) blood vessels. This is the mechanism believed to account for the finding that obesity is associated with an increased risk of blood clot formation. Occluded arteries may produce myocardial infarction (heart attack) or stroke. Overweight increases the risk for ischemic stroke (resulting from a clot or blockage) but does not appear to increase the risk for hemorrhagic stroke (bleeding inside the brain), which, in general, is associated with more fatality. Andrew B. Mitchell et al. report in "Obesity Increases Risk of Ischemic Stroke in Young Adults" (*Stroke*, vol. 46, no. 6, June 2015) that the risk of stroke in young adults aged 15 to 49 years increases with a BMI greater than 30. The researchers suggest that increased stroke risk may be mediated by hypertension, diabetes, and atherosclerosis (the deposit of fatty plaque in the walls of arteries that impede blood flow).

In "Inflammation, a Link between Obesity and Cardiovascular Disease" (*Mediators of Inflammation*, August 2010), Zhaoxia Wang and Tomohiro Nakayama confirm that obesity is associated with increased morbidity and mortality from cardiovascular disease (heart disease,

TABLE 2.7

Hypertension and elevated blood pressure among persons 20 years of age and older, by selected characteristics, selected years 1988–2012

[Data are based on interviews and physical examinations of a sample of the civilian noninstitutionalized population]

Sex, age, race and Hispanic origin[a], and percent of poverty level	Hypertension[b, c] (measured high blood pressure and/or taking antihypertensive medication)				Uncontrolled high blood pressure among persons with hypertension[d]			
	1988–1994	1999–2002	2003–2006	2009–2012	1988–1994	1999–2002	2003–2006	2009–2012
20 years and over, age-adjusted[e]				Percent of population				
Both sexes[f]	25.5	30.0	31.3	30.0	77.2	70.6	63.3	55.1
Male	26.4	28.8	31.8	30.6	83.2	73.3	65.0	62.0
Female	24.4	30.6	30.3	29.3	68.5	61.8	53.6	44.7
Not Hispanic or Latino:								
White only, male	25.6	27.6	31.2	29.6	82.6	70.3	63.3	58.7
White only, female	23.0	28.5	28.3	27.5	67.0	63.6	47.5	42.8
Black or African American only, male	37.5	40.6	42.2	42.5	84.0	74.3	70.2	68.9
Black or African American only, female	38.3	43.5	44.1	44.2	71.1	67.2	59.0	46.8
Mexican origin male	26.9	26.8	24.8	27.3	87.9	89.5	70.7	76.4
Mexican origin female	25.0	27.9	28.6	29.3	77.6	71.5	66.1	47.1
Percent of poverty level:[g]								
Below 100%	31.7	33.9	35.0	33.4	75.0	71.2	69.8	56.3
100%–199%	26.6	33.5	34.1	33.1	76.0	73.4	68.2	57.6
200%–399%	24.7	30.2	31.9	30.6	76.2	67.8	63.9	51.5
400% or more	22.6	26.4	28.9	27.3	81.5	70.3	56.8	60.2
20 years and over, crude								
Both sexes[f]	24.1	30.2	32.1	32.2	73.9	67.3	58.6	47.4
Male	23.8	27.6	31.3	31.6	79.3	67.1	58.4	50.7
Female	24.4	32.7	32.9	32.8	68.8	67.4	58.8	44.2
Not Hispanic or Latino:								
White only, male	24.3	28.3	32.4	33.1	78.0	64.0	56.2	47.2
White only, female	24.6	32.8	33.4	33.7	67.8	66.9	58.2	42.6
Black or African American only, male	31.1	35.9	38.8	39.9	83.3	71.3	65.9	60.5
Black or African American only, female	32.5	41.9	42.8	44.5	70.0	67.5	55.5	45.8
Mexican origin male	16.4	16.5	16.6	19.1	86.5	86.9	66.9	69.8
Mexican origin female	15.9	18.8	20.0	22.0	80.6	74.5	68.6	52.8
Percent of poverty level:[g]								
Below 100%	25.7	30.3	28.8	27.3	74.0	71.3	67.3	54.8
100%–199%	26.7	34.8	36.8	35.3	75.1	70.7	63.2	49.8
200%–399%	22.4	29.9	33.1	33.4	73.4	64.4	58.0	45.7
400% or more	22.0	26.8	29.2	31.5	74.3	63.8	53.4	43.1
Male								
20–44 years	10.9	12.1	14.2	11.2	90.5	79.7	71.1	70.3
20–34 years	7.1	*8.1	9.2	5.8	92.6	89.9	83.1	88.4
35–44 years	17.1	17.1	21.1	19.1	89.0	73.3	63.6	62.0
45–64 years	34.2	36.4	41.2	42.2	73.1	61.4	57.0	50.2
45–54 years	29.2	31.0	36.2	33.6	76.2	66.4	59.3	47.7
55–64 years	40.6	45.0	50.2	51.9	70.3	55.9	53.9	52.0
65–74 years	54.4	59.6	64.1	61.7	74.3	59.1	45.9	36.9
75 years and over	60.4	69.0	65.0	75.1	82.5	74.3	59.7	48.9
Female								
20–44 years	6.5	8.3	6.9	8.7	63.4	58.3	49.1	46.5
20–34 years	2.9	*2.7	*2.2	3.9	82.2	56.9	*47.9	49.0
35–44 years	11.2	15.1	12.6	15.5	56.8	58.6	49.4	45.5
45–64 years	32.8	40.0	43.4	39.5	62.1	60.5	55.5	36.5
45–54 years	23.9	31.8	36.2	29.5	58.5	61.1	57.4	36.2
55–64 years	42.6	53.9	54.4	51.0	64.3	60.0	53.6	36.8
65–74 years	56.2	72.7	70.8	66.7	68.7	73.5	58.5	45.4
75 years and over	73.6	83.1	80.2	79.3	81.9	78.1	70.3	57.8

stroke and other vascular disease, and atherosclerosis). The researchers posit that obesity induces inflammation, which accelerates atherosclerosis. Wang and Nakayama believe that advancing the understanding of inflammation and the relationship between obesity and cardiovascular disease will help enhance the biological, physical, and functional changes that are associated with obesity.

Figure 2.1 shows the process, known as a treatment algorithm, that is used to assess and treat overweight and obese individuals, based on their body weight, abdominal fat, and the risk factors for cardiovascular morbidity and mortality.

Type 2 Diabetes

Diabetes is a disease that affects the body's use of food, causing blood glucose (sugar levels in the blood) to become too high. Normally, the body converts sugars, starches, and proteins into a form of sugar called glucose.

TABLE 2.7

Hypertension and elevated blood pressure among persons 20 years of age and older, by selected characteristics, selected years 1988–2012 [CONTINUED]

[Data are based on interviews and physical examinations of a sample of the civilian noninstitutionalized population]

—Data not available.
*Estimates are considered unreliable. Data preceded by an asterisk have a relative standard error of 20%–30%.
[a]Persons of Mexican origin may be of any race. Starting with 1999 data, race-specific estimates are tabulated according to the 1997 *Revisions to the Standards for the Classification of Federal Data on Race and Ethnicity* and are not strictly comparable with estimates for earlier years. The two non-Hispanic race categories shown in the table conform to the 1997 Standards. Starting with 1999 data, race-specific estimates are for persons who reported only one racial group. Prior to data year 1999, estimates were tabulated according to the 1977 Standards. Estimates for single-race categories prior to 1999 included persons who reported one race or, if they reported more than one race, identified one race as best representing their race.
[b]Hypertension is defined as having measured high blood pressure and/or taking antihypertensive medication. High blood pressure is defined as having measured systolic pressure of at least 140 mm Hg or diastolic pressure of at least 90 mm Hg. Those with high blood pressure also may be taking prescribed medicine for high blood pressure. Those taking antihypertensive medication may not have measured high blood pressure but are still classified as having hypertension.
[c]Respondents were asked, "Are you now taking prescribed medicine for your high blood pressure?"
[d]Uncontrolled high blood pressure among persons with hypertension is defined as measured systolic pressure of at least 140 mm Hg or diastolic pressure of at least 90 mm Hg, among those with measured high blood pressure or reporting taking antihypertensive medication.
[e]Estimates are age-adjusted to the year 2000 standard population using five age groups: 20–34 years, 35–44 years, 45–54 years, 55–64 years, and 65 years and over. Age-adjusted estimates in this table may differ from other age-adjusted estimates based on the same data and presented elsewhere if different age groups are used in the adjustment procedure.
[f]Includes persons of all races and Hispanic origins, not just those shown separately.
[g]Percent of poverty level was calculated by dividing family income by the U.S. Department of Health and Human Services' poverty guideline specific to family size, as well as the appropriate year, and state. Persons with unknown percent of poverty level are excluded (7% in 2009–2012).
Notes: Percentages are based on the average of blood pressure measurements taken. In 2009–2012, 84% of participants had three systolic or diastolic blood pressure readings. Excludes pregnant women.

SOURCE: "Table 60. Hypertension among Adults Aged 20 and over, by Selected Characteristics: United States, Selected Years 1988–1994 through 2009–2012," in *Health, United States, 2014: With Special Feature on Adults Aged 55–64*, Centers for Disease Control and Prevention, National Center for Health Statistics, May 2015, http://www.cdc.gov/nchs/data/hus/hus14.pdf (accessed October 5, 2015)

The blood then carries glucose to all the cells throughout the body. In the cells, with the help of the hormone insulin, the glucose is either converted into energy for use immediately or stored for the future. Beta cells of the pancreas, a small organ located behind the stomach, manufacture the insulin. The process of turning food into energy via glucose (blood sugar) is important because the body depends on glucose for every function.

With diabetes, the body can convert food to glucose, but there is a problem with insulin. In one type of diabetes (insulin-dependent diabetes or type 1), the pancreas does not manufacture enough insulin, and in another type (noninsulin dependent or type 2), the body has insulin but cannot use the insulin effectively (this latter condition is called insulin resistance). When insulin is either absent or ineffective, glucose cannot get into the cells to be used for energy. Instead, the unused glucose builds up in the bloodstream and circulates through the kidneys. If a person's blood-glucose level rises high enough, the excess glucose "spills" over into the urine, causing frequent urination. This, in turn, leads to an increased feeling of thirst as the body tries to compensate for the fluid that is lost through urination.

Type 2 diabetes is most often seen in adults and is the most common type of diabetes in the United States. In this type, the pancreas produces insulin, but it is not used effectively because the body resists responding to it. Heredity may be a predisposing factor in the genesis of type 2 diabetes, but because the pancreas continues to produce insulin, the disease is considered more of a problem of insulin resistance, in which the body is not using the hormone efficiently.

Because diabetes deprives body cells of the glucose needed to function properly, several complications can develop to threaten the lives of diabetics. The healing process of the body is slowed or impaired and the risk of infection increases. Complications of diabetes include higher risk and rates of heart disease; circulatory problems, especially in the legs, are often severe enough to require surgery or even amputation; diabetic retinopathy, a condition that can cause blindness; kidney disease that may require dialysis; dental problems; and problems with pregnancy.

The NIH's Weight-Control Information Network observes in *Do You Know Some of the Health Risks of Being Overweight?* (December 2012, http://win.niddk.nih.gov/Publications/health_risks.htm) that about 80% of people with type 2 diabetes are overweight, and in people who are prone to type 2 diabetes, becoming overweight can trigger the onset of the disease. It is not known precisely how overweight contributes to the causation of this disease. One hypothesis is that being overweight causes cells to change, making them less effective at using glucose. This then stresses the cells that produce insulin, causing them to fail gradually. Maintaining a healthy weight and keeping physically fit can usually prevent or delay the onset of type 2 diabetes.

From 1997 to March 2015 the percentage of Americans diagnosed with diabetes rose from 5.1% to 9.3%. (See Figure 2.2.) These numbers may significantly underestimate the true prevalence of diabetes in the United States in view of National Health and Nutrition Examination Survey findings that show sizable numbers of adults have undiagnosed diabetes.

FIGURE 2.1

Overweight and obesity treatment algorithm

☐ Examination ☐ Treatment

Note: This algorithm applies only to the assessment for overweight and obesity and subsequent decisions based on that assessment. It does not include any initial overall assessment for cardiovascular risk factors or diseases that are indicated.
*BMI = Body mass index.

SOURCE: "Treatment Algorithm," in *Clinical Guidelines on the Identification, Evaluation, and Treatment of Overweight and Obesity in Adults: The Evidence Report*, National Institutes of Health, National Heart, Lung, and Blood Institute in cooperation with The National Institute of Diabetes and Digestive and Kidney Diseases, 1998, http://www.nhlbi.nih.gov/guidelines/obesity/ob_gdlns.pdf (accessed October 5, 2015)

"DIABESITY" AND "DOUBLE DIABETES." The recognition of obesity-dependent diabetes prompted scientists and physicians to coin a new term to describe this condition: diabesity. The term was first used during the 1990s and has gained widespread acceptance. Although diabesity is attributed to the same causes as type 2 diabetes (insulin resistance and pancreatic cell dysfunction), researchers are beginning to link the inflammation that is associated with obesity to the development of diabetes and cardiovascular disease.

Qudsia Anjum of the International Medical Center in Rabigh, Saudi Arabia, contends in "Diabesity—A Future Pandemic" (*Journal of Pakistan Medical Association*, vol. 61, no. 4, April 2011) that the diabesity epidemic is the "tip of the iceberg; the impending threat is yet to be dealt. The combination and interdependence of diabetes and obesity imposes a therapeutic challenge to the clinicians." Anjum observes that global estimates of diabetes project an increase from 171 million in 2000 to 366 million in 2030. The increasing prevalence of diabesity has prompted the development of new treatment strategies to address both problems. In "Emerging Therapies in the Treatment of 'Diabesity': Beyond GLP-1" (*Trends in Pharmacological Sciences*, vol. 32, no. 1, January 2011), George Tharakan, Tricia Tan, and Stephen Bloom of the Imperial College of London explain that although weight-loss surgery has proven to be an effective treatment for diabesity, "finding a pharmaceutical alternative that mimics the benefits of

FIGURE 2.2

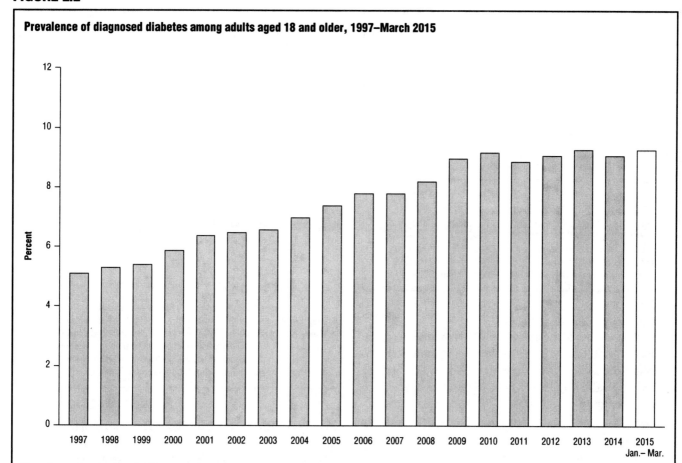

Prevalence of diagnosed diabetes among adults aged 18 and older, 1997–March 2015

Notes: Data are based on household interviews of a sample of the civilian noninstitutionalized population. Prevalence of diagnosed diabetes is based on self-report of ever having been diagnosed with diabetes by a doctor or other health professional. Persons reporting "borderline" diabetes status and women reporting diabetes only during pregnancy were not coded as having diabetes in the analyses. The analyses excluded persons with unknown diabetes status (about 0.1% of respondents each year).

SOURCE: Tainya C. Clarke et al., "Figure 14.1. Prevalence of Diagnosed Diabetes among Adults Aged 18 Years and over: United States, 1997–March 2015," in *Early Release of Selected Estimates Based on Data from the January–March 2015 National Health Interview Survey*, Centers for Disease Control and Prevention, National Center for Health Statistics, September 2015, http://www.cdc.gov/nchs/data/nhis/earlyrelease/earlyrelease201509_14.pdf (accessed September 25, 2015)

surgery without surgical complications has become the 'holy grail' of the twenty-first century."

Another recent phenomenon is the growing number of patients diagnosed with both type 1 and type 2 diabetes simultaneously. Dubbed "double diabetes," it has been reported in both children and adults. Paolo Pozzilli et al. explain in "Obesity, Autoimmunity, and Double Diabetes in Youth" (*Diabetes Care*, vol. 34, suppl. 2, May 2011) that the increase in double diabetes, also known as type 1.5, has gained the attention of the medical community. People with double diabetes have characteristics of both type 1 and type 2 diabetes. When children and adolescents with type 1 diabetes become overweight or obese, they are at increased risk for double diabetes. Pozzilli et al. do not believe that double diabetes is a new or emerging form of diabetes; they opine that it reflects the increasing prevalence of obesity.

Treatment for diabetes is individualized and may involve diet, exercise, orally administered medication,

and injected insulin or a combination of these measures. In general, people with type 1.5 diabetes require insulin within four years of diagnosis, compared with those with type 2 diabetes, who may not require it for more than 10 years after being diagnosed.

Osteoarthritis and Joint Injury

Being only 10 pounds overweight increases the force on the knee by 30–60 pounds with each step.... Even small amounts of weight loss reduce the risk of developing knee OA [osteoarthritis]. Preliminary studies suggest weight loss decreases pain substantially in those with knee OA.

—Susan Bartlett, "Osteoarthritis Weight Management" (2010)

The word *arthritis* literally means joint inflammation. The name applies to more than 100 related diseases that are known as rheumatic diseases. A joint is any point where two bones meet. When a joint becomes inflamed, swelling, redness, pain, and loss of motion occur. In the

FIGURE 2.3

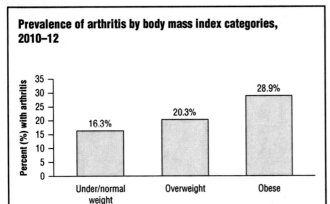

Prevalence of arthritis by body mass index categories, 2010–12

SOURCE: "Figure 4a. Age-Adjusted Arthritis Prevalence by Body Mass Index (BMI) Categories, 2010–2012," in *National Statistics*, National Center for Chronic Disease Prevention and Health Promotion, Division of Population Health, February 25, 2015, http://www.cdc.gov/arthritis/data_statistics/national-statistics.html (accessed October 5, 2015)

FIGURE 2.4

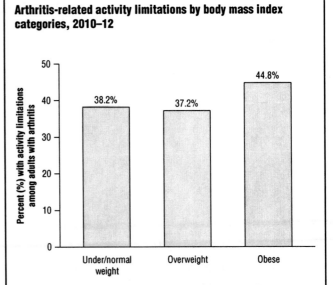

Arthritis-related activity limitations by body mass index categories, 2010–12

SOURCE: "Figure 4b. Age-Adjusted Arthritis-Attributable Activity Limitations among Adults with Arthritis by Body Mass Index (BMI) Categories, NHIS 2010–2012," in *National Statistics*, National Center for Chronic Disease Prevention and Health Promotion, Division of Population Health, February 25, 2015, http://www.cdc.gov/arthritis/data_statistics/national-statistics.html (accessed October 5, 2015)

most serious forms of the disease, the loss of motion can be physically disabling. Arthritis is the leading cause of disability and the leading cause of limitation of activity among working-age adults (aged 18 to 64 years) in the United States. According to the CDC, in "National Statistics" (January 25, 2016, http://www.cdc.gov/arthritis/data_statistics/national-statistics.html), an estimated 52.5 million adults in the United States suffer from arthritis.

People who are overweight or obese are at increased risk for osteoarthritis, which is not an inflammatory arthritis. (See Figure 2.3.) Osteoarthritis, sometimes called degenerative arthritis, causes the breakdown of bones and cartilage (connective tissue attached to bones) and usually causes pain and stiffness in the fingers, knees, feet, hips, and back. An estimated 20 million Americans suffer from osteoarthritis, and this number is expected to double by 2035. Extra weight places extra pressure on joints and cartilage, causing them to erode. Furthermore, people with more body fat may have higher blood levels of substances that cause inflammation. Inflammation at the joints may increase the risk for osteoarthritis. People who are obese are also more likely to experience arthritis-related activity limitations. (See Figure 2.4.)

In "Role of Body Weight in Osteoarthritis" (March 27, 2012, http://www.hopkinsarthritis.org/patient-corner/disease-management/role-of-body-weight-in-osteoarthritis/), Susan Bartlett of Johns Hopkins University indicates that obese women have about four times the risk of knee osteoarthritis, compared with women of healthy weight, and for obese men the risk is five times greater. The CDC observes that even modest weight loss of just 11 pounds (5 kg) can reduce the risk for knee osteoarthritis among women by 50% and may also reduce the mortality risk in people with osteoarthritis by half.

By 2016 the relationship between weight loss and improvements in the symptoms of knee pain due to arthritis was clear and definitive enough to warrant classifying it as an effective treatment for this condition. According to Robin Christensen et al., in "Effect of Weight Maintenance on Symptoms of Knee Osteoarthritis in Obese Patients: A Twelve-Month Randomized Controlled Trial" (*Arthritis Care and Research*, vol. 67, no. 5, May 2015), obesity is the strongest modifiable risk factor for knee osteoarthritis. Weight loss is one of the standard nonsurgical treatments for overweight and obese patients suffering from osteoarthritis of the knee because it acts to reduce pain and improve physical function.

Gallbladder Disease

Gallstones are small, hard pellets that can form when bile in the gallbladder (a muscular saclike organ that lies under the liver in the right side of the abdomen) precipitates (becomes solid out of the bile solution). Bile contains water, cholesterol, fats, bile salts, proteins, and bilirubin. The gallbladder stores and concentrates the bile produced in the liver that is not needed immediately for digestion. Bile is released from the gallbladder into the small intestine in response to food. The pancreatic duct joins the common bile duct at the small intestine, adding enzymes to aid in digestion. (See Figure 2.5.) If bile contains too much cholesterol, bile salts, or bilirubin, under certain conditions it can harden into stones. Most gallstones are formed primarily from cholesterol. Although some

FIGURE 2.5

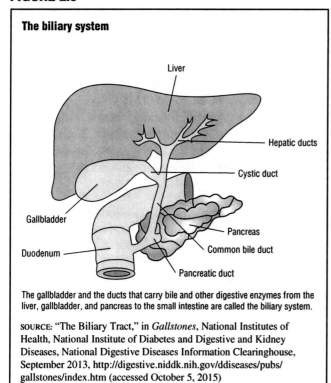

The biliary system

The gallbladder and the ducts that carry bile and other digestive enzymes from the liver, gallbladder, and pancreas to the small intestine are called the biliary system.

SOURCE: "The Biliary Tract," in *Gallstones*, National Institutes of Health, National Institute of Diabetes and Digestive and Kidney Diseases, National Digestive Diseases Information Clearinghouse, September 2013, http://digestive.niddk.nih.gov/ddiseases/pubs/gallstones/index.htm (accessed October 5, 2015)

gallstones produce no symptoms, others cause serious and even life-threatening medical conditions.

The National Digestive Diseases Information Clearinghouse of the National Institute of Diabetes and Digestive and Kidney Diseases explains in "Gallstones" (November 2013, http://www.niddk.nih.gov/health-information/health-topics/digestive-diseases/gallstones/Pages/facts.aspx) that when gallstones block the flow of bile they can produce inflammation in the gallbladder, liver, and pancreas. When blockage persists, the consequences may be severe infection, which if left untreated may not only be painful but also deadly. When gallstones produce such symptoms, the treatment is generally a surgical procedure, called cholecystectomy, in which the gallbladder is removed. People who are not candidates for surgery may be given prescription drugs to dissolve gallstones; however, it is likely that gallstones will recur in people treated with drugs.

People who are overweight have an increased risk for developing gallstones because the liver overproduces cholesterol and deposits it in the bile, which then becomes supersaturated. The National Digestive Diseases Information Clearinghouse indicates that the risk of gallstones is higher among people who are overweight or obese and among people who fast or lose a large amount of weight very quickly. Rapid weight loss or weight cycling (the repeated loss and regain of body weight) further increases cholesterol production in the liver, with resulting supersaturation and risk for gallstone formation.

In "Gallstone Disease and Obesity: A Population-Based Study on Abdominal Fat Distribution and Gender Differences" (*Annals of Hepatology*, vol. 14, no. 5, September–October 2015), Amir Reza Radmard et al. confirm that obesity increases the risk for development of cholesterol gallstones. The researchers theorize this occurs because there is increased secretion of cholesterol by the liver in response to activity of visceral fat, which surrounds organs and is more metabolically active than subcutaneous fat, which is directly below the skin. This condition creates an environment that is conducive to stone formation.

Fatty Liver Disease

Fatty liver is defined as an excess accumulation of fat in the liver, usually exceeding 5% of the total liver weight. More than 50% of the excess fat deposit in the liver is triglyceride. The enlargement of the liver is caused by the reduction of fatty acid oxidation (fat metabolism) in the liver, resulting in an excess accumulation of fat. It causes injury and inflammation in the liver and may lead to severe liver damage, cirrhosis (buildup of scar tissue that blocks proper blood flow in the liver), or liver failure. Arthur J. McCullough of the Cleveland Clinic in Cleveland, Ohio, observes in "Epidemiology of the Metabolic Syndrome in the USA" (*Journal of Digestive Diseases*, vol. 12, no. 5, October 2011) that nonalcoholic fatty liver disease (NAFLD) is recognized as a component of metabolic syndrome, which includes hypertension, diabetes, and elevated triglycerides. Metabolic syndrome is a major risk factor for the development of nonalcoholic steatohepatitis, the most severe form of NAFLD. McCullough estimates that 25% of people in the United States have metabolic syndrome and as such also suffer from NAFLD.

People with diabetes or with higher than normal blood sugar levels (but not yet in the diabetic range) are more likely to have fatty liver disease than those with normal blood sugar levels. It is not known why some people who are overweight or diabetic get fatty liver and others do not. Losing weight reduces the buildup of fat in the liver and prevents further injury; however, weight loss should not exceed 2.2 pounds (1 kg) per week because more rapid weight loss may exacerbate the disease.

In "Nonalcoholic Fatty Liver Disease and the Metabolic Syndrome: Clinical Implications and Treatment" (*Nutrition in Clinical Practice*, vol. 28, no. 1, February 2013), Robert S. Rahimi and Carmen Landaverde predict that the prevalence of NAFLD is anticipated to increase as the prevalence of obesity increases. They observe that along with obesity, specific nutritional trends such as increased consumption of high-fructose corn syrup and animal fats may also be implicated in the rise of NAFLD.

Cancer

Cancer encompasses a group of diseases that are characterized by the uncontrolled growth and spread of abnormal cells. These cells may grow into masses of tissue called malignant tumors. The dangerous aspect of cancer is that cancer cells invade and destroy normal tissue.

The spread of cancer cells occurs either by local growth of the tumor or by some of the cells becoming detached and traveling through the blood and lymph systems to start additional tumors in other parts of the body. Metastasis (the spread of cancer cells) may be confined to a region of the body, but if left untreated (and often despite treatment), the cancer cells can spread throughout the entire body, eventually causing death. It is perhaps the rapid, invasive, and destructive nature of cancer that makes it, arguably, the most feared of all diseases, although it is second to heart disease as the leading cause of death in the United States. (See Table 2.2.)

Melina Arnold et al. report in "Global Burden of Cancer Attributable to High Body-Mass Index in 2012: A Population-Based Study" (*Lancet Oncology*, vol. 16, no. 1, January 2015) that worldwide overweight and obesity are responsible for as much as 3% to 6% of all new cancers or 13% of high BMI-related cancers and about 9% of cancer deaths. These percentages are equivalent to nearly half a million cancer cases attributable to obesity in 2012. Nearly a quarter of obesity-related cancers—23% or 111,000 cases—occurred in North America. In "Breaking the Cancer-Obesity Link" (Scientist.com, November 1, 2015), Stephen D. Hursting, Ciara H. O'Flanagan, and Laura W. Bowers observe that in 2015, obesity overtook smoking as the leading preventable cause of cancer death in the United States, with an estimated 20% of the 600,000 cancer deaths per year attributed to obesity.

Overweight increases the risk of developing several types of cancer, including cancers of the colon, esophagus, gallbladder, kidney, pancreas, liver, and prostate, as well as uterine (specifically cancer of the lining of the uterus) and postmenopausal breast cancer. Excessive weight gain during adult life increases the risk for several of these cancers. For example, according to the American Cancer Society, in *Cancer Prevention and Early Detection: Facts and Figures, 2015–2016* (2015, http://www.cancer.org/acs/groups/content/@research/documents/webcontent/acspc-045101.pdf), overweight and obesity contributed an estimated 171,000 cancer-related deaths in 2015, and between a quarter and one-third of all cancer cases in the United States were attributed to poor diet, physical inactivity, overweight, and obesity. The American Cancer Society states that losing weight may reduce the risk of developing some cancers such as breast cancer and that diets high in processed and red meat and low in fruits, vegetables, and whole grains are associated with increased cancer risk.

In "Epidemiology: Obesity and Cancer—The Evidence Is Fattening Up" (*Nature Reviews Endocrinology*, vol. 10, no. 11, November 2014), Rudolf Kaaks and Tilman Kühn of the German Cancer Research Center in Heidelberg, Germany, report that a large-scale study with 5.2 million participants has found statistically significant associations between increased BMI and 17 of 22 frequently occurring cancers, including breast, esophageal, colorectal, pancreatic, and prostate cancers. The strongest associations were for cancers of the uterus, endometrium (lining of the uterus), kidney, and gallbladder.

It is not yet known exactly how being overweight increases cancer risk, recurrence, or mortality. It may be that fat cells make or influence hormones such as estrogen, progesterone, androgens, and insulin that affect cell growth and lead to cancer. It is also possible that eating habits—such as a high-fat, high-calorie diet—or physical inactivity that promote overweight contribute to cancer risk.

Sleep Apnea and Sleep Disorders

Sleep apnea is a condition in which breathing becomes shallow or stops completely for short periods during sleep. A pause in breathing can last about 10 to 20 seconds or longer, and pauses can occur 20 times or more an hour. Sleep apnea increases the risk of developing high blood pressure, heart attack, or stroke. Untreated sleep apnea can increase the risk of diabetes and daytime sleepiness, which can increase the risk for work-related and automobile accidents.

The most common type of sleep apnea, and the type that is linked to overweight and obesity, is obstructive sleep apnea. During sleep there is insufficient airflow into the lungs through the mouth and nose, and the amount of oxygen in the blood may drop because the airway is transiently occluded. The National Heart, Lung, and Blood Institute notes in "Who Is at Risk for Sleep Apnea?" (July 10, 2012, http://www.nhlbi.nih.gov/health/health-topics/topics/sleepapnea/atrisk.html) that millions of Americans have obstructive sleep apnea and that "about half of the people who have this condition are overweight."

Obesity, particularly upper-body obesity, is a risk factor for sleep apnea and is related to its severity. Most people with sleep apnea have a BMI greater than 30. In general, men whose neck circumference is 17 inches (43.2 cm) or greater and women with a neck circumference of 16 inches (40.6 cm) or greater are at higher risk for sleep apnea. Large neck girth in both men and women who snore is highly predictive of sleep apnea because people with large neck girth store more fat around their neck, which may compromise their airway. A smaller airway can make breathing difficult or stop it altogether. In addition, fat stored in the neck and throughout the body can produce substances that cause inflammation, and inflammation in the neck may be a risk factor for sleep apnea. Weight loss usually resolves or significantly improves sleep apnea by decreasing neck size and reducing inflammation.

Too little sleep is also linked to obesity. Anne G. Wheaton et al. of the CDC note in "Relationship between Body Mass Index and Perceived Insufficient Sleep among U.S. Adults: An Analysis of 2008 BRFSS Data" (*BMC Public Health*, vol. 10, no. 11, May 2011) that people who are overweight or obese report that they sleep less per week than their normal-weight counterparts. The researchers analyzed data from 384,541 participants in the 2008 Behavioral Risk Factor Surveillance System, which asked survey respondents, "During the past 30 days, for about how many days have you felt you did not get enough rest or sleep?" The researchers find a strong association between reported insufficient sleep and BMI-based weight categories from normal weight through obese class III among both men and women. For example, 35% of people with class III obesity said they had 14 or more days of insufficient sleep, compared with 25% of normal-weight people. Wheaton et al. suggest that "the possible effect of excess weight on sleep should be considered by developers of programs to address sleep disorders and that the possible effect of insufficient sleep on weight should be considered by developers of weight-reduction programs."

Other research suggests that sleep deprivation may be related to craving high-calorie foods that are most likely to promote weight gain. In "The Impact of Sleep Deprivation on Food Desire in the Human Brain" (*Nature Communications*, August 6, 2013), Stephanie M. Greer, Andrea N. Goldstein, and Matthew P. Walker compare food choices made by people who received adequate sleep and those who were sleep deprived. They find that high-calorie foods such as chocolate and potato chips were significantly more desirable when people were sleep-deprived and that, on average, sleep-deprived study subjects consumed about 600 more calories than well-rested subjects. Greer, Goldstein, and Walker opine that a "combination of altered brain activity and decision-making may help explain why people who sleep less also tend to be overweight or obese."

Women's Reproductive Health

Besides increased risk of breast cancer and cancer of the lining of the uterus, women who are overweight or obese may suffer from infertility (difficulty or inability to conceive a child) and other gynecological or pregnancy-related medical problems. Obesity is associated with menstrual irregularities such as abnormally heavy menstrual periods and amenorrhea (cessation of menstruation), and has been found to affect ovulation, response to fertility treatment, pregnancy rates, and pregnancy outcomes.

Lea S. Vilmann et al. note in "Development of Obesity and Polycystic Ovary Syndrome in Adolescents" (*Hormone Research in Pediatrics*, vol. 78, nos. 5–6, November 2012) that obesity is linked to polycystic ovarian syndrome (PCOS), an endocrine condition that afflicts approximately 15% of women of reproductive age. PCOS is characterized by the accumulation of cysts (fluid-filled sacs) on the ovaries, chronic anovulation (absent ovulation), and other metabolic disturbances. Symptoms include excess facial and body hair, acne, obesity, irregular menstrual cycles, insulin resistance, and infertility. A key characteristic of PCOS is hyperandrogenism (excessive production of male hormones [androgens], particularly testosterone, by the ovaries), which is responsible for the acne, male-pattern hair growth, and baldness seen in women with PCOS. Hyperandrogenism has been linked to insulin resistance and hyperinsulinemia, both of which are common in PCOS. Women with PCOS have an increased risk of early-onset heart disease, hypertension, diabetes, and reproductive cancers and a higher incidence of miscarriage and infertility. In overweight women, modest weight loss (as little as 5%) through diet and exercise may correct hyperandrogenism and restore ovulation and fertility.

Vilmann et al. report that between 18% and 26% of adolescent females have PCOS, and the risk of developing this condition is highest among obese adolescents. Signs of PCOS have even been observed in preadolescent girls who are obese. Vilmann et al. conclude that "it is of great importance to detect girls who are obese in adolescence (and even younger), because counseling and treatment in an early stage of the metabolic disturbances may prevent the future deleterious effects on their health."

Obesity during pregnancy is associated with increased morbidity for both the expectant mother and the unborn child. Obese pregnant women are significantly more likely to suffer from hypertension and gestational diabetes (glucose intolerance of variable severity that begins during pregnancy and generally resolves after birth) than normal-weight expectant mothers. Obesity is also associated with difficulties in managing labor and delivery, leading to premature births and higher rates of cesarean section (delivery of a fetus by surgical incision through the abdominal wall and uterus). Risks associated with anesthesia are higher in obese women because there is a greater tendency toward hypoxemia (abnormal lack of oxygen in the blood) and greater difficulty administering local or general anesthesia.

Children of women who are obese during pregnancy are at increased risk of birth defects—congenital malformations, particularly of neural tube defects. Neural tube defects are abnormalities of the brain and spinal cord that result from the failure of the neural tube to develop properly during early pregnancy. The neural tube is the embryonic nerve tissue that eventually develops into the brain and the spinal cord.

Babies born to overweight and obese women are also at greater risk of having heart defects. In "Association between Prepregnancy Body Mass Index and Congenital Heart Defects" (*American Journal of Obstetrics and Gynecology*, vol. 202, no. 1, January 2010), Suzanne M. Gilboa et al. report the results of a study of 6,440 infants born with congenital heart defects and 5,673 infants without birth defects. The researchers find that when compared with babies born to normal-weight women, there was a significant increase in many types of heart defects in babies born to overweight and obese women. Gilboa et al. looked at 25 types of heart defects and found associations with obesity for 10 of them. Five of these 10 types were also associated with overweight prior to pregnancy. Women who were overweight but not obese prior to and during pregnancy had approximately a 15% increased risk of delivering a baby with certain heart defects.

Women who are obese before pregnancy also appear to have a higher risk of stillbirth and of having an infant die soon after birth. Peter W. Tennant, Judith Rankin, and Ruth Bell of Newcastle University note in "Maternal Body Mass Index and the Risk of Fetal and Infant Death: A Cohort Study from the North of England" (*Human Reproduction*, vol. 26, no. 6, April 2011) that early pregnancy obesity (BMI greater than or equal to 30) carries significant health implications. The researchers find that obese mothers were at increased risk for gestational diabetes and that their infants were at increased risk for stillbirth, early infant death, and birth defects. It is not yet known how obesity increases the risk of stillbirth and early infant death, but one possible explanation may be that obesity influences the hormonal system and the metabolism of blood fats that in turn may compromise blood flow to the placenta (an organ that forms during pregnancy and functions as a filter between the mother and fetus).

WEIGHT GAIN DURING PREGNANCY. Weight gain during pregnancy is expected and beneficial. The fetus, expanded blood volume, the enlarged uterus, breast tissue growth, and other products of conception generate approximately 13 to 17 pounds (5.9 to 7.7 kg) of extra weight. Weight gain beyond this anticipated amount is largely maternal adipose tissue that is often retained after pregnancy. The challenge health professionals face when developing recommendations about weight gain during pregnancy is achieving a balance between gains intended to produce high-birth-weight infants, who may then require delivery by cesarean section, and low-birth-weight infants with a higher infant mortality rate. Analysis of data from the CDC's Pregnancy Nutrition Surveillance System shows that extremely overweight women benefit from reduced weight gain during pregnancy to help decrease the risk for high-birth-weight infants. Table 2.8 shows the recommended amount of weight gain during pregnancy based on prepregnancy BMI.

In "Obesity and Weight Gain in Pregnancy" (*Contemporary OB/GYN*, July 1, 2013), Raul Artal and Amy Flick opine that no pregnancy weight gain in women with a BMI of 30 or even modest weight loss may reduce some risks such as infants who are large for their gestational age, cesarean delivery, and preeclampsia (high blood pressure and excess protein in the urine). They assert, "Physical activity, weight maintenance, and even weight reduction have not proven harmful in obese pregnant patients according to studies in the recent literature." Artal and Flick also point out that infants of obese women are at significantly increased risk for being born with neural tube defects, congenital heart disease, and other anomalies.

Metabolic Syndrome

McCullough estimates that approximately 25% of Americans exhibit a cluster of medical conditions that are characterized by insulin resistance and the presence of obesity, abdominal fat, high blood sugar and triglycerides, high blood cholesterol, and high blood pressure.

TABLE 2.8

Recommended weight gain during pregnancy

Prepregnancy body mass index category	Mothers of singletons		Mothers of twins (provisional)
	Total weight gain (lb)	Rate of weight gain in the second and third trimesters (lb/wk)	Total weight gain at term (lb)
Underweight (<18.5 kg/m²)	28–40	1.0 (1.0–1.3)	No guideline available
Normal-weight (18.5–24.9 kg/m²)	25–35	1.0 (0.8–1.0)	37–54
Overweight (25.0–29.9 kg/m²)	15–25	0.6 (0.5–0.7)	31–50
Obese (≥30.0 kg/m²)	11–20	0.5 (0.4–0.6)	25–42

SOURCE: Kathleen M. Rasmussen, Patrick M. Catalano, and Ann L. Yaktine, "Table 2. 2009 IOM/NRC Guidelines for Weight Gain and Rate of Weight Gain during Pregnancy for Women with Singleton Fetuses and for Weight Gain for Women with Twin Fetuses," in "New Guidelines for Weight Gain during Pregnancy: What Obstetrician Gynecologists Should Know," *Current Opinion in Obstetrics and Gynecology*, vol. 21, no. 6, December 2009, http://www.ncbi .nlm.nih.gov/pmc/articles/PMC2847829/pdf/nihms180944.pdf (accessed October 5, 2015)

This constellation of symptoms, called metabolic syndrome, was first defined in *Third Report of the National Cholesterol Education Program (NCEP) Expert Panel on Detection, Evaluation, and Treatment of High Blood Cholesterol in Adults (Adult Treatment Panel III)* (September 2002, http://www.nhlbi.nih.gov/sites/www.nhlbi.nih.gov/files/Circulation-2002-ATP-III-Final-Report-PDF-3143.pdf). The report concludes that for most affected people, metabolic syndrome results from poor diet and insufficient physical activity.

The diagnosis of metabolic syndrome, which is also known as syndrome X, requires that people meet at least three of the following criteria:

- Waistline measurement (waist circumference) of 40 inches (102 cm) or more for men and 35 inches (89 cm) or more for women

- Blood pressure of 130/85 millimeters of mercury (mmHg) or higher

- Fasting blood glucose level greater than 100 mg/dL

- Serum triglyceride level above 150 mg/dL

- HDL level less than 40 mg/dL for men or under 50 mg/dL for women

According to the American Heart Association, three groups of people are the most likely to be diagnosed with metabolic syndrome: diabetics, people with hypertension and hyperinsulinemia, and people who have suffered heart attacks and have hyperinsulinemia without glucose intolerance.

Although research shows that the signs of metabolic syndrome are common among family members, until 2003 a definitive genetic link had not been identified. Ruth J. F. Loos et al. demonstrate in "Genome-Wide Linkage Scan for the Metabolic Syndrome in the HERITAGE Family Study" (*Journal of Clinical Endocrinology and Metabolism*, vol. 88, no. 12, December 2003) the existence of genetic regions that may signal a predisposition to metabolic syndrome. The researchers find evidence of genetic linkages to metabolic syndrome in both African American and white patients.

By 2015 additional genetic links had been identified. For example, Sadhbh O'Neill and Lorraine O'Driscoll report in "Metabolic Syndrome: A Closer Look at the Growing Epidemic and Its Associated Pathologies" (*Obesity Reviews*, vol. 16, no. 1, January 2015) that an evaluation of linkages for traits that are associated with metabolic syndrome finds multiple genes that correlate with these traits. Genome-wide association studies also provide some evidence of a genetic component of metabolic syndrome.

The exact origins of metabolic syndrome are not fully known; regardless, affected individuals experience a series of biochemical changes that, in time, lead to the development of potentially harmful medical conditions. The biochemical changes begin when insulin loses its ability to cause cells to absorb glucose from the blood (insulin resistance). As a result, glucose levels remain high after food is consumed and the pancreas, sensing a high glucose level in the blood, continues to secrete insulin. The loss of insulin sensitivity may be genetic or may be in response to high fat levels with fatty deposits in the pancreas.

Moderate weight loss, in the range of 5% to 10% of body weight, can help restore the body's sensitivity to insulin and greatly reduce the chance that the syndrome will progress into a more serious illness. Increased physical activity alone has also been shown to improve insulin sensitivity.

By 2016 it was widely accepted that metabolic syndrome included vascular risk factors that were associated with cognitive decline and even the development of dementia. In "Low Cerebral Blood Flow Is Associated with Lower Memory Function in Metabolic Syndrome" (*Obesity*, vol. 21, no. 7, July 2013), Alex C. Birdsill et al. assert that, although it is not understood how or why metabolic syndrome causes cognitive impairment, early identification and treatment of people at risk may offer new ways to delay the onset of cognitive decline and dementia syndromes or to prevent the progression of these syndromes. The researchers believe that reducing cardiovascular risk factors that compromise blood flow to the brain can reduce the risk of cognitive decline.

Bhumsoo Kim and Eva L. Feldman of the University of Michigan, Ann Arbor, suggest in "Insulin Resistance as a Key Link for the Increased Risk of Cognitive Impairment in the Metabolic Syndrome" (*Experimental and Molecular Medicine*, vol. 47, no. 3, March 2015) that the insulin resistance that is characteristic of metabolic syndrome may be the link between it and cognitive decline and Alzheimer's disease (AD). The researchers note that insulin plays a key role in learning and memory and that AD patients display impaired insulin signaling that is similar to what is observed in people with metabolic syndrome.

REDEFINING METABOLIC SYNDROME. In an effort to standardize diagnosis, prevention, screening, and treatment, the International Diabetes Federation presents in *The IDF Consensus Worldwide Definition of the Metabolic Syndrome* (2006, http://www.idf.org/webdata/docs/IDF_Meta_def_final.pdf) a new worldwide definition of metabolic syndrome. The diagnostic criteria are central obesity, which is defined as a waist circumference that is equal to or more than 37 inches (94 cm) for males and 31.5 inches (80 cm) for females of European descent, along with two of the following:

- Triglycerides of at least 150 mg/dL

- Low HDL cholesterol, which is defined as less than 40 mg/dL in males and less than 50 mg/dL in females

- Blood pressure of at least 130/85 mmHg

- Fasting hyperglycemia, which is defined as glucose that is equal to or greater than 100 mg/dL

- Previous diagnosis of diabetes

- Impaired glucose tolerance

This definition of metabolic syndrome, which includes diabetes or prediabetes, abdominal obesity, unfavorable lipid profile, and hypertension, triples the risk of myocardial infarction and stroke and doubles mortality from these conditions. It also increases the risk of developing type 2 diabetes, if not already present, fivefold.

Kim and Feldman present the following ethnic-specific waist circumference thresholds for abdominal obesity that is associated with metabolic syndrome:

- Equal to or more than 35.4 inches (90 cm) for males and 31.5 inches (80 cm) for females of South Asian, Chinese, Japanese, or Central and South American descent

- Equal to or more than 37 inches (94 cm) for males and 31.5 inches (80 cm) for females of Middle Eastern/ Mediterranean or sub-Saharan African descent

SOME QUESTION THE DIAGNOSIS OF METABOLIC SYNDROME. In 2010 the World Health Organization joined the American Diabetes Association and the European Association for the Study of Diabetes in questioning the utility of the diagnosis of metabolic syndrome. Representatives of these organizations say they feel the syndrome is neither a distinct disease nor well established by scientific research. Rakesh M. Parikh and Viswanathan Mohan state in "Changing Definitions of Metabolic Syndrome" (*Indian Journal of Endocrinology and Metabolism*, vol. 16, no. 1, January–February 2012) that there are different definitions of metabolic syndrome, which creates confusion when comparing prevalence rates. Parikh and Mohan propose a simple clinical definition and explain that metabolic syndrome should be considered a screening tool that is used "to identify people at high risk of metabolic complications and cardiovascular disease so that further detailed investigations can be performed. This definition translates into a very simple message to the community 'If your waist size is more than half of your height, you should consult your doctor.'"

Kim and Feldman add that prevention, timely diagnosis, and treatment of metabolic syndrome are vital for ensuring global population health and the global economy. They also exhort the medical community to standardize criteria for the disorder, asserting, "Given the current obesity epidemic among all ages and increased life expectancy, there is a critical need to understand the underlying causes of cognitive impairment due to [insulin resistance], which may be the key link for the increased incidence of AD in individuals with metabolic disorders."

CHAPTER 3
THE INFLUENCES OF MENTAL HEALTH AND CULTURE ON WEIGHT AND EATING DISORDERS

That diet and appetite are closely linked to psychological health and emotional well-being is widely recognized. Psychological factors often influence eating habits. Many people overeat when they are bored, stressed, angry, depressed, or anxious. Psychological distress can aggravate weight problems by triggering impulses to overeat. Emotional discomfort drives many people to overeat as a way to relieve anxiety and improve mood. Some people revert to the so-called comfort foods of their youth—the meals or treats that were offered to them when they were sick or the foods that evoke memories of the carefree days of childhood. Others rely on chocolate and other sweets, which actually contain chemicals that are known to have a soothing effect on mood. Over time, the associations between emotions, food, and eating can become firmly fixed.

Emotional arousal may also sabotage healthy self-care efforts such as resolutions to diet and exercise. Anxiety and depression can produce feelings of helplessness and hopelessness about efforts to lose weight that undermine the best intentions, prompt detrimental food choices and inactivity, and over time cause many people to give up trying entirely. Because overweight and obesity often contribute to emotional stress and psychological disorders, a cycle develops that couples increasing weight gain with progressively more severe emotional difficulties.

Emotional disturbance alone is rarely the causative factor of overweight or obesity. However, for people with a genetic susceptibility or predisposition to obesity and exposure to environmental factors that promote obesity, emotional and psychological stress can trigger or exacerbate the problem. Even efforts to lose weight can backfire, serving to increase rather than to alleviate emotional stress. For example, people who fail to lose weight or those who succeed in losing weight only to regain it may suffer from frustration and diminished feelings of competence and self-worth. Similarly, being overweight or

obese and feeling self-conscious about it or suffering from weight-based discrimination or prejudice can be ongoing sources of stress and frustration. Feelings of helplessness, frustration, and continuous emotional stress can cause or worsen mental health problems such as anxiety and depression.

Many mental health and medical professionals view overweight as both a cause and a consequence of disturbances in physical and mental health. Although it may be important to determine whether a metabolic disturbance caused an individual to become overweight or resulted from excessive weight gain, or whether depression triggered behaviors that led to obesity or resulted from problems associated with obesity, it is often impossible to distinguish whether overweight is a symptom of another disorder or the causative factor.

THE ORIGINS OF EATING DISORDERS

Despite the challenges of compromised self-esteem and societal prejudice, the National Institute of Diabetes and Digestive and Kidney Diseases indicates that most overweight people have about the same number of psychological problems as people of average weight. Nevertheless, the Weight-Control Information Network explains in "Binge Eating Disorder" (December 2012, http://win.niddk.nih.gov/publications/binge.htm) that although eating disorders affect normal-weight individuals, people who are mildly obese and try to lose weight repetitively may suffer from eating disorders such as binge eating, and most people with binge-eating disorder are overweight or obese. Binge-eating disorder is thought to be even more common in people who are severely obese. People with the most severe eating disorders are more likely to have symptoms of depression and low self-esteem.

Although depression and stress may contribute to a substantial percentage of cases of obesity, they are considered the leading causes of eating disorders. Most mental health professionals concur that the origins of eating disorders can be traced to behavioral or psychological difficulties. Anger and impulsive behavior have been associated with binge-eating disorder, but even mild mental health or social problems such as shyness or lack of self-confidence can lead to social withdrawal, isolation, and a sedentary lifestyle that promotes weight gain and ultimately obesity.

Jerica M. Berge et al. of the University of Minnesota report in "Family Life Cycle Transitions and the Onset of Eating Disorders: A Retrospective Grounded Theory Approach" (*Journal of Clinical Nursing*, vol. 21, nos. 9–10, May 2012) that eating disorders may be precipitated by transitional events in family life, such as school transitions, the death of a family member, relationship changes, illness or hospitalization, home or job changes, and abuse or sexual assault. The risk for eating disorders is greatest when there is a lack of needed support during these stressful life transitions.

At first glance, eating disorders appear to center on preoccupations with food and weight; however, mental health professionals believe these disorders are often about more than simply food. Besides psychological factors that may predispose people to eating disorders, including diminished self-esteem, depression, anxiety, loneliness, or feelings of lack of control, a variety of interpersonal and social factors have been implicated as causal factors for these disorders. Interpersonal factors that may increase the risk for developing eating disorders include troubled family and personal relationships; difficulty expressing emotions; a history of physical or sexual abuse; or the experience of being teased, taunted, or ridiculed about body size, shape, or weight.

Twin and family studies suggest that the predisposition to develop an eating disorder also has a genetic origin. In "The Genetics of Eating Disorders" (*Annual Review of Clinical Psychology*, vol. 9, March 2013), Sara E. Trace et al. report that genetic factors account for about 40% to 60% of eating disorders.

Social factors that may contribute to eating disorders include sharply restricted, rigid definitions of beauty that exclude people who do not conform to a particular body weight and shape; cultures that glorify thinness and overemphasize the importance of obtaining a "perfect body"; and cultures that judge and value people based on external physical appearance rather than on internal qualities such as character, intellect, generosity, and kindness. Appearance-driven concerns, rather than health needs, continue to motivate many obese individuals to lose weight. Societal pressures reinforce these appearance-driven concerns by portraying obese individuals in a negative manner.

A related consideration that further complicates pinpointing the origins of eating disorders is the extent to which temperament interacts with genetic predisposition and interpersonal and social factors to promote eating disorders. Researchers and mental health professionals observe that temperamental tendencies such as perfectionism, compulsivity, impulsivity, and other behavioral, cognitive, and emotional leanings seem to predispose to eating disorders.

Binge-Eating Disorder

Binge eating is a common problem among people who are overweight and obese. Besides consuming unusually large amounts of food in a single sitting, binge eaters generally suffer from low mood and low alertness, and experience uncontrollable compulsions to eat. They experience food cravings before binge episodes and feelings of discontent, dissatisfaction, and restlessness following binges.

An estimated 2.8% of adults will have a binge-eating disorder at some point during their lifetime. (See Figure 3.1.) In "Director's Blog: Spotlight on Eating Disorders" (February 24, 2012, http://www.nimh.nih.gov/about/director/2012/spotlight-on-eating-disorders.shtml), Thomas Insel, the director of the National Institute of Mental Health (NIMH), reports that the lifetime rate among women is higher (3.5%, compared with 2% among men). The NIMH indicates in "Eating Disorders among Adults—Binge Eating Disorder" (2015, http://www.nimh.nih.gov/health/statistics/prevalence/eating-disorders-among-adults-binge-eating-disorder.shtml) that binge-eating disorder is the most common eating disorder. The prevalence

FIGURE 3.1

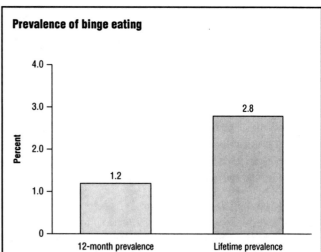

Prevalence of binge eating

- 12-month prevalence: 1.2% of U.S. adult population.
- Severe: Not reported.
- Lifetime prevalence: 2.8% of U.S. adult population.

SOURCE: "Prevalence," in *Eating Disorders among Adults—Binge Eating Disorder*, U.S. Department of Health and Human Services, National Institute of Mental Health, undated, http://www.nimh.nih.gov/health/statistics/prevalence/eating-disorders-among-adults-binge-eating-disorder.shtml (accessed October 7, 2015) of binge eating declines with advancing age; people aged 18 to 59 years are more likely to suffer from it than people aged 60 years and older.

Although the disorder is more common in people who are overweight or obese, normal-weight people also develop the disorder. People who suffer from binge eating often:

- Feel that eating is out of their ability to control
- Eat amounts of food most people would think are unusually large
- Eat much more quickly than usual during binge episodes
- Eat until the point of physical discomfort
- Consume large amounts of food, even when they are not hungry
- Eat alone because they feel embarrassed about the amount of food they eat
- Feel disgusted, depressed, or guilty after overeating

Until recently some eating disorders were not officially recognized as mental disorders. For example, whereas anorexia nervosa was included in the first edition of the *Diagnostic and Statistical Manual of Mental Disorders* (*DSM*; the definitive manual that classifies and establishes criteria for mental disorders) in 1952, binge-eating disorder was not included until the fifth edition of the *DSM* in 2012. Inclusion in the *DSM* is important because it promotes awareness, recognition, and treatment of the disorder.

Some Dieters Are Consumed by Eating Disorders

In the 21st century Americans are preoccupied with body image. They are constantly bombarded with images of thin, beautiful women and lean, muscular men in magazines, on billboards, on the Internet, on television, and in movies. Advertising implies that to be thin and beautiful is to be happy. Many prominent weight-loss programs reinforce this suggestion. Well-balanced, low-fat food plans or other diets that restrict carbohydrates or calories combined with exercise can help many overweight people achieve a healthier weight and lifestyle. Dieting to achieve a healthy weight is quite different from dieting obsessively to become "model thin," which can have consequences that range from mildly harmful to life-threatening. Table 3.1 enumerates the health consequences of eating disorders.

According to the NIMH, dieting plays a role in the onset of two serious eating disorders: anorexia nervosa and bulimia. Preteens, teens, and college-age women are at special risk. However, researchers are beginning to report rising rates of anorexia and bulimia among men. In "Eating-Disordered Behavior in Adolescent Boys: Eating Disorder Examination Questionnaire Norms" (*International Journal*

TABLE 3.1

Health consequences of eating disorders

- Eating disorders are serious, potentially life-threatening conditions that affect a person's emotional and physical health.
- Eating disorders are not just a "fad" or a "phase." People do not just "catch" an eating disorder for a period of time. They are real, complex, and devastating conditions that can have serious consequences for health, productivity, and relationships.
- People struggling with an eating disorder need to seek professional help. The earlier a person with an eating disorder seeks treatment, the greater the likelihood of physical and emotional recovery.

Health consequences of anorexia nervosa: In anorexia nervosa's cycle of self-starvation, the body is denied the essential nutrients it needs to function normally. Thus, the body is forced to slow down all of its processes to conserve energy, resulting in serious medical consequences:

- Abnormally slow heart rate and low blood pressure, which mean that the heart muscle is changing. The risk for heart failure rises as the heart rate and blood pressure level sink lower and lower.
- Reduction of bone density (osteoporosis), which results in dry, brittle bones.
- Muscle loss and weakness.
- Severe dehydration, which can result in kidney failure.
- Fainting, fatigue, and overall weakness.
- Dry hair and skin; hair loss is common.
- Growth of a downy layer of hair called lanugo all over the body, including the face, in an effort to keep the body warm.

Health consequences of bulimia nervosa: The recurrent binge-and-purge cycles of bulimia can affect the entire digestive system and can lead to electrolyte and chemical imbalances in the body that affect the heart and other major organ functions. Some of the health consequences of bulimia nervosa include:

- Electrolyte imbalances that can lead to irregular heartbeats and possibly heart failure and death. Electrolyte imbalance is caused by dehydration and loss of potassium and sodium from the body as a result of purging behaviors.
- Potential for gastric rupture during periods of bingeing.
- Inflammation and possible rupture of the esophagus from frequent vomiting.
- Tooth decay and staining from stomach acids released during frequent vomiting.
- Chronic irregular bowel movements and constipation as a result of laxative abuse.
- Peptic ulcers and pancreatitis.

Health consequences of binge eating disorder: Binge eating disorder often results in many of the same health risks associated with clinical obesity. Some of the potential health consequences of binge eating disorder include:

- High blood pressure.
- High cholesterol levels.
- Heart disease as a result of elevated triglyceride levels.
- Secondary diabetes.
- Gallbladder disease.

SOURCE: "Health Consequences of Eating Disorders," National Eating Disorders Association, 2002, http://www.nationaleatingdisorders.org/health-consequences-eating-disorders (accessed October 7, 2015)

of *Eating Disorders*, vol. 47, no. 4, May 2014), Jonathan Mond et al. report that in their study of boys aged 12 to 18 years, nearly 10% reported regular episodes of lost control of eating, 6% reported binge eating, 5.3% reported regular excessive exercise, and 4.9% reported overvaluation of weight or shape. As observed in girls, eating disorders are more common among older male adolescents than among younger male adolescents.

A 2013 survey of high school students found that 18.7% of teenaged girls and 7.4% of teenaged boys said they had not eaten for 24 or more hours to keep from gaining weight. (See Table 3.2.) Furthermore, 6.6% of teenaged girls and 3.4% of teenaged boys said they took diet pills, powders, or liquids without a doctor's advice to lose weight, and 6.6% of teenaged girls and 2.2% of teenaged boys admitted that they vomited or took laxatives to lose or maintain their weight. (See Table 3.2 and Table 3.3.)

TABLE 3.2

Percentage of high school students engaging in dangerous dieting behaviors, 2013

	Did not eat for ≥24 hours to lose weight or to keep from gaining weight				Took diet pills, powders, or liquids to lose weight or to keep from gaining weight		
	Female	Male	Total		Female	Male	Total
Category	%	%	%		%	%	%
Race/ethnicity							
White*	18.2	5.6	11.8		6.1	3.0	4.6
Black*	16.6	9.8	13.3		4.7	2.9	3.8
Hispanic	22.8	9.5	16.2		10.0	4.1	7.1
Grade							
9	20.9	7.2	14.0		4.8	2.1	3.4
10	20.5	7.1	13.7		6.8	2.5	4.6
11	17.2	7.7	12.5		6.6	4.3	5.5
12	15.8	7.5	11.7		8.6	5.1	6.8
Total	**18.7**	**7.4**	**13.0**		**6.6**	**3.4**	**5.0**

*Non-Hispanic.

Notes: Engaged in dangerous dieting behavior to lose weight or to keep from gaining weight without a doctor's advice during the 30 days before the survey.

SOURCE: Adapted from Laura Kann et al., "Table 109. Percentage of Students Who Did Not Eat for 24 or More Hours and Who Took Diet Pills, Powders, or Liquids, by Sex, Race/Ethnicity, and Grade—United States, Youth Risk Behavior Survey, 2013," in "Youth Risk Behavior Surveillance—United States, 2013," *MMWR*, vol. 63, no. 4, June 13, 2014, http://www.cdc.gov/mmwr/pdf/ss/ss6304.pdf (accessed October 7, 2015)

TABLE 3.3

Percentage of high school students who vomited or took laxatives to lose or maintain weight, 2013

	Female	Male	Total
Category	%	%	%
Race/ethnicity			
White*	6.1	1.3	3.7
Black*	4.1	3.2	3.7
Hispanic	10.3	3.0	6.7
Grade			
9	6.7	1.7	4.2
10	6.4	2.2	4.3
11	6.1	2.0	4.1
12	6.9	2.7	4.8
Total	**6.6**	**2.2**	**4.4**

*Non-Hispanic.

Note: Vomited or took laxatives to lose weight or to keep from gaining weight during the 30 days before the survey.

SOURCE: Adapted from Laura Kann et al., "Table 111. Percentage of High School Students Who Vomited or Took Laxatives, by Sex, Race/Ethnicity, and Grade—United States, Youth Risk Behavior Survey, 2013," in "Youth Risk Behavior Surveillance—United States, 2013," *MMWR*, vol. 63, no. 4, June 13, 2014, http://www.cdc.gov/mmwr/pdf/ss/ss6304.pdf (accessed October 7, 2015)

Anorexia Nervosa

Anorexia nervosa involves severe weight loss (a minimum of 15% below normal body weight). Anorexic people literally starve themselves, although they may be very hungry. For reasons that researchers do not yet fully understand, anorexics become terrified of gaining weight. Both food and weight become obsessions. They often develop strange eating habits, refuse to eat with other people, and exercise strenuously to burn calories and prevent weight gain. Anorexic individuals continue to believe they are overweight even when they are dangerously thin.

This condition often begins when a young woman who is slightly overweight or normal weight starts to diet to lose weight. After achieving the desired weight loss, she redoubles her efforts to lose more weight, and dieting becomes an obsession that may eclipse other interests. Affected individuals take pleasure in how well they can avoid food consumption and measure their self-worth by their ability to lose weight. Eating and weight gain are perceived as weaknesses and personal failures.

The medical complications of anorexia are similar to starvation. When the body attempts to protect its most vital organs, the heart and the brain, it goes into "slow gear." Menstrual periods stop, and breathing, pulse, blood pressure, and thyroid function slow down. The nails and hair become brittle, the skin dries, and the lack of body fat produces an inability to withstand cold temperatures. Depression, weakness, and a constant obsession with food are also symptoms of the disease. In addition, personality changes may occur. The person suffering from anorexia may have outbursts of anger and hostility or may withdraw socially. In the most serious cases, death can result.

Scientists often describe eating disorders as addictions, and Mario Speranza et al. support this notion in "An Investigation of Goodman's Addictive Disorder Criteria in Eating Disorders" (*European Eating Disorders Review*, vol. 20, no. 3, May 2012). The researchers find that common addictive personality traits are present in many people suffering from eating disorders and substance use–related disorders. Speranza et al. conclude that "a subgroup of individuals with an eating disorder experiences their disorder as an addiction and may deserve specific therapeutic attention."

Bulimia

People who suffer from bulimia eat compulsively and then purge (get rid of the food) through self-induced vomiting, use of laxatives or diuretics, strict diets, fasts, exercise, or a combination of several of these compensatory behaviors. Bulimia often begins when a person is disgusted with the excessive amount of "bad" food consumed and vomits to rid the body of the calories.

Many bulimics are at a normal body weight or above because of their frequent binge-purge behavior, which can occur from once or twice per week to several times per day. Those bulimics who maintain normal weight may manage to keep their eating disorder a secret for years. As with anorexia, bulimia usually begins during adolescence or early adulthood. According to the NIMH, the average age of onset is 20, but many bulimics do not seek help until they are in their 30s or 40s. Figure 3.2 shows the prevalence and demographics of bulimia nervosa as well as the utilization of treatment and services.

Binge eating and purging are dangerous. In rare cases bingeing can cause esophageal ruptures, and purging can result in life-threatening cardiac (heart) conditions because the body loses vital minerals. The acid in vomit wears down tooth enamel and the lining of the esophagus, throat, and mouth and can cause scarring on the hands when fingers are pushed down the throat to induce vomiting. The esophagus may become inflamed, and glands in the neck may become swollen.

Bulimics often talk of being "hooked" on certain foods and needing to feed their "habits." This addictive behavior carries over into other areas of their life, including the likelihood of alcohol and drug abuse. Many bulimics suffer from coexisting medical or mental health problems, such as severe depression, which increases their risk for suicide.

CAUSES OF EATING DISORDERS

As described earlier, research indicates there is a genetic component to susceptibility to eating disorders. For example, in the general population the chance of developing anorexia is about one out of 200, but when a family member has the disorder, the risk increases to one out of 30. Twin studies demonstrate that when one twin is affected, there is a 50% chance the other will develop an eating disorder. Cynthia M. Bulik et al. calculated heritability estimates for anorexia nervosa and bulimia nervosa and published the estimates of their genetic correlation in "Understanding the Relation between Anorexia Nervosa and Bulimia Nervosa in a Swedish National Twin Sample" (*Biological Psychiatry*,

FIGURE 3.2

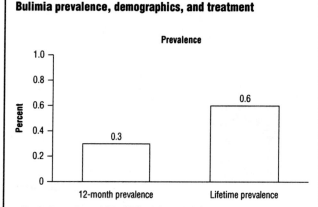

Bulimia prevalence, demographics, and treatment

Prevalence

- 12-month prevalence: 0.3% of U.S. adult population.
- Severe: Not reported.
- Lifetime prevalence: 0.6% of U.S. adult population.

Average age-of-onset: 20 years old.

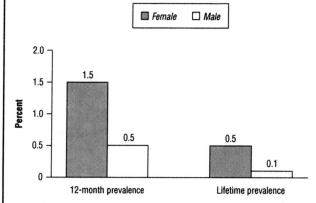

Demographics (for lifetime prevalence)

- Sex:

- Race: Not reported.
- Age: People ages 18–29, 30–44, and 45–59 were all significantly more likely than 60+ year olds to suffer from bulimia nervosa.

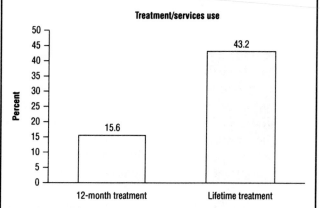

Treatment/services use

- 12-month treatment for bulimia nervosa: 15.6% of those with disorder are receiving treatment.
- Lifetime treatment for bulimia nervosa: 43.2% of those with disorder are receiving treatment.

SOURCE: "Bulimia Nervosa," in *Eating Disorders among Adults—Bulimia Nervosa*, U.S. Department of Health and Human Services, National Institute of Mental Health, undated, http://www.nimh.nih.gov/health/statistics/prevalence/file_148097.pdf (accessed October 7, 2015) vol. 67, no. 1, January 1, 2010). Consistent with the findings of other researchers, Bulik et al. find an overlap of genetic and unique environmental factors that influence the development of both eating disorders.

Besides a genetic predisposition, bulimics and anorexics seem to have different temperaments. Bulimics are likely to be impulsive (acting without thought of the consequences) and are more likely to abuse alcohol and drugs. Anorexics tend to be perfectionists, good students, and competitive athletes. They usually keep their feelings to themselves and rarely disobey their parents. However, bulimics and anorexics do share certain traits: they lack self-esteem, have feelings of helplessness, and fear gaining weight. In both disorders, the eating problems appear to develop as a way of handling stress and anxiety.

Eating disorders are maladaptive coping strategies for blunting uncomfortable feelings, maintaining a false sense of control, and attempting to cope with past trauma. Bulimics consume huge amounts of food (often junk food) in search of comfort and stress relief. The bingeing, however, results in feelings of guilt and depression. By contrast, anorexics restrict food to gain a sense of control and mastery over some aspect of their life. Controlling their weight seems to offer two advantages: they can take control of their body, and they can gain approval from others.

Psychological theories that explain the origins of bulimia include conflicted relationships between mothers and daughters, attempts to control one's own body in the face of seemingly uncontrollable family or other interpersonal relationships, or ambivalence about sexual development and attention. The latter theory has also been used to explain overweight and obesity in teenage girls and young women—as protection from or defense against attention from males who make them fearful or uncomfortable.

In one study, Pamela K. Keel and K. Jean Forney of Florida State University considered risk factors for developing eating disorders and reported their findings in "Psychosocial Risk Factors for Eating Disorders" (*International Journal of Eating Disorders*, vol. 46, no. 5, July 2013). The researchers find that idealizing thinness, coupled with negativity and perfectionism, contributes to the development of eating disorders, as do peer influences. In another study, "Adolescent Eating Disorder Behaviours and Cognitions: Gender-Specific Effects of Child, Maternal and Family Risk Factors" (*British Journal of Psychiatry*, vol. 207, no. 4, October 2015), Nadia Micali et al. note that risk factors for eating disorders vary by sex. For example, body dissatisfaction in childhood was associated with eating disorders in girls but not in boys in the study. Female adolescents with mothers who had eating disorders were more likely to express dissatisfaction with their weight and shape, whereas adolescent males were more likely to diet.

OCCURRENCE OF EATING DISORDERS

Sonia A. Swanson et al. of the NIMH analyzed eating disorders using data from the National Comorbidity Survey Replication Adolescent Supplement, a nationally representative sample of adolescents aged 13 to 18 years in the United States. In "Prevalence and Correlates of Eating Disorders in Adolescents: Results from the National Comorbidity Survey Replication Adolescent Supplement" (*Archives of General Psychiatry*, vol. 68, no. 7, July 2011), the researchers note that the lifetime prevalence rates of anorexia nervosa, bulimia nervosa, and binge-eating disorder were 0.3%, 0.9%, and 1.6%, respectively, and their 12-month prevalence rates were 0.2%, 0.6%, and 0.9%, respectively. The majority of adolescents with an eating disorder also met criteria for at least one other mental disorder, and nearly all adolescents with anorexia nervosa reported social problems. Adolescents with eating disorders were also at increased risk for other self-destructive and suicidal behavior. Swanson et al. conclude that "the prevalence of these disorders is higher than previously expected in this age range, and the patterns of comorbidity, role impairment, and suicidality indicate that eating disorders represent a major public health concern."

The Eating Disorders Coalition for Research, Policy, and Action notes in the fact sheet "Facts about Eating Disorders: What the Research Shows" (September 2014, http://eatingdisorderscoalition.org.s208556.gridserver.com/couch/uploads/file/Eating%20Disorders%20Fact%20Sheet.pdf) that at least 30 million Americans are affected by eating disorders and that anorexia is the third most common illness among adolescents. The coalition observes that the incidence of eating disorders is increasing in younger age groups and is becoming more common in diverse ethnic and sociocultural groups. Eating disorders account for 4% of children's hospitalizations.

According to Swanson et al., the prevalence of eating disorders among adults ranges from 0.5% to 1% for anorexia nervosa and from 0.5% to 3% for bulimia nervosa. In *Textbook of Psychiatric Epidemiology* (2011), Ming T. Tsuang, Mauricio Tohen, and Peter B. Jones observe that the lifetime prevalence of anorexia nervosa across studies from North America, Europe, Australia, and New Zealand ranges from 0.9% to 2.2%; for bulimia nervosa the range is from 1.5% to 4.6%; and for binge-eating disorder the range is from 0.6% to 3.5%. Research reveals that males are much less likely to suffer from eating disorders, with their lifetime prevalence of anorexia nervosa ranging from 0.1% to 0.4% and bulimia nervosa of about 0.5%. When all other eating disorders are added, between 8.7% and 15.9% of women will suffer from an eating disorder during their lifetime.

Eating disorders are often associated with various impulsive behaviors. Leonardo F. Fontenelle et al. examine in "Obsessive-Compulsive Disorder, Impulse Control Disorders, and Drug Addiction: Common Features and Potential Treatments" (*Drugs*, vol. 71, no. 7, May 7, 2011) the relationship between compulsive, impulsive, and addictive behaviors. They find a relationship between these behaviors and posit that impulsive or addictive features of eating disorders might be effectively treated with drugs that address the quality of the underlying drives and the involvement of neural systems such as those that act to reduce or prevent relapse of addiction. In "Weight Gain, Executive Functioning, and Eating Behaviors among Girls" (*Pediatrics*, vol. 136, no. 4, October 2015), Andrea B. Goldschmidt et al. assessed 2,450 girls and find that girls who were impulsive and had difficulties planning at age 10 tended to gain more weight as they entered puberty and were more prone to binge eating. Similar patterns have been observed in boys in the same age group.

According to Walter Kaye et al., in "Does a Shared Neurobiology for Foods and Drugs of Abuse Contribute to Extremes of Food Ingestion in Anorexia and Bulimia Nervosa?" (*Biological Psychiatry*, vol. 73, no. 9, May 1, 2013), there is a significant association between eating disorders and substance use disorders, in that high rates of substance abuse (alcohol and illicit drugs) are reported by people with bulimia, while those with anorexia appear to be protected from substance abuse. The researchers explain that people with bulimia may share vulnerabilities to specific chemicals in the brain. Kaye et al. report that imaging studies of the brain provide insights into the inhibition and self-control characteristic of anorexia and the diminished self-control in bulimia that may also increase the risk of substance abuse.

TREATMENT OF EATING DISORDERS

Generally, physicians treat the medical complications of the disorder, whereas nutritionists advise the affected individuals about specific diet and eating plans. Psychotherapy is usually necessary to help people with eating disorders face their underlying problems and emotional issues. The initial challenge is to convince them to seek and obtain treatment; after they start treatment, the challenge then becomes helping them to stay in treatment. Many anorexics deny their illness, and getting and keeping anorexic patients in treatment can be difficult. Treating bulimia is also difficult. Many bulimics are easily frustrated and want to leave treatment if their symptoms are not quickly relieved.

Several approaches are used to treat eating disorders. Cognitive-behavioral therapy (CBT) teaches people how to monitor their eating and change unhealthy eating habits. It also teaches them how to change the way they respond to stressful situations. CBT is based on the premise that thinking influences emotions and behavior—that feelings and actions originate with thoughts. CBT posits that it is possible to change the way people feel and act even if their circumstances do not change. It teaches the advantages of feeling calm when faced with undesirable situations. CBT clients learn that they will confront undesirable events and circumstances whether they become troubled about them or not. When they are troubled about events or circumstances, they have two problems: the troubling event or circumstance, and the troubling feelings about the event or circumstance. Clients learn that when they do not become troubled about trying events and circumstances, they can reduce the number of problems they face by half.

Interpersonal psychotherapy (IPT) helps people look at their relationships with friends and family and make changes to resolve problems. IPT is short-term therapy that has demonstrated effectiveness for the treatment of depression. According to the International Society for Interpersonal Psychotherapy, IPT emphasizes that mental health and emotional problems occur within an interpersonal context. For this reason the therapy aims to intervene specifically in social functioning to relieve symptoms.

Group therapy has been found helpful for bulimics, who are relieved to find that they are not alone or unique in their eating behavior. A combination of behavioral therapy and family systems therapy is often the most effective with anorexics. Family systems therapy considers the family as the unit of treatment and focuses on relationships and communication patterns within the family rather than on the personality traits or symptoms displayed by individual family members. Problems are addressed by modifying the system rather than by trying to change an individual family member. People with eating disorders who also suffer from depression may benefit from antidepressant and antianxiety medications to help relieve coexisting mental health problems.

Recovery from eating disorders is uneven and the lack of consensus about the criteria for recovery further confounds efforts to assess how people fare as a result of treatment. Greta Noordenbos of Leiden University explains in "When Have Eating Disordered Patients Recovered and What Do the DSM-IV Criteria Tell about Recovery?" (*Eating Disorders*, vol. 19, no. 3, May 2011) that varying criteria result in a wide range of estimates of recovered patients. Noordenbos laments that "outcome studies not only use different criteria for recovery, but also quite different instruments, rendering their results incomparable. The same problem occurs among studies of predictors for recovery from eating disorders. Without consensus on criteria for recovery, it is not clear which goals of treatment are important to realize full recovery."

In "Facts about Eating Disorders," the Eating Disorders Coalition for Research, Policy, and Action characterizes recovery as a process that frequently entails multiple rehospitalizations, limited ability to work or attend school, and limited capacity for interpersonal relationships. With treatment, which can take months to years, about one-third of people with an eating disorder recover after an initial episode, one-third fluctuates between recovery and relapse, and the remaining third suffer chronic deterioration.

Eating disorders are difficult to treat effectively because many sufferers resist entering treatment and/or fail to complete treatment programs. Because attrition (dropping out of treatment) is a known problem, Karen Farchaus Stein et al. report in "An Eating Disorder Randomized Clinical Trial and Attrition: Profiles and Determinants of Dropout" (*International Journal of Eating Disorders*, vol. 44, no. 4, May 2011) their efforts to determine whether attrition is related to changes in symptoms during treatment, including participants' perceptions of dissatisfaction with their body. To do this, the researchers compared the perceptions of dropouts to those of participants who remained in treatment for six months.

Stein et al. find that both dropouts and those who remained in treatment experienced decreases in the drive for thinness, body dissatisfaction, and bulimia during the treatment phase, but that women who dropped out of treatment had a greater decrease in body dissatisfaction after one month of treatment than those who remained. The researchers theorize that a decrease in symptoms along with changes in self-perception, such as diminished body dissatisfaction, discourage participants from continuing in treatment. Stein et al. opine that "attention to treatment response from the earliest phases of intervention through follow-up may help to identify those at greatest risk of dropping and lead to strategies for promoting participant retention."

New Directions in Research and Treatment

According to the NIMH, in "Eating Disorders among Adults—Binge Eating Disorder," the results of its research are aiding both the understanding of eating disorders and their treatment. Research on intervening in the binge-eating cycle demonstrates that initiating structured patterns of eating enables people with eating disorders to experience less hunger, less deprivation, and fewer negative feelings about food and eating. When the two key predictors of bingeing (hunger and negative feelings) are reduced, the frequency of binges declines.

Continued study of the human genome promises the identification of additional susceptibility genes (genes that indicate an individual's increased risk for developing eating disorders) that will help develop more effective treatments for these disorders. Other research is investigating the relationship between brain functions and emotional and social behavior related to eating disorders and the role of the brain in feeding behavior. Scientists have learned that both appetite and energy expenditure are regulated by a highly complex network of nerve cells and intercellular messengers called neuropeptides. The role of sex hormones, known as gonadal steroids, in the development of eating disorders is suggested by the onset of puberty as a risk for these disorders. These discoveries provide insight into the biochemical mechanisms of eating disorders and offer potential direction for the development of new drugs and treatments for these disorders.

The considerable proportion of people with eating disorders who do not fare well in treatment, along with the high mortality rates that are associated with these disorders, prompts questions about factors that may influence recovery. In view of the genetic component in the genesis and progression of eating disorders, it seems likely that there may be genetic variants that contribute to the prospects for recovery. Identifying these variants may lead to more personalized treatment that includes more effective psychotherapies and/or pharmacological interventions for the most treatment-resistant patients.

In "Genetic Association of Recovery from Eating Disorders: The Role of GABA Receptor SNPs" (*Neuropsychopharmacology*, vol. 36, no. 11, October 2011), Cinnamon S. Bloss et al. tested more than 5,000 single nucleotide polymorphisms (SNPs) in approximately 350 genes to determine whether any of these SNPs were associated with recovery from eating disorders. SNPs associated with g-aminobutyric acid (a neurotransmitter that acts to inhibit the central nervous system, exerting a calming effect) were overrepresented among people with eating disorders. Bloss et al. conclude that their findings "could provide new insights into the development of more effective interventions for the most treatment-resistant patients." Giovanni Castellini et al. of the University of Florence find in "Association between Serotonin Transporter Gene Polymorphism and Eating Disorders Outcome: A 6-Year Follow-Up Study" (*American Journal of Medical Genetics*, vol. 159B, no. 5, July 2012) that a specific variant of the serotonin transporter (5-HTT) gene not only increases the risk of suffering from both eating disorders and depression but also influences the long-term outcomes of patients with anorexia.

In "Virtual Reality for Enhancing the Cognitive Behavioral Treatment of Obesity with Binge Eating Disorder: Randomized Controlled Study with One-Year Follow-Up" (*Journal of Medical Internet Research*, vol. 15, no. 6, June 2013), Gian Luca Cesa et al. look at how people suffering from obesity and binge-eating disorder fared following treatment with CBT that included a virtual reality program. The virtual reality presented environments and situations related to the triggering of disordered eating or relapse, such as home, supermarket, pub, and restaurant, enabling patients to practice eating and emotional management as well as decision-making and problem-solving skills. By practicing these skills in the virtual reality environment, patients learned to develop specific strategies for avoiding and/or coping with triggering situations. When Cesa et al. compare this novel approach to CBT alone, they find it was more effective in terms of preventing weight regain and improving weight loss after one-year follow-up.

Walter H. Kaye et al. describe in "Temperament-Based Treatment for Anorexia Nervosa" (*European Eating Disorders Review*, vol. 23, no. 1, January 2015) the development of treatment that addresses temperamental traits, such as anxiety, inflexibility, and rigidity, that are associated with anorexia nervosa. Temperament-based treatment aims to build "awareness of temperament tendencies and teaching constructive ways to make use of and manage associated traits to target [anorexia nervosa] behaviour, rather than attempting to change or work against temperament." Kaye et al. report that this approach to treatment is well accepted by patients and may help improve their symptoms.

PREVENTING EATING DISORDERS

Conventional public health definitions describe primary prevention as the prevention of new cases and secondary prevention as the prevention of recurrence of a disease or prevention of its progression. Primary prevention measures fall into two categories: actions to protect against disease and disability and actions to promote health such as good nutrition and hygiene, adequate exercise and rest, and avoidance of environmental and health risks. Health promotion also includes education about other interdependent dimensions of health known as wellness. Examples of health promotion programs aimed at preventing eating disorders include programs to enhance self-esteem, nutrition education classes, and programs that support children and teens to resist unhealthy pressures to conform to unrealistic body weight.

Secondary prevention programs are intended to identify and detect disease in its earliest stages, when it is most likely to be successfully treated. With early detection and diagnosis, it may be possible to cure the disease, slow its progression, prevent or minimize complications, and limit disability. Secondary prevention of eating disorders includes efforts to identify affected individuals to intervene early and prevent the development of serious and potentially life-threatening consequences.

Tertiary prevention programs aim to improve the quality of life for people with various diseases by limiting complications and disabilities, reducing the severity and progression of the disease, and providing rehabilitation (therapy to restore function and self-sufficiency). Unlike primary and secondary prevention, tertiary prevention involves actual treatment for the disease, and in the case of eating disorders it is conducted primarily by medical and mental health practitioners rather than by public health or social service agencies. An example of tertiary prevention is a program that monitors people with eating disorders to ensure that they maintain appropriate body weight and adhere to healthy diets and other prescribed medication or treatment. Because the treatment of eating disorders is not always effective or lasting, many health professionals contend that initiatives directed at controlling or eliminating the disorders by treating each affected individual or by training enough professionals as interventionists are ill advised. Instead, they advocate redirecting time, energy, and resources to primary and secondary prevention efforts.

Table 3.4 lists the basic principles for the prevention of eating disorders prepared by the National Eating Disorders Association (NEDA). These principles underscore the complexity of addressing eating disorders and the need for comprehensive, community-wide prevention programs that address the social and cultural issues promoting the rise of these disorders. The NEDA also urges parents to spearhead efforts to prevent eating disorders by practicing positive, healthy attitudes and behaviors and

TABLE 3.4

Eating disorders prevention

What is eating disorders prevention?

Prevention is any systematic attempt to change the circumstances that promote, initiate, sustain, or intensify problems like eating disorders.

- **Primary prevention** refers to programs or efforts that are designed to prevent the occurrence of eating disorders before they begin. Primary prevention is intended to help promote healthy development.
- **Secondary prevention** (sometimes called "targeted prevention") refers to programs or efforts that are designed to promote the early identification of an eating disorder—to recognize and treat an eating disorder before it spirals out of control. The earlier an eating disorder is discovered and addressed, the better the chance for recovery.

Basic principles for the prevention of eating disorders

1. Eating disorders are serious and complex problems. We need to be careful to avoid thinking of them in simplistic terms, like "anorexia is just a plea for attention," or "bulimia is just an addiction to food." Eating disorders arise from a variety of physical, emotional, social, and familial issues, all of which need to be addressed for effective prevention and treatment.
2. Eating disorders are not just a "woman's problem" or "something for the girls." Males who are preoccupied with shape and weight can also develop eating disorders as well as dangerous shape control practices like steroid use. In addition, males play an important role in prevention. The objectification and other forms of mistreatment of women by others contribute directly to two underlying features of an eating disorder: obsession with appearance and shame about one's body.
3. Prevention efforts will fail, or worse, inadvertently encourage disordered eating, if they concentrate solely on warning the public about the signs, symptoms, and dangers of eating disorders. Effective prevention programs must also address:
   - Our cultural obsession with slenderness as a physical, psychological, and moral issue.
   - The roles of men and women in our society.
   - The development of people's self-esteem and self-respect in a variety of areas (school, work, community service, hobbies) that transcend physical appearance.
4. Whenever possible, prevention programs for schools, community organizations, etc., should be coordinated with opportunities for participants to speak confidentially with a trained professional with expertise in the field of eating disorders, and, when appropriate, receive referrals to sources of competent, specialized care.

SOURCE: Michael Levine and Margo Maine, "Eating Disorders Can Be Prevented!" National Eating Disorders Association, 2005, https://www.chapman.edu/students/health-and-safety/psychological-counseling/_files/eating-disorder-files/10.50eds-Pprev.pdf (accessed October 7, 2015) encouraging children to resist media stereotypes about body shape and weight. Furthermore, it outlines the philosophies and actions parents can adopt and the behaviors they can model to help their children cultivate healthy attitudes about food, eating, exercise, and body weight. Table 3.5 outlines 10 steps parents can take to help prevent eating disorders, and Table 3.6 presents 10 steps family, friends, and the public-at-large can take to help prevent eating disorders.

Changing Social and Cultural Norms

The cultural idealization of thinness as a standard of female beauty and worth and the societal acceptance of dieting as a female ritual have been widely cited as sociocultural causes of eating disorders. The widespread misperception that the body is readily reshaped and that one can, and should, strive to change its size and form to correspond with aesthetic preferences also contributes to distorted perceptions and unrealistic expectations.

Media images that create, reflect, communicate, and reinforce cultural definitions of attractiveness, especially female beauty, are often acknowledged as factors that contribute to the rise of eating disorders. They exert powerful influences on values, attitudes, and practices for body image, diet, and activity. The role of the media, in conjunction with the fashion and entertainment industries, in promoting unrealistic standards of female beauty and unhealthy eating habits has been named as a causative factor for body dissatisfaction, unhealthy dieting behavior, and the rise of eating disorders.

Media messages portraying thinness as a desirable attribute do not directly cause eating disorders, but they do help create the context in which people learn to place a value on the size and shape of their body. To the extent that media advertising defines cultural values about that which is beautiful and desirable, the media have potent power over the development of self-esteem and body image. Although the media have begun to present more diverse and realistic images of people, this change is not expected to immediately reduce or eliminate eating disorders. However, many observers believe it will, over time, reduce the pressures to conform to one ideal, lessen feelings of body dissatisfaction, and ultimately decrease the potential for eating disorders.

EMPHASIS ON REALISTIC BODIES IN ADVERTISING CAMPAIGNS. In 2005 Dove, a skin and hair care division of Unilever, launched the groundbreaking "Campaign for Real Beauty," which featured a purportedly unretouched photo of six smiling women of various sizes and ethnicities posing in plain white underwear to promote a skin-firming cream. The women, who were not professional models, ranged from a slim size 6 to a curvy size 14 and graced print advertisements and billboards. The campaign generated considerable discussion and debate in the media.

According to the article "Dove Ads with 'Real' Women Get Attention" (Associated Press, July 29, 2005), Philippe Harousseau, the Dove marketing director, described the campaign as responsive to "our belief that beauty comes in different shapes, sizes, and ages. Our mission is to make more women feel beautiful every day by broadening the definition of beauty." Industry observers wondered whether the company was in fact broadening the definition of beauty and improving women's body image and self-esteem or simply launching a provocative advertising campaign. Although the company did not disclose just how much the advertisements helped promote its products, it conceded that the campaign was beneficial for all Dove products, not just the firming creams.

TABLE 3.5

Ten things parents can do to prevent eating disorders

1. Consider your thoughts, attitudes, and behaviors toward your own body and the way that these beliefs have been shaped by the forces of weightism and sexism. Then educate your children about
   (a) the genetic basis for the natural diversity of human body shapes and sizes, and
   (b) the nature and ugliness of prejudice.
   • Make an effort to maintain positive, healthy attitudes & behaviors. Children learn from the things you say and do!
2. Examine closely your dreams and goals for your children and other loved ones. Are you overemphasizing beauty and body shape, particularly for girls?
   • Avoid conveying an attitude which says in effect, "I will like you more if you lose weight, don't eat so much, look more like the slender models in ads, fit into smaller clothes, etc."
   • Decide what you can do and what you can stop doing to reduce the teasing, criticism, blaming, staring, etc. that reinforce the idea that larger or fatter is "bad" and smaller or thinner is "good."
3. Learn about and discuss with your sons and daughters (a) the dangers of trying to alter one's body shape through dieting, (b) the value of moderate exercise for health, and (c) the importance of eating a variety of foods in well-balanced meals consumed at least three times a day.
   • Avoid categorizing foods into "good/safe/no-fat or low-fat" vs. "bad/dangerous/fattening."
   • Be a good role model in regard to sensible eating, exercise, and self-acceptance.
4. Make a commitment not to avoid activities (such as swimming, sunbathing, dancing, etc.) simply because they call attention to your weight and shape. Refuse to wear clothes that are uncomfortable or that you don't like but wear simply because they divert attention from your weight or shape.
5. Make a commitment to exercise for the joy of feeling your body move and grow stronger, not to purge fat from your body or to compensate for calories eaten.
6. Practice taking people seriously for what they say, feel, and do, not for how slender or "well put together" they appear.
7. Help children appreciate and resist the ways in which television, magazines, and other media distort the true diversity of human body types and imply that a slender body means power, excitement, popularity, or perfection.
8. Educate boys and girls about various forms of prejudice, including weightism, and help them understand their responsibilities for preventing them.
9. Encourage your children to be active and to enjoy what their bodies can do and feel like. Do not limit their caloric intake unless a physician requests that you do this because of a medical problem.
10. Do whatever you can to promote the self-esteem and self-respect of all of your children in intellectual, athletic, and social endeavors. Give boys and girls the same opportunities and encouragement. Be careful not to suggest that females are less important than males, e.g., by exempting males from housework or child care. A well-rounded sense of self and solid self-esteem are perhaps the best antidotes to dieting and disordered eating.

SOURCE: Michael Levine, "10 Things Parents Can Do to Help Prevent Eating Disorders," National Eating Disorders Association, 2002, http://dillarddrivems.wcpss.net/wp-content/uploads/10tipsforparents-eating-disorders.pdf (accessed October 7, 2015)

TABLE 3.6

Ten ways family and friends can help to prevent eating disorders

- Learn all you can about anorexia nervosa, bulimia nervosa, and binge eating disorder. Genuine awareness will help you avoid judgmental or mistaken attitudes about food, weight, body shape, and eating disorders.
- Discourage the idea that a particular diet, weight, or body size will automatically lead to happiness and fulfillment.
- Choose to challenge the false belief that thinness, weight loss and/or muscularity are desirable, while body fat and weight gain are shameful, or indicate laziness, worthlessness, or immorality.
- Avoid categorizing foods as "good/safe" vs. "bad/dangerous." Remember, we all need to eat a balanced variety of foods.
- Decide to avoid judging others and yourself on the basis of body weight or shape. Turn off the voices in your head that tell you that a person's body weight or muscularity says anything about their character, personality, or value as a person.
- Avoid conveying an attitude that says, "I will like you better if you lose weight, don't eat so much, or change your body shape."
- Become a critical viewer of the media and its messages about self-esteem and body image. Talk back to the television when you hear a comment or see an image that promotes a certain body ideal at all costs. Rip out (or better yet, write to the editor about) advertisements or articles in magazines that make you feel bad about your body shape or size.
- If you think someone has an eating disorder, express your concerns in a forthright, caring manner. Gently but firmly encourage the person to seek trained professional help.
- Be a model of healthy self-esteem and body image. Recognize that others pay attention and learn from the way you talk about yourself and your body. Choose to talk about yourself with respect and appreciation. Choose to value yourself based on your goals, accomplishments, talents, and character. Refrain from letting the way you feel about your body weight and shape determine the course of your day. Embrace the natural diversity of human bodies and celebrate your body's unique shape and size.
- Support local and national nonprofit eating disorders organizations—like the National Eating Disorders Association—by volunteering your time or giving a tax-deductible donation.

SOURCE: "What Can You Do To Help Prevent Eating Disorders?" National Eating Disorders Association, 2013, http://www.nationaleatingdisorders.org/what-can-you-do-help-prevent-eating-disorders (accessed October 7, 2015)

The article notes that the ads were not, however, universally well received. For example, the *Chicago Sun-Times* columnist Richard Roeper characterized the women as "chunky," which earned him angry letters from about a thousand readers. Some skeptics asserted that although they endorsed the notion of the ads featuring real women who felt good about their body, they believed the ads sent contradictory messages (e.g., promoting a product to reduce the curves the models were flaunting). The most impassioned detractors accused the company of appearing hypocritical because the ads aimed to profit from "improving" the same curves the campaign exhorted women to celebrate.

Since then, other groups have sought to promote acceptance of a wide range of body types. For example, the magazine *Wear Your Voice* launched the #DropTheTowel campaign (http://www.wearyourvoicemag.com/dropthetowel-this-summer/) during the summer of 2015 to combat body shaming and encourage people of all body shapes and sizes to feel confident about wearing swimsuits. Butterfly (http://thebutterflyfoundation.org.au/), an Australian foundation that supports people with eating disorders, has launched the Don't Dis My Appearance, Fat Talk Free February, and Change the Conversation campaigns to increase awareness of practices that reinforce negative body images.

Be Real (2016, http://www.berealcampaign.co.uk/the-campaign.html), a national campaign in the United Kingdom, is a partnership with Dove and is sponsored by bareMinerals, Facebook, the Government Equalities Office, N Brown Group PLC, New Look, Superdrug, and YMCA, with All Walks beyond the Catwalk as its lead ambassador. The campaign aims to promote healthy living rather than weight and appearance and calls on "businesses, publishers, editors and advertisers to act responsibly by positively promoting different body shapes and sizes, people with and without disabilities, and all ages, genders and ethnicities." It also encourages consumers to choose brands that promote body confidence and confront those that do not.

Social media campaigns are also working to combat sizeism and help people foster healthy relationships with their body. For example, Love Your Body (http://now.org/now-foundation/love-your-body/), a movement started by the National Organization for Women, named October 14 "Love Your Body Day" to encourage women to ignore narrow, unrealistic, and oppressive beauty standards in favor of a definition of beauty that is realistic and includes health and diversity.

Another social media campaign, #LessIsMore (2016, http://www.rawbeautytalks.com/get-involved/less-is-more/), aims to reduce photo editing and retouching because it promotes unrealistic and often unattainable images of men and women. The campaign asserts that "the beauty ideal represented in the images in magazines is detrimental to our health. It perpetuates low self-confidence, depression, anxiety, over-spending and eating disorders." The campaign asks consumers to tag images they consider overly retouched with the hashtag #LessIsMore and to post photos of themselves without makeup and unretouched.

ATTEMPTS TO ADOPT HEALTHY STANDARDS IN THE MODELING INDUSTRY. After the deaths of the dangerously thin models Luisel Ramos (1984–2006) and Ana Carolina Reston (1985–2006) in late 2006, Spain banned the use of models with a body mass index (BMI; body weight in kilograms divided by height in meters squared) of less than 18, and according to Eric Wilson, in "Health Guidelines Suggested for Models" (NYTimes.com, January 6, 2007), the Chamber of Fashion in Milan proposed that models be at least 16 years old with a minimum BMI of 18.5 (a BMI below 18.5 is considered underweight). (See Table 1.4 in Chapter 1.) In 2010 Isabelle Caro, a French fashion model who suffered from anorexia, died after posing for a campaign to raise awareness about the disorder.

In 2007 the Council of Fashion Designers of America proposed a series of actions intended to safeguard models' health. The recommendations included developing workshops for models and their families about eating disorders and supplying healthy meals, snacks, and water backstage and at shoots and provide nutrition and fitness education.

Despite efforts to encourage designers to use models of a healthy weight, models that appeared abnormally thin continued to dominate runways in 2016. However, Emile Picy reports in "France Bans Super-Skinny Models in Anorexia Clampdown" (Reuters, April 3, 2015) that Israel banned excessively thin models in 2013 and France followed in 2015. France's campaign is more stringent than other countries' because violations may result in prison terms and hefty fines. France not only prohibits the use of models with BMIs of less than 18 but also makes it illegal to condone anorexia and requires retouched photographs to be identified as manipulated images.

In "What 5 Models Really Think about France Banning Extremely Skinny Models" (Cosmopolitan.com, March 20, 2015), Helin Jung and Charles Manning find that models generally support the ban on excessively thin models and believe the public wants to see "natural women who work out and eat healthy and are not frail." However, some warn that using BMI exclusively may overlook models with eating disorders who have normal BMIs and exclude naturally thin but healthy young women.

CHAPTER 4
DIET, NUTRITION, AND WEIGHT ISSUES AMONG CHILDREN AND ADOLESCENTS

One of the most disturbing observations about overweight and obesity in the United States is the epidemic of supersized (overweight and obese) kids. The National Center for Health Statistics (NCHS) reports in *Health, United States, 2014* (May 2015, http://www.cdc.gov/nchs/data/hus/hus14.pdf) that in 2009–12 nearly 40% of American children aged six to 11 years and teenagers aged 12 to 19 years were obese, compared with 22% of young people in 1988–94. (See Table 4.1.) Between 1988–94 and 2009–12 the prevalence of obesity among children and adolescents increased from 7.2% to 10.2% for children aged two to five years and from 11.3% to 17.9% for children aged six to 11 years. Among teenagers aged 12 to 19 years, the percentage nearly doubled, from 10.5% to 19.4%.

With children and teens as well as with adults, the body mass index (BMI; body weight in kilograms divided by height in meters squared) is used to determine underweight, healthy weight, overweight, and at risk for overweight. Children's body fatness changes over the years as they grow, and girls and boys differ in their body fatness as they mature. In light of these differences, the BMI for children (also referred to as BMI-for-age) is gender and age specific. For example, Figure 4.1 shows BMI percentiles for boys aged two to 20 years and demonstrates how different BMI numbers are interpreted for a 10-year-old boy. Figure 4.2 shows that children of different ages (and gender) may have the same BMI number, but that number will fall into a different percentile for each child, classifying a 10-year-old boy as overweight and a 15-year-old boy as at a healthy weight.

Overweight is defined as at or above the age- and gender-specific 95th percentile on the BMI. (See Table 4.2.) Still, even children at the 85th percentile are considered at risk for overweight- and obesity-induced illnesses and overweight throughout their adult life.

Joan Lo et al. find in "PS3-20: Prevalence of Obesity and Extreme Obesity in Children Aged Three to Five Years" (*Clinical Medicine and Research*, vol. 11, no. 3, September 2013) that obesity, and even severe obesity, is evident in children as young as three to five years of age. A review of the medical records of nearly 43,000 children finds that 12.4% of boys and 10% of girls had a BMI equal to or greater than the 95th percentile. The 3.9% of young children with a BMI equal to or greater than the 99th percentile were considered extremely obese.

The Centers for Disease Control and Prevention (CDC) reports in "New CDC Vital Signs: Obesity Declines among Low-Income Preschoolers" (January 8, 2014, http://www.cdc.gov/media/dpk/2013/dpk-vs-child-obesity.html) that there may be some progress in reversing the rising tide of childhood obesity. Between 2008 and 2011, 19 states and territories had significant decreases in obesity among low-income preschoolers. (See Figure 4.3.) Another promising trend is the observed decline in obesity among this group of children. Figure 4.4 shows that obesity rates among low-income preschoolers rose to 14.9% in 2007 but decreased between 2008 and 2011 to 14.4%.

In "Prevalence of Childhood and Adult Obesity in the United States, 2011–2012" (*Journal of the American Medical Association*, vol. 311, no. 8, February 26, 2014), Cynthia L. Ogden et al. of the NCHS report that although substantial decreases in obesity were reported among low-income preschoolers participating in federal nutrition programs and among low-income children, overall, the prevalence of obesity among children remains high and 17% of youth are obese. Sabrina Tavernise observes in "Obesity Rate for Young Children Plummets 43% in a Decade" (NYTimes.com, February 25, 2014) that experts are unsure about why obesity among children aged two to five years decreased 43% between 2002 and 2012. The decrease may be attributable to reduced consumption of sugary beverages, an increase in breast-feeding (which may

TABLE 4.1

Obesity among children and teens, selected years 1988–2012

[Data are based on measured height and weight of a sample of the civilian noninstitutionalized population]

Sex, age, race and Hispanic origin[a], and percent of poverty level	1988–1994	1999–2002	2003–2006	2009–2012
2–5 years		Percent of population		
Both sexes[b]	7.2	10.3	12.5	10.2
Not Hispanic or Latino:				
White only	5.2	8.7	10.8	6.4
Black or African American only	7.7	8.8	14.9	14.7
Mexican origin	12.3	13.1	16.7	15.7
Boys	6.1	10.0	12.8	12.0
Not Hispanic or Latino:				
White only	4.5*	8.2*	11.1	9.3*
Black or African American only	7.7	8.0*	13.3	14.3*
Mexican origin	12.4	14.1	18.8	17.6
Girls	8.2	10.6	12.2	8.4
Not Hispanic or Latina:				
White only	5.9	9.0*	10.4	*
Black or African American only	7.6	9.6	16.6	15.3
Mexican origin	12.3	12.2*	14.5	13.8*
Percent of poverty level:[c]				
Below 100%	9.7	10.9	14.3	12.3
100%–199%	7.2	13.8*	12.7	11.6
200%–399%	5.6	7.6*	11.9	11.0
400% or more	*	*	10.0*	5.0*
6–11 years				
Both sexes[b]	11.3	15.9	17.0	17.9
Boys	11.6	16.9	18.0	18.3
Not Hispanic or Latino:				
White only	10.7	14.0	15.5	12.9
Black or African American only	12.3	17.0	18.6	27.6
Mexican origin	17.5	26.5	27.5	25.0
Girls	11.0	14.7	15.8	17.4
Not Hispanic or Latina:				
White only	9.8*	13.1	14.4	14.2
Black or African American only	17.0	22.8	24.0	24.8
Mexican origin	15.3	17.1	19.7	23.1
Percent of poverty level:[c]				
Below 100%	11.4	19.1	22.0	24.6
100%–199%	11.1	16.4	19.2	18.5
200%–399%	11.7	15.3	16.7	15.8
400% or more	*	12.9	9.2	12.2*
12–19 years				
Both sexes[b]	10.5	16.0	17.6	19.4
Boys	11.3	16.7	18.2	20.0
Not Hispanic or Latino:				
White only	11.6	14.6	17.3	17.9
Black or African American only	10.7	18.8	18.4	22.0
Mexican origin	14.1	24.7	22.1	27.0
Girls	9.7	15.3	16.8	18.9
Not Hispanic or Latina:				
White only	8.9	12.6	14.5	17.8
Black or African American only	16.3	23.5	27.7	23.7
Mexican origin	13.4*	19.6	19.9	20.2
Percent of poverty level:[c]				
Below 100%	15.8	19.8	19.3	23.2
100%–199%	11.2	15.1	18.4	22.5
200%–399%	9.4	15.7	19.3	17.9
400% or more	*	13.9	12.6	13.8

promote healthier weight gain in children), and an overall decrease in the number of calories children consume. Other possible explanations are increased emphasis on fruits and vegetables in the federally funded Special Supplemental Nutrition Program for Women, Infants, and Children and the effects of federal, state, and local initiatives aimed at preventing and reducing obesity.

TABLE 4.1

Obesity among children and teens, selected years 1988–2012 [CONTINUED]

[Data are based on measured height and weight of a sample of the civilian noninstitutionalized population]

*Estimates are considered unreliable.

[a]Persons of Mexican origin may be of any race. Starting with 1999 data, race-specific estimates are tabulated according to the 1997 *Revisions to the Standards for the Classification of Federal Data on Race and Ethnicity* and are not strictly comparable with estimates for earlier years. The two non-Hispanic race categories shown in the table conform to the 1997 Standards. Starting with 1999 data, race-specific estimates are for persons who reported only one racial group. Prior to data year 1999, estimates were tabulated according to the 1977 Standards. Estimates for single-race categories prior to 1999 included persons who reported one race or, if they reported more than one race, identified one race as best representing their race.

[b]Includes persons of all races and Hispanic origins, not just those shown separately.

[c]Percent of poverty level was calculated by dividing family income by the U.S. Department of Health and Human Services' poverty guideline specific to family size, as well as the appropriate year, and state. Persons with unknown percent of poverty level are excluded (7% in 2009–2012).

Notes: Obesity is defined as body mass index (BMI) at or above the sex- and age-specific 95th percentile from the 2000 CDC Growth Charts: United States. Kuczmarski RJ, Ogden CL, Guo SS, Grummer-Strawn LM, Flegal KM, Mei Z, Wei R, Curtin LR, Roche AF, Johnson CL. 2000 CDC Growth Charts for the United States: methods and development. Vital Health Stat 11. 2002 May;(246):1–190. In *Health, United States* the NHANES variable, Body Mass Index, is used to assign persons to BMI categories. Starting with *Health, United States, 2010*, the terminology describing weight for height among children changed from prior editions. The term "obesity" now refers to children who were formerly labeled as overweight. This is a change in terminology only and not measurement; the previous definition of overweight is now the definition of obesity. Ogden CL, Flegal KM. Changes in terminology for childhood overweight and obesity. National health statistics report; no. 25. Hyattsville, MD: NCHS; 2010. Age is at time of examination at the mobile examination center. Crude rates, not age-adjusted rates, are shown. Height was measured without shoes. Excludes pregnant females.

SOURCE: "Table 65. Obesity among Children and Adolescents Aged 2–19 Years, by Selected Characteristics: United States, Selected Years 1988–1994 through 2009–2012," in *Health, United States, 2014: With Special Feature on Adults Aged 55–64*, Centers for Disease Control and Prevention, National Center for Health Statistics, May 2015, http://www.cdc.gov/nchs/data/hus/hus14.pdf (accessed October 5, 2015)

The prevalence of overweight and obesity among adolescents is of particular concern because overweight and obese adolescents are at even greater risk than overweight children of becoming overweight or obese adults. The Federal Interagency Forum on Child and Family Statistics observes in *America's Children: Key National Indicators of Well-Being, 2015* (July 2015, http://www.childstats.gov/pdf/ac2015/ac_15.pdf) that obesity in adolescence continues into adulthood, along with increased risk for diabetes, stroke, heart disease, arthritis, and certain cancers.

In "The Utility of Childhood and Adolescent Obesity Assessment in Relation to Adult Health" (*Medical Decision Making*, vol. 33, no. 2, February 2013), Jeremy D. Goldhaber-Fiebert et al. sought to identify the portion of adult obesity and related chronic conditions associated with childhood obesity and the usefulness of assessing childhood obesity at different ages. The researchers find that consistent with other studies, most obese adults were normal-weight children, and many obese children become nonobese adults. The predictive value of BMI assessment in younger children is relatively poor; however, BMI stabilizes in preteen and teen years, so using childhood BMI as an indicator of future obesity risk may be more useful in older children. The CDC reports in "Childhood Obesity Causes & Consequences" (June 19, 2015, http://www.cdc.gov/obesity/childhood/causes.html) that among five- to 17-year-olds, "70% of obese children had at least one [cardiovascular disease] risk factor, and 39% had two or more."

PREVALENCE OF OVERWEIGHT AND OBESE TEENS BY SEX, GRADE, RACE, AND ETHNICITY

The Youth Risk Behavior Surveillance System (YRBSS) is a national school-based survey conducted by the CDC. It examines health-risk behaviors among youth and young adults, including unhealthy dietary behaviors, physical inactivity, and overweight.

The 2013 YRBSS found that throughout the United States, 31.1% of students described themselves as overweight. (See Table 4.3.) The prevalence of overweight was higher among female (36.3%) than among male (25.9%) students, and higher among non-Hispanic African American female (33.4%), non-Hispanic white female (35.8%), and Hispanic female (40.3%) students than among non-Hispanic African American male (18.3%), Hispanic male (27.1%), and non-Hispanic white male (27.8%) students.

The prevalence of self-described overweight was higher among 11th-grade students (32.5%) than among ninth- (30.2%), 10th- (30.4%), and 12th-grade (31.5%) students and higher among 11th-grade females (39.3%) than among 9th-grade (34.5%), 10th-grade (34.3%), and 12th-grade (37.5%) females. (See Table 4.3.)

The 2013 YRBSS found that 16.6% of high school students were overweight and 13.7% were obese. (See Table 4.4.) The prevalence of overweight was about the same for males and females (16.5% and 16.6%, respectively), and obesity was higher among male students (16.6%) than among female students (10.8%). Overweight and obesity were also higher among non-Hispanic African American females (22.8% and 16.7%, respectively) and Hispanic females (19.2% and 11.2%, respectively) than among non-Hispanic white females (14.3% and 9.7%, respectively). Overweight and obesity were higher among Hispanic males (17.4% and 19%, respectively) and non-Hispanic African American males (15.2% and 14.8%, respectively) than among non-Hispanic white males (16.9% and 16.5%, respectively). Overall, there were

FIGURE 4.1

Body mass index percentiles for boys, ages 2–20

A 10-year-old boy with a BMI of 23 would be in the overweight category (95th percentile or greater).

A 10-year-old boy with a BMI of 21 would be in the at-risk-of-overweight category (85th to less than 95th percentile).

A 10-year-old boy with a BMI of 18 would be in the healthy weight category (5th percentile to less than 85th percentile).

A 10-year-old boy with a BMI of 13 would be in the underweight category (less than 5th percentile).

95th percentile
90th
85th percentile
75th
50th
25th
10th
5th percentile

SOURCE: "Body Mass Index-for-Age Percentiles: Boys, 2 to 20 Years," in *About Child and Teen BMI*, Centers for Disease Control and Prevention, National Center for Chronic Disease Prevention and Health Promotion, Division of Nutrition, Physical Activity, and Obesity, May 15, 2015, http://cdc.gov/nccdphp/dnpa/bmi/childrens_BMI/about_childrens_BMI.htm (accessed October 12, 2015)

FIGURE 4.2

The interpretation of body mass index (BMI) varies by age

A 10-year-old boy with a BMI of 23 would be in the overweight category (95th percentile or greater).

A 15-year-old boy with a BMI of 23 would be in the healthy weight category (5th percentile to less than 85th percentile).

95th percentile

90th

85th percentile

75th

50th

25th

10th

5th percentile

Age (years)

SOURCE: "Weight Status Category," in *About Child and Teen BMI*, Centers for Disease Control and Prevention, National Center for Chronic Disease Prevention and Health Promotion, Division of Nutrition, Physical Activity, and Obesity, May 15, 2015, http://www.cdc.gov/nccdphp/dnpa/bmi/childrens_BMI/about_childrens_BMI.htm (accessed October 12, 2015) higher rates of obesity among non-Hispanic African American (15.7%) and Hispanic (15.1%) students than among non-Hispanic white (13.1%) students.

TABLE 4.2

Weight status categories by BMI-for-age percentiles

Weight status category	Percentile range
Underweight	Less than the 5th percentile
Healthy weight	5th percentile to less than the 85th percentile
At risk of overweight	85th to less than the 95th percentile
Overweight	Equal to or greater than the 95th percentile

BMI = Body mass index.

SOURCE: "Weight Status Category," in *About Child and Teen BMI*, Centers for Disease Control and Prevention, National Center for Chronic Disease Prevention and Health Promotion, Division of Nutrition, Physical Activity, and Obesity, May 15, 2015, http://www.cdc.gov/nccdphp/dnpa/bmi/childrens_BMI/about_childrens_BMI.htm (accessed October 12, 2015)

The prevalence of obesity was higher among 11th-grade males (17.6%) than among ninth-grade males (16.2%), 10th-grade males (17.2%), 12th-grade males (15.3%), ninth-grade females (10.2%), 10th-grade females (10.1%), 11th-grade females (11.4%), and 12th-grade females (11.8%). (See Table 4.4.)

The 2013 YRBSS finding of significant percentages of overweight and obese teens suggests the likelihood of yet another generation of overweight adults who may be at risk for subsequent overweight- and obesity-related health problems. According to Y. Claire Wang et al., in "Health and Economic Burden of the Projected Obesity Trends in the USA and the UK" (*Lancet*, vol. 378, no. 9793, August 2011), forecasts based on the National Health and Nutrition Examination Surveys predict that if the current trends continue, three out of four Americans will be overweight or obese by 2020 and by 2030 there

FIGURE 4.3

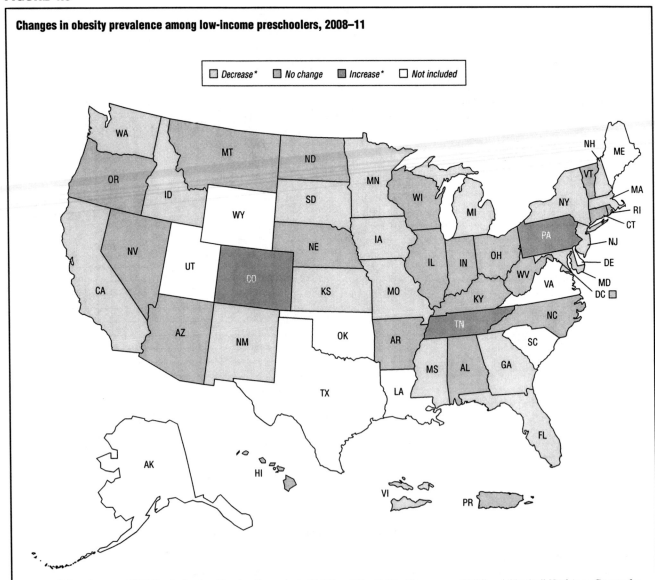

Changes in obesity prevalence among low-income preschoolers, 2008–11

☐ Decrease*   ☐ No change   ☐ Increase*   ☐ Not included

SOURCE: "Many States and U.S. Territories Are Showing Decreases in Childhood Obesity," in "Progress on Childhood Obesity," *Vitalsigns*, Centers for Disease Control and Prevention, August 2013, http://www.cdc.gov/VitalSigns/ChildhoodObesity/index.html#infographic (accessed October 16, 2015)

FIGURE 4.4

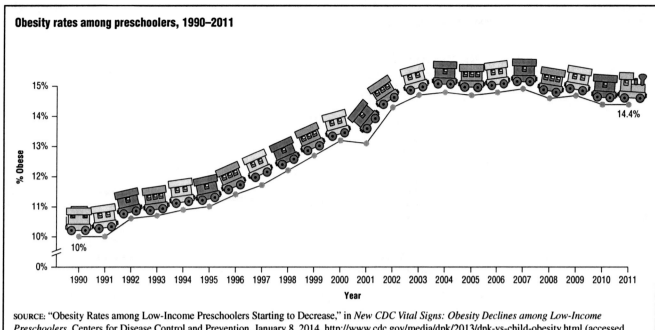

Obesity rates among preschoolers, 1990–2011

SOURCE: "Obesity Rates among Low-Income Preschoolers Starting to Decrease," in *New CDC Vital Signs: Obesity Declines among Low-Income Preschoolers*, Centers for Disease Control and Prevention, January 8, 2014, http://www.cdc.gov/media/dpk/2013/dpk-vs-child-obesity.html (accessed October 12, 2015)

TABLE 4.3

Percentage of high school students who described themselves as overweight by sex, race/ethnicity, and grade, 2013

	Described themselves as overweight			Were trying to lose weight		
	Female	Male	Total	Female	Male	Total
Category	%	%	%	%	%	%
Race/ethnicity						
White*	35.8	27.8	31.8	63.1	31.4	47.1
Black*	33.4	18.3	26.0	54.9	26.3	40.9
Hispanic	40.3	27.1	33.8	66.9	41.8	54.5
Grade						
9	34.5	26.1	30.2	60.5	37.1	48.7
10	34.3	26.7	30.4	62.8	31.2	46.7
11	39.3	25.4	32.5	64.7	32.1	48.6
12	37.5	25.4	31.5	62.6	31.2	47.0
Total	**36.3**	**25.9**	**31.1**	**62.6**	**33.0**	**47.7**

*Non-Hispanic.

SOURCE: Adapted from Laura Kann et al., "Table 107. Percentage of High School Students Who Described Themselves as Slightly or Very Overweight and Who Were Trying to Lose Weight, by Sex, Race/Ethnicity and Grade—United States, Youth Risk Behavior Survey, 2013," in "Youth Risk Behavior Surveillance—United States, 2013," *MMWR*, vol. 63, no. 4, June 13, 2014, http://www.cdc.gov/mmwr/pdf/ss/ss6304.pdf (accessed October 7, 2015)

will be 65 million more obese American adults. In children, at the current rate, the prevalence of overweight is likely to nearly double by 2030.

WHY ARE SO MANY CHILDREN AND TEENS OVERWEIGHT?

Most children are overweight for the same reason as their adult counterparts: they consume more calories than they expend. Infants and toddlers appear to be effective regulators of caloric consumption, taking in only the calories needed for growth and development. By the time children are school age, this self-regulatory mechanism has weakened and when offered larger portions, they will eat them.

Heredity and environment play key roles in determining a child's risk of becoming overweight or obese. The American Academy of Child and Adolescent Psychiatry notes in "Obesity in Children and Teens" (March 2011, https://www.aacap.org/App_Themes/AACAP/docs/facts_for_families/79_obesity_in_children_and_teens.pdf) that if one parent is obese, then there is a 50%

TABLE 4.4

Percentage of high school students who were overweight or obese, by sex, race/ethnicity, and grade, 2013

	Obese			Overweight		
	Female	Male	Total	Female	Male	Total
Category	%	%	%	%	%	%
Race/ethnicity						
White*	9.7	16.5	13.1	14.3	16.9	15.6
Black*	16.7	14.8	15.7	22.8	15.2	19.1
Hispanic	11.2	19.0	15.1	19.2	17.4	18.3
Grade						
9	10.2	16.2	13.2	17.9	18.6	18.2
10	10.1	17.2	13.6	16.5	15.7	16.1
11	11.4	17.6	14.4	15.8	15.5	15.6
12	11.8	15.3	13.5	16.2	16.1	16.2
Total	**10.8**	**16.6**	**13.7**	**16.6**	**16.5**	**16.6**

*Non-Hispanic.

SOURCE: Adapted from Laura Kann et al., "Table 105. Percentage of High School Students Who Were Obese and Who Were Overweight, by Sex, Race/Ethnicity and Grade—United States, Youth Risk Behavior Survey, 2013," in "Youth Risk Behavior Surveillance—United States, 2013," *MMWR*, vol. 63, no. 4, June 13, 2014, http://www.cdc.gov/mmwr/pdf/ss/ss6304.pdf (accessed October 7, 2015)

chance that a child will be obese, and when both parents are obese, a child has an 80% chance of being obese. Although there is mounting evidence of genetic predisposition and susceptibility to overweight and obesity, childhood obesity is still considered largely an environmental problem—the result of behaviors, attitudes, and preferences learned early in life. Children's relationships with food develop in response to family and cultural values and practices as well as to the influences of school, peers, and the media.

The question remains: Which environmental factors have given rise to the increasing prevalence of overweight children and teens during the past three decades? Many observers point to a reliance on fat-laden convenience and fast foods, along with time spent watching television, playing video games, and surfing the Internet, instead of being outdoors and getting physical activity.

The Federal Interagency Forum on Child and Family Statistics reports in *America's Children: Key National Indicators of Well-Being, 2015* that between 2009 and 2012 the diet quality score, which is a measure of how well children's diets meet federal diet quality standards, for children aged two to 17 years was 52 out of a possible 100. The forum asserts that children's diet scores would improve by increasing consumption of vegetables, especially dark greens and beans, replacing refined grains with whole grains, substituting some meat and poultry with seafood, and decreasing the intake of salt, solid fats, and added sugars.

In "Patterns of Physical Activity, Sedentary Behavior, and Diet in U.S. Adolescents" (*Journal of Adolescent Health*, vol. 53, no. 2, August 2013), Ronald J. Iannotti and Jing Wang of the National Institute of Child Health and Human Development (NICHD) report the results of a

survey of more than 9,000 adolescents aged 11 to 16 years. Participants were asked about their physical activity, the amount of time they spent in front of a computer screen or other electronic screen, and the amount of healthful and unhealthful foods they consumed. They were also asked about symptoms of depression and their satisfaction with their body.

Based on their responses, Iannotti and Wang classified participants as unhealthful (26%), healthful (27%), and typical (47%). They find that the typical adolescents were the least likely to exercise five or more days each week or to eat fruits and vegetables at least once a day. They were more likely to spend time in front of screens than the healthful group, and less likely to do so than the unhealthful group. They occasionally ate fruits and vegetables but also infrequently consumed sweets, chips, fries, and soft drinks. These typical adolescents were more likely than those in the other two groups to be overweight or obese and to be dissatisfied with their body.

Not surprisingly, the unhealthful group consumed the most sweets, chips, fries, and soft drinks. It was more likely than the other two groups to spend more than two hours per day in front of screens. Adolescents in the unhealthful group were more likely to be underweight and to report needing to put on weight. They were also more likely to report symptoms of depression and of poor physical health.

Nearly two-thirds of youth in the healthful group said they exercised at least five days per week. These students were the least likely to spend time in front of a screen and were the most likely to report eating fruits and vegetables at least once a day. They were also the least likely to consume sweets, soft drinks, chips, and fries. They reported the fewest depressive symptoms and had the highest scores in life satisfaction.

The 2013 YRBSS found that more than four out of 10 (41.3%) high school students used computers or played video games for three or more hours per day and that 32.5% watched television for three or more hours per day. (See Table 4.5.)

Eating alone, in front of a television or computer, children are more likely to overeat because they are lonely, bored, or susceptible to advertising cues. Overcome with guilt because they are not home to prepare meals, some working parents may intensify the problem by indulging their children with too many food treats. However, stay-at-home parents do not necessarily convey healthier attitudes about food, eating, and nutrition than parents who work outside the home. Both groups may use food, especially sweets, to reward good behavior or may pressure children to clean their plates. Although these suppositions remain unproven, it is known that parents with eating disorders, obsessive dieters, and those with unhealthful eating habits are powerful, negative role models for children.

Another factor that may contribute to adolescents' weight gain may be late bedtimes and lack of sleep. Lauren D. Asarnow, Eleanor McGlinchey, and Allison G. Harvey analyze in "Evidence for a Possible Link between Bedtime and Change in Body Mass Index" (*Sleep*, vol. 38, no. 10, October 1, 2015) data from the National Longitudinal Study of Adolescent Health and find that the later the average bedtime during the week, the higher the teens' BMI over time, with each additional hour later prompting a 2.1% increase in BMI.

HOW HIGH SCHOOL STUDENTS EAT

The 2013 YRBSS found that 33.2% of students had eaten fruit or drank 100% fruit juice two or more times per day during the seven days preceding the survey and that just 21.9% consumed fruit or 100% fruit juice three or more times per day. (See Table 4.6.). More than six out of 10 (61.5%) students ate vegetables one or more times per day, and 6.6% did not eat any vegetables. (See Table 4.7.) Just 15.7% of students ate vegetables three or more times per day. (See Table 4.8.)

Even fewer students (12.5%) had drunk at least three glasses of milk per day than had eaten the recommended servings of fruits and vegetables during the seven days preceding the survey. (See Table 4.9.) The prevalence of having consumed at least three glasses of milk per day was more than two times higher among male (16.9%) than among female (8.1%) students.

Is Fast Food to Blame?

In "Trends in Energy Intake among U.S. Children by Eating Location and Food Source, 1977–2006" (*Journal of the American Dietetic Association*, vol. 111, no. 8, August 2011), Jennifer M. Poti and Barry M. Popkin of the University of North Carolina, Chapel Hill, indicate that children's increased food consumption between 1977 and 2006 was associated with a major increase in food that was eaten away from home. The researchers analyzed data from 29,217 children aged two to 18 years from the 1977–78 Nationwide Food Consumption Survey, the 1989–91 and 1994–98 Continuing Survey of Food Intakes by Individuals, and the 2003–06 National Health and Nutrition Examination Surveys. They find

TABLE 4.5

Percentage of high school students who used computers, played video games, or watched television for three hours or more/day, by sex, race/ethnicity and grade, 2013

| | Used computers 3 or more hours/day | | | Watched television 3 or more hours/day | | |
| | Female | Male | Total | Female | Male | Total |
Category	%	%	%	%	%	%
Race/ethnicity						
White*	35.6	39.1	37.4	24.3	25.7	25.0
Black*	46.6	51.9	49.1	52.2	55.3	53.7
Hispanic	44.8	42.0	43.4	39.0	36.5	37.8
Grade						
9	46.5	43.0	44.8	35.3	34.6	34.9
10	41.0	44.9	42.9	32.2	32.4	32.3
11	37.6	42.4	40.0	30.4	32.3	31.3
12	35.4	38.4	36.9	30.6	31.9	31.3
Total	**40.4**	**42.3**	**41.3**	**32.2**	**32.8**	**32.5**

*Non-Hispanic.
Note: Used computers, played video games, or watched television on an average school day for something that was not school work.

SOURCE: Adapted from Laura Kann et al., "Table 99. Percentage of High School Students Who Played Video or Computer Games or Used a Computer for 3 or More Hours/Day and Who Watched 3 or More Hours/Day of Television, by Sex, Race/Ethnicity and Grade—United States, Youth Risk Behavior Survey, 2013," in "Youth Risk Behavior Surveillance—United States, 2013," *MMWR*, vol. 63, no. 4, June 13, 2014, http://www.cdc.gov/mmwr/pdf/ss/ss6304.pdf (accessed October 7, 2015)

TABLE 4.6

Percentage of high school students who ate fruit or drank fruit juice two or more times/day, by sex, race/ethnicity, and grade, 2013

	Ate fruit or drank 100% fruit juices two or more times/day			Ate fruit or drank 100% fruit juices three or more times/day		
	Female	Male	Total	Female	Male	Total
Category	%	%	%	%	%	%
Race/ethnicity						
White*	27.9	32.1	30.0	16.0	20.0	18.0
Black*	33.9	42.3	38.0	27.0	31.5	29.1
Hispanic	33.6	40.3	36.9	23.2	29.1	26.1
Grade						
9	30.2	37.0	33.6	19.7	25.3	22.5
10	30.7	37.1	33.9	20.3	24.3	22.3
11	31.0	34.4	32.7	20.6	24.3	22.4
12	30.7	34.1	32.4	18.9	21.1	20.0
Total	**30.6**	**35.9**	**33.2**	**19.9**	**24.0**	**21.9**

*Non-Hispanic.
Note: Ate fruit or drank fruit juice two or more times during the 7 days before the survey.

SOURCE: Adapted from Laura Kann et al., "Table 79. Percentage of High School Students Ate Fruit or Drank 100% Fruit Juice Two of More Times/Day and Who Ate Fruit or Drank 100% Fruit Juices Three of More Times/Day, by Sex, Race/Ethnicity, and Grade—United States, Youth Risk Behavior Survey, 2013," in "Youth Risk Behavior Surveillance—United States, 2013," *MMWR*, vol. 63, no. 4, June 13, 2014, http://www.cdc.gov/mmwr/pdf/ss/ss6304.pdf (accessed October 7, 2015)

TABLE 4.7

Percentage of high school students who ate no vegetables and who ate vegetables one or more times/day, by sex, race/ethnicity, and grade, 2013

	Did not eat vegetables			Ate vegetables one or more times/day		
	Female	Male	Total	Female	Male	Total
Category	%	%	%	%	%	%
Race/ethnicity						
White*	3.3	5.7	4.5	66.0	63.5	64.8
Black*	12.1	10.5	11.3	48.5	55.4	51.9
Hispanic	8.5	10.2	9.3	55.8	58.0	56.9
Grade						
9	6.8	8.0	7.4	57.8	60.4	59.1
10	6.9	7.5	7.2	61.1	61.0	61.1
11	4.7	7.9	6.2	63.0	62.5	62.8
12	4.3	6.7	5.5	64.5	61.8	63.1
Total	**5.7**	**7.5**	**6.6**	**61.3**	**61.5**	**61.5**

*Non-Hispanic.
Notes: Vegetables include green salad, potatoes (excluding French fries, fried potatoes, or potato chips), carrots, or other vegetables. Eaten in during the 7 days before the survey.

SOURCE: Adapted from Laura Kann et al., "Table 81. Percentage of High School Students Who Did Not Eat Vegetables and Who Ate Vegetables One or More Times/Day, by Sex, Race/Ethnicity, and Grade—United States, Youth Risk Behavior Survey, 2013," in "Youth Risk Behavior Surveillance—United States, 2013," *MMWR*, vol. 63, no. 4, June 13, 2014, http://www.cdc.gov/mmwr/pdf/ss/ss6304.pdf (accessed October 7, 2015)

that the percentage of daily energy (as measured in calories) children ate away from home increased from 23.4% to 33.9% between 1977 and 2006. During the same period there were significant increases in children's consumption of fast food eaten at home and store-bought food eaten away from home. Poti and Popkin conclude that "foods prepared away from home, including fast food eaten at home and store-prepared food eaten away from home, are fueling the increase in total energy intake."

Echoing the sentiments of many health professionals, the Committee on Nutrition of the European Society for Paediatric Gastroenterology, Hepatology, and Nutrition named fast-food consumption as a contributing factor to childhood obesity. Carlo Agostino et al. observe in "Role of Dietary Factors and Food Habits in the Development of Childhood Obesity: A Commentary by the ESPGHAN Committee on Nutrition" (*Journal of Pediatric Gastroenterology and Nutrition*, vol. 52, no. 6, June 2011) that fast foods offer large portions of high-energy-dense foods that are low in fiber and high in saturated and trans fats, glycemic load (a ranking system for carbohydrate content in food based on its glycemic index [a measure of a food's ability to raise blood glucose] and portion size), and tastiness, which may promote not only a lifelong preference for foods high in fat, salt, and sugar but also

TABLE 4.8

Percentage of high school students who ate vegetables two or three or more times/day, by sex, race/ethnicity, and grade, 2013

	Ate vegetables two or more times/day			Ate vegetables three or more times/day		
	Female	Male	Total	Female	Male	Total
Category	%	%	%	%	%	%
Race/ethnicity						
White*	28.0	28.7	28.4	13.3	15.0	14.2
Black*	23.2	29.4	26.2	15.1	20.4	17.6
Hispanic	25.7	30.2	27.9	15.0	18.8	16.9
Grade						
9	23.7	27.6	25.7	13.6	15.7	14.6
10	27.4	28.9	28.1	13.7	16.8	15.3
11	28.6	29.4	29.0	15.6	18.0	16.8
12	29.2	32.2	30.7	14.5	17.7	16.1
Total	**27.1**	**29.6**	**28.4**	**14.3**	**17.0**	**15.7**

*Non-Hispanic.
Note: Vegetables include green salad, potatoes (excluding French fries, fried potatoes, or potato chips), carrots, or other vegetables. Eaten during the 7 days before the survey.

SOURCE: Adapted from Laura Kann et al., "Table 83. Percentage of High School Students Who Ate Vegetables Two or More Times/Day and Who Ate Vegetables Three or More Times/Day, by Sex, Race/Ethnicity, and Grade—United States, Youth Risk Behavior Survey, 2013," in "Youth Risk Behavior Surveillance—United States, 2013," *MMWR*, vol. 63, no. 4, June 13, 2014, http://www.cdc.gov/mmwr/pdf/ss/ss6304.pdf (accessed October 7, 2015)

TABLE 4.9

Percentage of students who drank two or three glasses of milk per day, by sex, race/ethnicity, and grade, 2013

	Drank two or more glasses/day of milk			Drank three or more glasses/day of milk		
	Female	Male	Total	Female	Male	Total
Category	%	%	%	%	%	%
Race/ethnicity						
White*	21.6	36.8	29.2	9.8	18.4	14.1
Black*	9.7	23.8	16.5	4.1	14.5	9.1
Hispanic	17.8	32.0	24.8	7.3	14.7	10.9
Grade						
9	21.2	35.1	28.2	9.4	17.6	13.5
10	18.3	36.0	27.2	7.8	17.2	12.6
11	16.7	32.0	24.1	8.2	17.4	12.7
12	17.6	29.2	23.3	6.8	14.5	10.6
Total	**18.5**	**33.4**	**25.9**	**8.1**	**16.9**	**12.5**

*Non-Hispanic.
Note: Drank two or three glasses of milk per day during the 7 days before the survey.

SOURCE: Adapted from Laura Kann et al., "Table 87. Percentage of High School Students Who Drank Two or more Glasses/Day of Milk, and Who Drank Three or More Glasses/Day of Milk, by Sex, Race/Ethnicity, and Grade—United States, Youth Risk Behavior Survey, 2013," in "Youth Risk Behavior Surveillance—United States, 2013," *MMWR*, vol. 63, no. 4, June 13, 2014, http://www.cdc.gov/mmwr/pdf/ss/ss6304.pdf (accessed October 7, 2015)

excessive weight gain. Agostino et al. reviewed the relevant literature and conclude that increasing consumption of fast food is associated with excess weight gain and recommend that "regular consumption of fast food with large portion sizes and high energy density should be avoided."

However, research suggests that fast-food consumption may not directly increase weight in children and adolescents. Jennifer M. Poti, Kiyah J. Duffey, and Barry M. Popkin of the University of North Carolina, Chapel Hill, looked at the relationship between fast-food consumption, the balance of children's diets, and childhood obesity and reported their findings in "The Association of Fast Food Consumption with Poor Dietary Outcomes and Obesity among Children: Is It the Fast Food or the Remainder of Diet?" (*American Journal of Clinical Nutrition*, vol. 99, no. 1, 2013). The researchers find that high fast-food consumption was associated with a lower intake of milk, dairy, and vegetables and a higher intake of sugar-sweetened beverages (SSBs) outside of the fast-food restaurant and that low and high fast-food consumption was associated with having a Western diet (higher intake of SSBs, salty snacks, high-fat sandwiches, candy, and french fries), which is independently associated with overweight and obesity, for the remainder of intake. Poti, Duffey, and Popkin conclude, "Fast food consumers may have less healthy dietary patterns outside the fast food restaurant. We provide evidence that a Western dietary pattern for the remainder of intake may be more strongly

TABLE 4.10

Percentage of students who did not drink soda and drank soda at least once a day, 2013

	Did not drink soda or pop			Drank soda or pop one or more times/day		
	Female	Male	Total	Female	Male	Total
Category	%	%	%	%	%	%
Race/ethnicity						
White*	26.1	18.1	22.1	25.0	32.9	29.0
Black*	19.8	21.2	20.4	28.8	31.5	30.2
Hispanic	22.4	20.4	21.4	20.5	24.8	22.6
Grade						
9	22.5	17.7	20.1	26.6	32.0	29.3
10	25.1	19.8	22.4	23.2	27.6	25.4
11	27.1	21.0	24.1	22.9	30.9	26.9
12	25.2	20.9	23.0	23.0	29.1	26.0
Total	**24.8**	**19.8**	**22.3**	**24.1**	**29.9**	**27.0**

*Non-Hispanic.
Notes: Not including diet soda or diet pop. Students who did not drink soda and drank soda at least once a day during the 7 days before the survey.

SOURCE: Adapted from Laura Kann et al., "Table 89. Percentage of High School Students Who Did Not Drink a Can, Bottle, or Glass of Soda or Pop, and Who Drank a Can, Bottle, or Glass of Soda or Pop One or More Times/Day—United States, Youth Risk Behavior Survey, 2013," in "Youth Risk Behavior Surveillance—United States, 2013," *MMWR*, vol. 63, no. 4, June 13, 2014, http://www.cdc.gov/mmwr/pdf/ss/ss6304.pdf (accessed October 7, 2015)

associated with overweight/obesity than fast food consumption itself."

Increased consumption of SSBs in childhood is linked to an increased risk of obesity. In "Substituting Sugar-Sweetened Beverages with Water or Milk Is Inversely Associated with Body Fatness Development from Childhood to Adolescence" (*Nutrition*, vol. 31, no. 1, January 2015), Miaobing Zheng et al. examine the relationship between SSBs by children and bodyweight, substitution of SSBs with water, milk, or 100% fruit juice, and changes in body fatness. The researchers analyzed SSB and other beverage consumption of 590 nine-year-olds for six years and tracked their body fat. Zheng et al. find that SSB intake at age nine, but not other beverages including water, milk, fruit juice, or coffee/tea, was directly related to subsequent six-year changes in body fatness. The researchers find that substitution of SSBs with other beverage alternatives—water, coffee/tea, or milk but not 100% fruit juice—was also significantly associated with less body fatness gain.

The 2013 YRBSS confirmed that soda remains popular with high school students. More than a quarter (27%) of students reported drinking at least one soda per day. (See Table 4.10.) More males (29.9%) than females (24.1%) drank one or more sodas per day, and female students (24.8%) were more likely than male students (19.8%) to report having had no soda during the previous week. For both male and female students, ninth graders were more likely to report drinking soda at least once per day than were students in any other grade.

Children's and Teens' Calorie Consumption Has Decreased

R. Bethene Ervin and Cynthia L. Ogden of the NCHS report in *Trends in Intake of Energy and Macronutrients*

in Children and Adolescents from 1999–2000 through 2009–2010 (February 2013, http://www.cdc.gov/nchs/data/databriefs/db113.pdf) that the average caloric intake for children and teens decreased between 1999–2000 and 2009–10. During this period, the average energy intake for boys decreased from 2,258 calories to approximately 2,100 calories, and the average energy intake for girls fell from 1,831 calories to 1,755 calories. (See Figure 4.5.)

In "Turning Point for US Diets? Recessionary Effects or Behavioral Shifts in Foods Purchased and Consumed" (*American Journal of Clinical Nutrition*, vol. 99, no. 3, March 2014), Shu Wen Ng, Meghan M. Slining, and Barry M. Popkin observe that between 2003 and 2011 there was a reduction in energy intake and caloric purchases, especially among households with children, and that during this period obesity declined for low-income preschoolers and leveled off for children. The researchers wanted to determine whether the reduction in energy intake and the leveling off and decline in obesity suggest a longer-term shift in dietary behavior that is unrelated to the effects of the Great Recession (which lasted from late 2007 to mid-2009). Ng, Slining, and Popkin find that shifts in food purchases began in 2003 and continued independent of the recession. They conclude that antiobesity measures, including an emphasis on reducing consumption of SSBs, along with revision of the Special Supplemental Nutrition Program for Women, Infants, and Children and school lunch programs, contributed to the decreased intake. They also suggest that efforts by food manufacturers and retailers to reduce the caloric content of their products and offer healthier products may have played a role in reducing caloric intake and purchases.

FIGURE 4.5

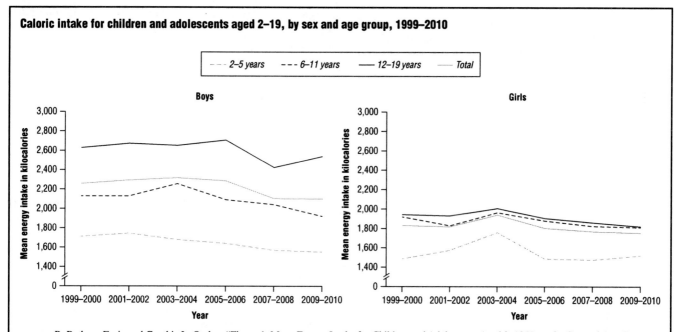

Caloric intake for children and adolescents aged 2–19, by sex and age group, 1999–2010

······· 2–5 years   - - - 6–11 years   ——— 12–19 years   ········ Total

SOURCE: R. Bethene Ervin and Cynthia L. Ogden, "Figure 1. Mean Energy Intake for Children and Adolescents Aged 2–19 Years, by Sex and Age Group, 1999–2010," in "Trends in Intake of Energy and Macronutrients in Children and Adolescents from 1999–2000 through 2009–2010," *NCHS Data Brief,* no. 113, National Center for Health Statistics, February 2013, http://www.cdc.gov/nchs/data/databriefs/db113.pdf (accessed October 16, 2015)

The Role of the Media

Despite television and print media antiobesity campaigns, many industry observers condemn corporate marketing efforts and media for continuing to assault children with unhealthy messages that encourage them to eat junk foods. The CDC defines junk foods as those that provide calories primarily through fats or added sugars and have minimal amounts of vitamins and minerals.

The Interagency Working Group (IWG) on Food Marketed to Children, with representation from the CDC, the Federal Trade Commission, the U.S. Department of Agriculture (USDA), and the U.S. Food and Drug Administration (FDA), was formed in 2009 and tasked with recommending principles for the marketing of food to children to help the food industry self-regulate its marketing and advertising practices. In April 2011 the IWG released the fact sheet "Food for Thought: Interagency Working Group Proposal on Food Marketing to Children" (http://cspinet.org/new/pdf/FTC_foodmarket _factsheet110428%20.pdf) to discuss its principles for food marketing to children aged two to 16 years. The first principle is that the foods "make a meaningful contribution to a healthful diet" and contain fruits, vegetables, whole grains, fat-free or low-fat (1%) milk products, fish, extra lean meat or poultry, eggs, nuts and seeds, or beans. The second principle is that the foods should "contain limited amounts of nutrients that have a negative impact on health or weight," which is defined as a saturated fat content of 1 gram or less per serving or less than 15% of calories, 0 grams of trans-fat per serving, no

more than 13 grams of added sugars per serving, and no more than 210 milligrams of sodium per serving. The principles are simply guidelines, and although they went into effect in 2016, adherence to them is entirely voluntary.

The Trust for America's Health (TFAH; a nonprofit, nonpartisan organization working to make disease prevention a national priority) and the Robert Wood Johnson Foundation observe in *The State of Obesity 2015: Better Policies for a Healthier America* (September 2015, http:// healthyamericans.org/assets/files/TFAH-2015-Obesity Report-final.22.pdf) that, to date, the largest voluntary effort is the Children's Food and Beverage Advertising Initiative (CFBAI), which adopted in 2014 a set of nutrition criteria with stricter limits on the calories, sugar, fats, and sodium in the foods marketed to children. Although the guidelines are an improvement over earlier, company-specific standards, they still allow companies to market some low-nutritional-value foods and beverages to children, such as popsicles, marshmallow treats, and sugary cereals.

Rebecca M. Schermbeck and Lisa M. Powell of the University of Illinois, Chicago, compared the CFBAI's new nutrition criteria with the federal IWG recommendations for such advertising and reported their findings in "Nutrition Recommendations and the Children's Food and Beverage Advertising Initiative's 2014 Approved Food and Beverage Product List" (*Preventing Chronic Disease*, vol. 12, April 23, 2015). The researchers find that more than half (52.5%) of the CFBAI products failed to meet the IWG nutrition guidelines. (See Figure 4.6.)

FIGURE 4.6

Percentage of food and beverages on the Children's Food and Beverage Advertising Initiative's April 2014 list that exceed the Interagency Working Group's recommended nutrients to limit, 2015

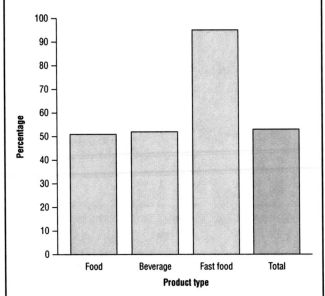

SOURCE: Rebecca M. Schermbeck and Lisa M. Powell, "Figure. Percentage of Food, Beverage, Fast-Food Products, and Total Products on the Children's Food and Beverage Advertising Initiative's April 2014 List That Exceed the Interagency Working Group's (IWG's) Recommended Nutrients to Limit (Saturated Fat, *Trans* Fat, Sugar, and Sodium)," in "Nutrition Recommendations and the Children's Food and Beverage Advertising Initiative's 2014 Approved Food and Beverage Product List," *Preventing Chronic Disease*, vol. 12, April 2015, http://www.cdc.gov/pcd/issues/2015/pdf/14_0472.pdf (accessed October 12, 2015)

Schermbeck and Powell note that "if companies choose to advertise products from the CFBAI's list of approved food products that meet the IWG recommendations more often than products that do not, children's exposure to food and beverage advertising could improve substantially." They call for "continued monitoring of child-directed marketing by public health researchers and that the public encourage the food and beverage industry to market their healthiest products to young consumers."

Many researchers and industry observers concur that the obesity epidemic cannot be effectively combated without dramatic changes in food marketing that is aimed at children. In "New Media but Same Old Tricks: Food Marketing to Children in the Digital Age" (*Current Obesity Reports*, vol. 4, no. 1, March 2015), Bridget Kelly et al. report that new media (the Internet and digital devices) offer food companies new ways to influence children's food preferences and choices. New media marketing includes promotions on company-owned and other websites, social media, e-mail, and marketing via text messages, applications (apps), and branded games. The researchers report that by 2009 spending on new media marketing had outpaced radio and print advertising.

According to Kelly et al., new media offers the prospect of viral messaging (rapid spread of commercial messages through social media) to increase peer-group acceptance. It also enables peer endorsement of products and personal communication with brands. Some new media, such as branded online gaming, expose children to messages for extended periods of time. Research demonstrates that "advergaming" influences children's food product choices and consumption. Advanced analytics enable marketers to track young consumers' online activities and social media use, which enhances their ability to target and personalize messages. Kelly et al. note that because parents may be unaware of food marketing on new media, they are unable to help children critically analyze marketing messages.

According to Kelly et al., it is challenging to monitor new media marketing and to regulate it because these media and marketing techniques evolve rapidly. The researchers suggest that restricting the content of online marketing communications that target children and adolescents and improving educational campaigns to strengthen children's understanding of food marketing may help reduce advergaming's impact. Kelly et al. assert, "While traditional media remain important promotional platforms for food brands, research and policy actions need to consider the reality of contemporary marketing environments, which are multiplatform, integrated and mutable. For this reason, regulatory provisions to protect children from unhealthy food marketing should apply to all forms of commercial communication directed to children, not just for distinct media."

The Role of Schools

In *State of Obesity 2015*, the TFAH and the Robert Wood Johnson Foundation note that because children spend a great deal of time at school and in before- and after-school programs, eating as many as two meals and snacks and up to half their daily calories in school settings, school programs have the potential to prevent and reduce obesity.

In many parts of the country students have healthier beverage and food options in school. Updated national standards for school meal programs took effect in late 2012. The new standards call for more fruits and vegetables, whole grains, and low-fat dairy products and less sugar and fat. Figure 4.7 compares snacks offered in schools before and after the new standards were enacted. Janna Raudenbush of the USDA's Food and Nutrition Service notes in "Celebrate National School Lunch Week 2015" (October 13, 2015, http://blogs.usda.gov/2015/10/13/celebrate-national-school-lunch-week-2015/) that by October 2015, 96% of schools were meeting the revised standards.

In "New School Meal Regulations Increase Fruit Consumption and Do Not Increase Total Plate Waste"

FIGURE 4.7

Snacks offered by schools before and after Smart Snacks in School nutrition standards, 2012 and 2014

● Equals 1 calorie   ○ Shows empty calories*

Before the new standards

	Chocolate sandwich cookies (6 medium)	Fruit flavored candies (2.2 oz. pkg.)	Donut (1 large)	Chocolate bar (1 bar–1.6 oz.)	Regular cola (12 fl. oz.)
Total calories	286	249	242	235	136
Empty calories	182	177	147	112	126

After the new standards

	Peanuts (1 oz.)	Light popcorn (Snack bag)	Low-fat tortilla chips (1 oz.)	Granola bar (oats, fruit, nuts) (1 bar–0.8 oz.)	Fruit cup (w/100% juice) (Snack cup 4 oz.)	No-calorie flavored water (12 fl. oz.)
Total calories	170	161	118	95	68	0
Empty calories	0	17	0	32	0	0

*Calories from food components such as added sugars and solid fats that provide little nutritional value. Empty calories are part of total calories.

SOURCE: "Smart Snacks in School," in *Healthier School Day*, U.S. Department of Agriculture Food and Nutrition Service, August 27, 2015, http://www.fns.usda.gov/sites/default/files/allfoods_infographic.pdf (accessed October 12, 2015)

(*Childhood Obesity*, vol. 11, no. 3, June 2015), Marlene B. Schwartz et al. compare students' food consumption before and after the updated standards were implemented. The researchers find that students responded favorably to the healthier meals by consuming more fruit and discarding less of their entrees and vegetables.

Some Schools Still Offer Unhealthful Food Choices

Food manufacturers and marketers know that schools are ideal sites to promote their products to children and teens. Nearly all youth attend school and spend many of their waking hours at school. Furthermore, the presence of foods in schools allows food companies to benefit from the implied endorsement of the schools and teachers. According to Zewditu Demissie et al., in *School Health Profiles 2012: Characteristics of Health Programs among Secondary Schools* (2013, http://www.cdc.gov/healthyyouth/profiles/2012/profiles_report.pdf), many schools have vending machines, stores, or snack bars on campus that sell "competitive foods[, which] are any foods or beverages sold or served at school separately from the USDA school meal programs." Competitive foods are usually low in nutrients and high in fat, sugar, and calories.

Until the 2014–15 school year the sale of competitive foods was essentially unregulated, and students often purchased these foods instead of, or in addition to, school meals. In December 2011 the USDA issued federal nutrition standards for competitive foods sold on school grounds, and in June 2013 the department issued its "Smart Snacks in Schools" nutrition standards, which limit calories, fat, sugar, and sodium content of foods and beverages sold in school vending machines, cafeterias, and snack bars.

Besides selling food in schools, food manufacturers advertise on vending machines, posters, book covers, scoreboards, and banners and offer schools educational materials, contests in which children receive prizes or food rewards for achievement, and fund-raising opportunities. Some critics, including the Center for Science in the Public Interest, assert that the manufacturers are taking unfair advantage of cash-strapped school districts.

In "Salty or Sweet? Nutritional Quality, Consumption, and Cost of Snacks Served in Afterschool Programs" (*Journal of School Health*, vol. 85, no. 2, February 2015), Michael W. Beets et al. analyze snacks served to more than 1,700 children in 20 after-school programs in South Carolina. The researchers observe that the snacks served were largely high-sugar and artificially flavored food products that failed to meet the Healthy Eating Standards, which were endorsed by the National Afterschool Association in April 2011. Beets et al. note that adhering to snack policies is voluntary rather than mandated by law but urge after-school-program providers "to carefully evaluate the types of foods and beverages served as snack and determine whether they promote the healthy eating of the children enrolled. In cases where improvements are required and price barriers preclude purchasing healthier foods, programs will need to develop innovative partnerships with foods sellers to lower food prices."

Food for Thought Has New Meaning at Many Schools

The second week of October is designated National School Lunch Week, and Raudenbush indicates that in the three years since the revised nutrition standards were implemented school lunch revenue has increased and teachers report that students are more attentive. Likewise, Juliana F. W. Cohen et al. confirm in "Impact of the New U.S. Department of Agriculture School Meal Standards on Food Selection, Consumption, and Waste" (*American Journal of Preventive Medicine*, vol. 46, no. 4, April 2014) that students are consuming more fruits and vegetables.

In "School Lunches Becoming Healthier, Statistics Indicate" (NYTimes.com, August 27, 2015), Sabrina Tavernise reports that industry experts have seen the effects of the updated standards firsthand. Deb Bentzel, a senior associate at the Food Trust in Philadelphia, which works to improve access to nutritious food in schools and communities, explained, "The way the school lunch line looks is different. It's brighter, it's healthier-looking, it's fresher." Margo Wootan, the director of nutrition policy at the Center for Science in the Public Interest, described the changes as profound, asserting, "The improvement to school foods in the last three years is much more than had been done in the last three decades."

One approach to improving school nutrition is the growing farm-to-school movement, which encourages purchasing locally grown products. For example, according to the Mississippi Farm to School Interagency Council, in *Progress Report to the Mississippi Legislature on Farm to School in Mississippi* (December 2014, http://www.mdac.ms.gov/wp-content/uploads/fts_report.pdf), the Vicksburg Warren School District in Mississippi has developed a purchasing model for locally grown produce. The district also integrates school gardening, farm visits, and culinary classes into its curricula.

Another example of a school district working to improve nutrition, as described by Emily Richmond in "Are Healthier School Lunches Doomed" (Atlantic.com, September 28, 2015), is the Detroit Public School district's move to remove all deep-fat fryers from campus cafeterias and to grow fresh greens in the district's gardens.

The Media Can Deliver Powerful Nutrition and Health Education

Greater emphasis on children's diets has inspired the media to offer nutrition education. The children's classic, *Sesame Street* (2015, http://www.sesamestreet.org/parents/topicsandactivities/toolkits/food), produces programs aimed at families with children aged two to eight years on a wide range of nutrition topics: eating well on a budget, trying new foods, preparing and eating a healthful breakfast, healthful snacks, and how food arrives at the market and dinner table.

Children's television programming such as Disney's *Tasty Time with ZeFronk* offers easy-to-prepare recipes and aims to inspire young viewers to choose healthful meals and snacks in three-minute animated shorts. The Travel Channel's *Bizarre Foods America* exposes older children, teens, and adults to different cultures and foods. The Public Broadcasting Service's *Arthur* is an animated series that teaches children about nutrition, healthy eating, and fitness.

Blending fitness and entertainment, video game makers have developed a genre of active rhythm games, including *Dance Dance Revolution*, which features a workout mode that can track how many calories the user burns while playing. *In the Groove* and *Pump It Up: Exceed* are video games in which players try to match the onscreen action by stepping on different sections of a floor pad, and *Yourself!Fitness* and *Kinetic* offer teens exercise routines in video game formats. Nintendo's *Wii Fit* instructs and coaches users in yoga, balance games, strength training, aerobics, and simulated sports. *Just Dance 4* is a music video game that enables up to four players dance to on-screen choreography.

Increasingly, tech-savvy children can learn about nutrition using an expanding array of apps. For example, Eat & Move-O-Matic explains the relationship between calories consumed and burned with exercise and encourages healthy alternatives to high-calorie foods. Smash Your Food gives children the opportunity to smash images of foods to determine their sugar, salt, and oil content to see how they compare with nutritional guidelines, and Veggie Circus Farm teaches toddlers and preschoolers to recognize vegetables.

A DECADE OF EFFORTS TO IMPROVE FOOD AND BEVERAGE MARKETING PRACTICES. In 2005 the National Academies of Sciences, Engineering, and Medicine's Institute of Medicine (IOM) published the report *Food Marketing to Children and Youth: Threat or Opportunity?* (http://www.iom.edu/Reports/2005/Food-Marketing-to-Children-and-Youth-Threat-or-Opportunity.aspx) to evaluate the influence of food marketing on the health of American children and teens. The IOM found that marketing practices, particularly television advertising, did not support a healthful diet and called on food and beverage companies and the media to promote programs and practices to support healthful eating. The IOM Committee on Progress in Preventing Childhood Obesity followed up with the publications *Food Marketing and the Diets of Children and Youth* (2006, http://www.iom.edu/Activities/Children/KidsFoodMarketing.aspx), which included a framework to guide the development of marketing and advertising

strategies to foster healthful food choices among children and teens, and *Progress in Preventing Childhood Obesity: How Do We Measure Up?* (2007, http://books.nap.edu/openbook.php?record_id=11722), which described the challenges of balancing corporate goals with promoting children's health.

In November 2012 the IOM Standing Committee on Childhood Obesity Prevention held a workshop to assess progress made on food and beverage marketing aimed at children and youth and published the presenters' findings in *Challenges and Opportunities for Change in Food Marketing to Children and Youth—Workshop Summary* (March 4, 2013, http://www.iom.edu/Reports/2013/Challenges-and-Opportunities-for-Change-in-Food-Marketing-to-Children-and-Youth.aspx). Presenters observed that limited to modest progress has been made toward implementing the recommendations in the IOM's 2006 report. They observed that integrated marketing communications, which use multiple media (videos on the Internet, ads on mobile phones, and advergames) to deliver and reinforce messages, are powerful. Marketing is often disguised as entertainment, and social networks provide additional marketing opportunities. Despite progress in limiting food advertising to children, youth are still targeted by advertisers of unhealthful foods.

In "Evaluating Industry Self-Regulation of Food Marketing to Children" (*American Journal of Preventive Medicine*, vol. 49, no. 2, August 2015), Dale L. Kunkel, Jessica S. Castonguay, and Christine R. Filer compare food advertisements aired during children's television programming between 2007 and 2013. The researchers find that the majority (80.5%) of foods advertised were for products in the poorest nutritional category, which increase children's risk for overweight and obesity. Kunkel, Castonguay, and Filer observe that there was no improvement in advertising content between 2007 and 2013, which they attribute to the fact that many food marketers do not practice self-regulation. The researchers conclude, "The lack of success achieved by self-regulation indicates that other policy actions are needed to effectively reduce children's exposure to obesogenic [obesity-causing] food advertising."

Physical Activity

School physical education programs, especially at the high school level, have been found lacking, and too few youth are physically active. The 2013 YRBSS found that in 2013 fewer than one-third (27.1%) of high school students were physically active every day for at least 60 minutes, and that about half (51.7%) of students participated in muscle strengthening exercises on three or more days. (See Table 4.11.)

TABLE 4.11

Percentages of high school students who met recommended levels of physical activity by sex, race/ethnicity, and grade, 2013

	Physically active at least 60 minutes/day on all 7 days			Participated in muscle strengthening activities on 3 or more days		
	Female	Male	Total	Female	Male	Total
Category	%	%	%	%	%	%
Race/ethnicity						
White*	18.7	37.5	28.2	42.8	61.7	52.4
Black*	16.0	37.2	26.3	34.7	64.1	48.8
Hispanic	17.4	33.9	25.5	44.4	62.6	53.3
Grade						
9	20.1	40.5	30.4	44.3	65.1	54.8
10	20.5	34.6	27.6	46.1	61.9	54.0
11	14.4	37.0	25.5	38.4	61.2	49.5
12	15.3	33.5	24.3	36.9	58.6	47.7
Total	**17.7**	**36.6**	**27.1**	**41.6**	**61.8**	**51.7**

*Non-Hispanic.

Note: Because of changes in question context starting in 2011, national YRBS prevalence estimates derived from the 60 minutes of physical activity question in 2011 and 2013 are not comparable to those reported in 2009 or earlier. On the 2005–2009 national YRBS questionnaire, physical activity was assessed with three questions (in the following order) that asked the number of days students participated in 1) at least 20 minutes of vigorous physical activity; 2) at least 30 minutes of moderate physical activity; and 3) at least 60 minutes of aerobic (moderate and vigorous) physical activity. On the 2011 and 2013 national YRBS questionnaire, only the 60 minutes of aerobic physical activity question was included. Students doing any kind of physical activity (such as, push-ups, sit-ups, or weight lifting) during the 7 days before the survey that increased their heart rate and made them breathe hard some of the time during the 7 days before the survey.

SOURCE: Adapted from Laura Kann et al., "Table 97. Percentage of High School Students Who Were Physically Active at Least 60 Minutes/Day on All 7 Days and Who Participated in Muscle Strengthening Activities on 3 or More Days, by Sex, Race/Ethnicity, and Grade—United States, Youth Risk Behavior Survey, 2013," in "Youth Risk Behavior Surveillance—United States, 2013," *MMWR*, vol. 63, no. 4, June 13, 2014, http://www.cdc.gov/mmwr/pdf/ss/ss6304.pdf (accessed October 7, 2015)

HEALTH RISKS AND CONSEQUENCES

The harmful health consequences of overweight and obesity can begin during childhood and adolescence. Furthermore, health risks increase with increasing obesity. In "Cardiometabolic Risks and Severity of Obesity in Children and Young Adults" (*New England Journal of Medicine*, vol. 373, October 1, 2015), Asheley C. Skinner et al. analyze National Health and Nutrition Examination Survey data for 8,579 overweight and obese children and young adults between the ages of three and 19 years and find that of those with a BMI at the 85th percentile or higher, 46.9% were overweight, while 36.4% had class I obesity, 11.9% had class II obesity, and 4.8% had class III obesity. The researchers also note that cardiometabolic risk factors such as high blood pressure and high triglycerides were all greater among children and young adults with class III obesity compared with those with class I obesity.

The most frequently occurring medical consequences of overweight and obesity among children and adolescents are:

- Elevated blood lipids—overweight children and adolescents display the same elevated levels of cholesterol, triglycerides (a fatty substance found in the blood), and/or low-density lipoproteins as overweight adults. These hyperlipidemias are linked to an increased risk for cardiovascular disease and premature mortality (death) in adulthood.

- Glucose intolerance and type 2 diabetes—glucose intolerance, a carbohydrate intolerance that varies in severity, is a forerunner of diabetes. The incidence of type 2 diabetes among adolescents is increasing in response to the national rise of overweight teens. A skin condition known as acanthosis nigricans (velvety thickening and darkening of skinfold areas at the neck, elbow, and behind the knee) often coexists with glucose intolerance in youth.

- Fatty liver disease—high concentrations of liver enzymes are associated with fatty degeneration of the liver (also called hepatic steatosis) and have been found in overweight children and adolescents. Excessively high blood insulin levels (hyperinsulinemia) may contribute to the genesis of this disease.

- Gallstones—although gallstones occur less frequently among children and adolescents who are overweight than in obese adults, nearly half of the cases of inflammation of the gallbladder (also called cholecystitis) in adolescents may be associated with overweight. Like adults, the risk for cholecystitis and gallstones in adolescents may decrease with weight reduction.

Another common health consequence of overweight is early maturation, a condition in which the skeletal age is more than three months greater than the chronological age. Early maturation is linked to overweight in adulthood and is also associated with the distribution of fat—it predicts that the fat will be predominantly located on the abdomen and trunk, which is in turn predictive of increased disease risk.

Less frequently occurring health consequences include hypertension (high blood pressure), a condition that is nine times more frequent among children who are overweight, compared with children who have a healthy weight; obstructive sleep apnea (breathing becomes shallow or stops completely for short periods during sleep), a condition that afflicts an estimated 7% of overweight children; and orthopedic problems resulting from excessive stress on the feet, legs, and hips. Hypertension for children and adolescents aged one to 17 years is defined as average blood pressure readings at or above the 95th percentile (based on age, sex, and height) on at least three separate occasions. (See Table 4.12 and Table 4.13 for blood pressures by age and sex that are considered indicative of hypertension or at risk for hypertension; children and adolescents between the 90th and 95th percentiles for their age, sex, and height are at risk for developing hypertension.)

Metabolic Syndrome

The metabolic syndrome is a group of risk factors for atherosclerotic cardiovascular disease and type 2 diabetes mellitus in adults that include insulin resistance, obesity, hypertension, and hyperlipidemia. (Atherosclerosis is a hardening of the walls of the arteries caused by the buildup of fatty deposits on the inner walls of the arteries that interferes with blood flow.) Atherosclerotic cardiovascular disease is the leading cause of death among adults, but it rarely occurs in young people. Recently, however, the risk factors—high blood pressure, elevated triglycerides, obesity, and low levels of the "good" high-density lipoprotein cholesterol—that are associated with the development of metabolic syndrome have been appearing during childhood. Gerald S. Berenson et al. indicate in "Glycemic Status, Metabolic Syndrome, and Cardiovascular Risk in Children" (*Medical Clinics of North America*, vol. 95, no. 2, March 2011) that in the United States more than 17% of children with a BMI greater than the 95th percentile are considered to have all the conditions that are associated with metabolic syndrome.

Mental Health Consequences

One of the most immediate, distressing, and widespread consequences of being overweight as described by children themselves is social discrimination and low self-esteem. Overweight and obese children and adolescents are at risk for psychological and social adjustment problems, such as considering themselves less competent than normal-weight youth in social, athletic, and appearance arenas, and for suffering from overall diminished self-worth.

In "Development of Mental Health Problems and Overweight between Ages 4 and 11 Years: A Population-Based Longitudinal Study of Australian Children" (*Academic Pediatrics*, vol. 13, no. 2, March–April 2013), Pauline W. Jansen et al. look at the relationship between mental health and overweight in children. The researchers find an association between overweight and mental health problems beginning at ages eight and nine and increasing among children ages 10 and 11. Overweight children had more problems with peers and emotional difficulties than did their healthy-weight peers. Jansen et al. conclude that "in childhood, it appears that overweight precedes mental health problems, particularly peer problems."

SCREENING AND ASSESSMENT OF OVERWEIGHT CHILDREN AND ADOLESCENTS

In view of the rising prevalence of overweight youth, screening children and adolescents for overweight and risk for overweight has assumed a prominent place in pediatric practice (the medical specialty devoted to the diagnosis and treatment of children) and public health programs. The Recommendations for Preventive Pediatric Health Care by the American Academy of Pediatrics advise a frequent schedule of accurate weight and height measurements to determine whether children require further assessment or treatment for overweight. Screening distinguishes between youths who are not at risk of overweight, at risk of overweight, and overweight. Those deemed to be overweight receive an in-depth medical assessment; those considered at risk are assessed for changes in BMI, blood pressure, and cholesterol levels; and annual screening is advised for those who are not at risk of being overweight.

The comprehensive assessment that is performed on overweight children and adolescents generally includes obtaining a detailed medical history to identify any underlying medical conditions that may contribute to overweight and analyzing family history for the presence of familial risks for overweight or obesity. Relevant familial factors include the occurrence of obesity, eating disorders, type 2 diabetes, heart disease, high blood pressure, and abnormal lipid profiles such as high cholesterol among immediate family members. The assessment may also involve:

- A dietary evaluation to consider the quantity, quality, and timing of food consumed to identify foods and patterns of eating that may lead to excessive calorie intake. A food record or food diary may be used to assess eating habits.

- An evaluation of daily activities. This assessment involves an estimate of time that is devoted to exercise and activity as well as time spent on sedentary behaviors such as television, video games, and computer use.

- A physical examination to provide information about the extent of overweight and any complications of overweight, including high blood pressure. Children

TABLE 4.12

Blood pressure levels for the 90th and 95th percentiles of blood pressure for boys aged 1 to 17 years

Age	BP percentile*	Systolic BP (mm Hg), by height percentile from standard growth curves							Diastolic BP (mm Hg), by height percentile from standard growth curves						
		5%	10%	25%	50%	75%	90%	95%	5%	10%	25%	50%	75%	90%	95%
1	90th	94	95	97	98	100	102	102	50	51	52	53	54	54	55
	95th	98	99	101	102	104	106	106	55	55	56	57	58	59	59
2	90th	98	99	100	102	104	105	106	55	55	56	57	58	59	59
	95th	101	102	104	106	108	109	110	59	59	60	61	62	63	63
3	90th	100	101	103	105	107	108	109	59	59	60	61	62	63	63
	95th	104	105	107	109	111	112	113	63	63	64	65	66	67	67
4	90th	102	103	105	107	109	110	111	62	62	63	64	65	66	66
	95th	106	107	109	111	113	114	115	66	67	67	68	69	70	71
5	90th	104	105	106	108	110	112	112	65	65	66	67	68	69	69
	95th	108	109	110	112	114	115	116	69	70	70	71	72	73	74
6	90th	105	106	108	110	111	113	114	67	68	69	70	70	71	72
	95th	109	110	112	114	115	117	117	72	72	73	74	75	76	76
7	90th	106	107	109	111	113	114	115	69	70	71	72	72	73	74
	95th	110	111	113	115	116	118	119	74	74	75	76	77	78	78
8	90th	107	108	110	112	114	115	116	71	71	72	73	74	75	75
	95th	111	112	114	116	118	119	120	75	76	76	77	78	79	80
9	90th	109	110	112	113	115	117	117	72	73	73	74	75	76	77
	95th	113	114	116	117	119	121	121	76	77	78	79	80	80	81
10	90th	110	112	113	115	117	118	119	73	74	74	75	76	77	78
	95th	114	115	117	119	121	122	123	77	78	79	80	80	81	82
11	90th	112	113	115	117	119	120	121	74	74	75	76	77	78	78
	95th	116	117	119	121	123	124	125	78	79	79	80	81	82	83
12	90th	115	116	117	119	121	123	123	75	75	76	77	78	78	79
	95th	119	120	121	123	125	126	127	79	79	80	81	82	83	83
13	90th	117	118	120	122	124	125	126	75	76	76	77	78	79	80
	95th	121	122	124	126	128	129	130	79	80	81	82	83	83	84
14	90th	120	121	123	125	126	128	128	76	76	77	78	79	80	80
	95th	124	125	127	128	130	132	132	80	81	81	82	83	84	85
15	90th	123	124	125	127	129	131	131	77	77	78	79	80	81	81
	95th	127	128	129	131	133	134	135	81	82	83	83	84	85	86
16	90th	125	126	128	130	132	133	134	79	79	80	81	82	82	83
	95th	129	130	132	134	136	137	138	83	83	84	85	86	87	87
17	90th	128	129	131	133	134	136	136	81	81	82	83	84	85	85
	95th	132	133	135	136	138	140	140	85	85	86	87	88	89	89

*Blood pressure percentile determined by a single measurement.
BP = blood pressure. mm Hg = millimeters of mercury.

SOURCE: "Table 16. Blood Pressure Levels for the 90th and 95th Percentiles of Blood Pressure for Boys Ages 1 to 17 Years," in *Overweight Children and Adolescents: Screen, Access, and Manage,* Centers for Disease Control and Prevention, National Center for Chronic Disease Prevention and Promotion, Division of Nutrition, Physical Activity and Obesity, May 2000, http://www.cdc.gov/nccdphp/dnpa/growthcharts/training/modules/module3/text/hypertension_tables.htm (accessed October 14, 2015)

TABLE 4.13

Blood pressure levels for the 90th and 95th percentiles of blood pressure for girls aged 1 to 17 years

Age	BP percentile*	Systolic BP (mm Hg), by height percentile from standard growth curves							Diastolic BP (mm Hg), by height percentile from standard growth curves						
		5%	10%	25%	50%	75%	90%	95%	5%	10%	25%	50%	75%	90%	95%
1	90th	97	98	99	100	102	103	104	53	53	53	54	55	56	56
	95th	101	102	103	104	105	107	107	57	57	57	58	59	60	60
2	90th	99	99	100	102	103	104	105	57	57	58	58	59	60	61
	95th	102	103	104	105	107	108	109	61	61	62	62	63	64	65
3	90th	100	100	102	103	104	105	106	61	61	61	62	63	63	64
	95th	104	104	105	107	108	109	110	65	65	65	66	67	67	68
4	90th	101	102	103	104	106	107	108	63	63	64	65	65	66	67
	95th	105	106	107	108	109	111	111	67	67	68	69	69	70	71
5	90th	103	103	104	106	107	108	109	65	66	66	67	68	68	69
	95th	107	107	108	110	111	112	113	69	70	70	71	72	72	73
6	90th	104	105	106	107	109	110	111	67	67	68	69	69	70	71
	95th	108	109	110	111	112	114	114	71	71	72	73	73	74	75
7	90th	106	107	108	109	110	112	112	69	69	69	70	71	72	72
	95th	110	110	112	113	114	115	116	73	73	73	74	75	76	76
8	90th	108	109	110	111	112	113	114	70	70	71	71	72	73	74
	95th	112	112	113	115	116	117	118	74	74	75	75	76	77	78
9	90th	110	110	112	113	114	115	116	71	72	72	73	74	74	75
	95th	114	114	115	117	118	119	120	75	76	76	77	78	78	79
10	90th	112	112	114	115	116	117	118	73	73	73	74	75	76	76
	95th	116	116	117	119	120	121	122	77	77	77	78	79	80	80
11	90th	114	114	116	117	118	119	120	74	74	75	75	76	77	77
	95th	118	118	119	121	122	123	124	78	78	79	79	80	81	81
12	90th	116	116	118	119	120	121	122	75	75	76	76	77	78	78
	95th	120	120	121	123	124	125	126	79	79	80	80	81	82	82
13	90th	118	118	119	121	122	123	124	76	76	77	78	78	79	80
	95th	121	122	123	124	126	127	128	80	80	81	82	82	83	84
14	90th	119	120	121	122	124	125	126	77	77	78	79	79	80	81
	95th	123	124	125	126	128	129	130	81	81	82	83	83	84	85
15	90th	121	121	122	124	125	126	127	78	78	79	79	80	81	82
	95th	124	125	126	128	129	130	131	82	82	83	83	84	85	86
16	90th	122	122	123	125	126	127	128	79	79	79	80	81	82	82
	95th	125	126	127	128	130	131	132	83	83	83	84	85	86	86
17	90th	122	123	124	125	126	128	128	79	79	79	80	81	82	82
	95th	126	126	127	129	130	131	132	83	83	83	84	85	86	86

*Blood pressure percentile determined by a single measurement.

BP = blood pressure. mm Hg = millimeters of mercury.

SOURCE: "Table 17. Blood Pressure Levels for the 90th and 95th Percentiles of Blood Pressure for Girls Ages 1 to 17 Years," in *Overweight Children and Adolescents: Screen, Access, and Manage,* Centers for Disease Control and Prevention, National Center for Chronic Disease Prevention and Promotion, Division of Nutrition, Physical Activity and Obesity, May 2000, http://www.cdc.gov/nccdphp/dnpa/growthcharts/training/modules/module3/text/hypertension_tables.htm (accessed October 14 2015) and adolescents with a BMI-for-age at or above the 95th percentile and who are athletic and muscular may be further assessed using the triceps skinfold measurement to assess body fat. A measurement of greater than the 95th percentile indicates that the child has excess fat rather than increased lean body mass or a large frame.

- Laboratory tests, such as cholesterol screening, are dictated by the degree of overweight, family history, and the results of the physical examination. Table 4.14 shows the range of values for total blood cholesterol and low-density lipoprotein cholesterol that are considered acceptable, borderline, and high.

- A mental health evaluation to determine the readiness of children and adolescents to change behaviors and to identify a history of eating disorders or depression that may require treatment. An assessment of the family's ability to support a child's weight-loss or weight-management efforts may also be performed.

INTERVENTION AND TREATMENT OF OVERWEIGHT AND OBESITY

In the absence of acute medical necessity, such as with children who are dangerously obese, most health professionals concur that drastic caloric restriction is an inappropriate weight-loss strategy for children who are still growing. Instead, they advise efforts to stabilize body weight with a healthful, balanced diet, increased physical activity, and education about nutrition, food choices, and preparation. This approach is especially effective for children who are just slightly overweight, because maintaining body weight often allows them to outgrow overweight and become normal-weight adults.

When active weight loss is indicated, it is generally for children with a BMI greater than the 95th percentile

TABLE 4.14

Classification of cholesterol levels in high-risk children and adolescents

	Total cholesterol, ng/dL	LDL cholesterol, ng/dL
Acceptable	<170	<110
Borderline	170–199	110–129
High	Greater than or equal to 200	Greater than or equal to 130

Note: High-risk children are defined as those from families with hypercholesterolemia or premature cardiovascular disease.
LDL = low density lipoprotein. ng/dL = nanograms per deciliter.

SOURCE: "Table 15. Classification of Cholesterol Levels in High-Risk Children and Adolescents," in *Overweight Children and Adolescents: Screen, Assess, and Manage*, Centers for Disease Control and Prevention, National Center for Chronic Disease Prevention and Promotion, Division of Nutrition, Physical Activity and Obesity, 2000, http://www.cdc.gov/nccdphp/dnpa/growthcharts/training/modules/module3/text/cholesterol.htm (accessed October 14, 2015)

or those experiencing complications of overweight or obesity. Among children aged two to seven years, gradual weight loss of about 1 pound (0.5 kg) per month is advised. Older children with serious health risks who are severely overweight (BMI greater than 35) may be advised to lose between 1 and 2 pounds (0.5 and 0.9 kg) per week.

In "Pediatric Obesity: Etiology and Treatment" (*Pediatric Clinics of North America*, vol. 58, no. 5, October 2011), Melissa K. Crocker and Jack A. Yanovski of the NICHD observe that pediatric childhood obesity has a tremendous impact on later health, even independent of adult weight. The researchers consider lifestyle modification and restricting energy intake to be the foundation of successful treatment of obesity in children. They explain that interventions for overweight and obese children range from basic diets and lifestyle interventions to more intensive very-low-energy diets, medications, and surgery. These methods achieve varying levels of success and all are optimally successful when the child and family are motivated and educated. Crocker and Yanovski assert that "the participation and cooperation of the entire family is critical regardless of the mode of therapy employed."

Crocker and Yanovski observe that dietary changes alone may benefit children who are overweight but are relatively ineffective for children and adolescents with severe obesity. Similarly, exercise without dietary intervention is relatively ineffective. Comprehensive approaches to weight loss that involve behavior modification to reduce screen time, increase physical activity, motivate children to improve their eating behavior, and engage the school system and family to support weight-loss goals appear to be more effective than diet alone.

Pharmacotherapy (drug treatment to support weight loss) has shown limited success when combined with diet and exercise. As of 2016, only one weight-loss drug, orlistat (a drug that induces weight loss by blocking the absorption of about one-third of the fat contained in a meal) was approved for use in children aged 16 years and younger. However, many physicians believe that in view of orlistat's limited effectiveness and potential side effects, it should be limited to children and adolescents with a BMI over the 95th percentile who also have significant obesity-related medical complications.

Some adolescents who are obese may be treated with weight-loss surgery. The National Institutes of Health criteria for adolescents aged 13 to 17 years are the same as those applied to adults: a BMI greater than or equal to 40 or a BMI greater than or equal to 35 with at least one coexisting serious medical condition such as type 2 diabetes, hypertension, or obstructive sleep apnea. Valerio Nobili et al. observe in "Indications and Limitations of Bariatric Intervention in Severely Obese Children and

Adolescents with and without Nonalcoholic Steatohepatitis: ESPGHAN Hepatology Committee Position Statement" (*Journal of Pediatric Gastroenterology and Nutrition*, vol. 60, no. 4, April 2015) that although bariatric surgery is increasingly performed in adolescents, there are few standards of care and little consensus about when surgery is indicated. The researchers state that Roux-en-Y gastric bypass "is considered a safe and effective option for adolescents with extreme obesity, as long as appropriate long-term follow-up is provided." Other types of surgery and temporary devices that are placed in the gastrointestinal tract to promote weight loss have not been approved by the FDA for use in adolescents.

Innovative interventions such as Internet-based programs and cell phone apps may also help adolescents lose weight. In "Design and Implementation of a Randomized Controlled Social and Mobile Weight Loss Trial for Young Adults (Project SMART)" (*Contemporary Clinical Trials*, vol. 37, no.1, January 2014), Kevin Patrick et al. report the design of a two-year study of an intervention for overweight or obese college students that used multiple channels of communication, including Facebook, text messaging, smartphone apps, blogs, and e-mail. The researchers posit that use of multiple intervention will increase participants' "adoption and maintenance of improved health behaviors."

Educating Parents

Researchers agree that primary prevention is the strategy with the greatest potential for reversing the alarming rise in overweight and obesity among children and teens. Public health educators recommend counseling parents and caregivers about healthy eating habits for children. They advise offering children a variety of healthful foods, in reasonable quantities, to assist children to make wise food choices. Children should be encouraged, but not forced, to sample new foods and should not be pressured to clean their plates. No foods or food groups should be entirely off-limits, or children may become fixated on obtaining the forbidden foods.

Although it is difficult to impress on children the future health risks that are associated with excess weight, parents should be informed that obese children are more likely to suffer from diabetes, heart disease, and joint diseases such as osteoarthritis, as well as breast and colon cancer. Adults should model healthy habits by consuming no more than 30% of calories from fat, exercising regularly, and limiting time spent in front of the television. Health educators are especially eager to reduce children's television viewing, with its destructive blend of junk-food advertising and enforced inactivity. Finally, health professionals caution that food should not be used to punish or reward behavior or as a way to comfort or console children. The undivided attention of a parent or caregiver

or an expression of sympathy, reassurance, or encouragement may satisfy a child's need better than an ice cream cone or an order of french fries.

Multidisciplinary Treatment for Children and Teens

The MassGeneral Hospital for Children's Weight Center in Boston, Massachusetts (2016, http://www.mass general.org/children/services/treatmentprograms.aspx?id= 1655) recognizes that treating obesity in children requires a novel approach, one that addresses the many lifelong physical and mental health problems associated with it as well as family and social concerns. The MassGeneral program includes parents and other family members in the child's treatment, and an array of practitioners are used to deliver this family-centered care. The program uses a wide range of age-appropriate approaches to meet children's changing needs and has an established weight-loss surgery program for adolescents. It also collaborates with researchers who are investigating the genetics of obesity and the outcomes of weight-loss surgery.

Let's Move! National Program to Improve Children's Health

In 2010 First Lady Michelle Obama (1964–) launched Let's Move! (http://www.letsmove.gov/), a comprehensive set of strategies aimed at combating childhood obesity. The antiobesity initiative involves private- and public-sector resources in alliances with states, local communities, athletic organizations, and schools. The ambitious program aims to:

- Inform parents to enable them to make healthy choices for their family

- Assist retailers and manufacturers to implement new nutritionally sound and user-friendly front-of-package labeling

- Educate health professionals about obesity to ensure they regularly monitor children's BMI, provide counseling for healthy eating, and write prescriptions for parents detailing the steps they can take to increase healthy eating and physical activity

- Use the media to enhance public awareness of the need to combat obesity through public service announcements, special programming, and marketing

- Promote use of the Food Environment Atlas, a USDA interactive database that helps identify communities with diet and obesity-related problems such as high incidences of diabetes; this information should prove useful for parents, educators, government, and businesses

- Improve food choices in schools by doubling the number of schools that participate in the Healthier U.S. School Challenge, which sets rigorous standards for schools' food quality, participation in meal programs, and physical activity and nutrition education

- Encourage food suppliers to decrease the amount of sugar, fat, and salt in school meals; increase whole grains; and double the amount of produce they serve within 10 years

- Improve Americans' access to healthful affordable foods by bringing grocery stores to underserved areas, helping places such as convenience stores and bodegas carry healthier food options, and investing in farmers' markets

- Increase physical activity by challenging children and adults to commit to physical activity five days per week for six weeks and supporting efforts to get children physically active in and outside of school

According to Kevin Liptak, in "Michelle Obama's Let's Move Turns 5; Is It Working?" (CNN.com, April 6, 2015), in the five years since its launch the program has endured criticism from food companies, school cafeteria workers, Republicans, and even students, who protest the program's emphasis on eating vegetables. Although it is unclear how much the program has contributed to the leveling off of obesity among children and teens, the First Lady asserts that the program has not only increased awareness of the problem of childhood obesity but has also catalyzed a culture shift characterized by improvements in school lunches, salad bars in school cafeterias, healthier foods on grocers' shelves, and an emphasis on physical activity.

EATING DISORDERS

Overweight and obesity are among the most stigmatizing and least socially acceptable conditions in childhood and adolescence. Society, culture, and the media send children powerful messages about body weight and shape ideals. For girls these messages include the "thin ideal" and encouragement to diet and exercise. Messages to boys emphasize a muscular body and pressure to body build and even use potentially harmful dietary supplements and steroids. Gender has not been identified as a specific risk factor for obesity in children, but the pressure placed on girls to be thin may put them at a greater risk for developing eating-disordered behaviors. Although society presents boys with a wider range of acceptable body images, they are also at risk for developing disordered eating and body image disturbances.

Adolescence is a developmental period marked by great physical changes, and it is a time when many teens subject themselves to painful scrutiny. Uneven growth, puberty, and sexual maturation may make teens feel awkward and self-conscious about their body. Teenaged girls are especially susceptible to developing negative body images, ignoring other qualities and focusing exclusively

on appearance to measure their self-worth. This single-minded, and often distorted, destructive focus can result in lowered self-esteem and increased risk for mental health problems, including eating disorders. For example, the 2013 YRBSS found that 6.6% of female high school students engaged in dangerous dieting behaviors (vomiting or taking laxatives). (See Table 3.3 in Chapter 3.)

Who Is at Risk?

Although there are biological, genetic, and familial factors that predispose certain people to eating disorders such as anorexia nervosa (intense fear of becoming fat even when dangerously underweight) and bulimia nervosa (recurrent episodes of binge eating followed by purging to prevent weight gain), the emergence of these disorders is triggered by environmental factors. Chief among the environmental triggers is body image. Many researchers and health professionals believe that teenaged girls who identify with the idealized body images projected throughout U.S. culture are at an increased risk for eating disorders.

Other risk factors are peer group pressures and sociocultural forces such as the fashion and entertainment industries and the media. The National Eating Disorders Association identifies media definitions of attractiveness, beauty, and health as among the myriad factors that contribute to the rise of eating disorders.

Historically, most adolescents with eating disorders have been first- or second-born white females from middle- to upper-class families. Girls who suffer from anorexia are often academically successful, with athletic prowess or training in dance. They tend to be perfectionists, well behaved, emotionally dependent, socially anxious, and intent on receiving approval from others. Adolescent girls with bulimia are generally more extroverted and socially involved.

Research reveals that the incidence of eating disorders in young children is relatively high. In "Eating Disorders in Children and Adolescents: State of the Art Review" (*Pediatrics*, vol. 134, no. 3, September 2014), Kenisha Campbell and Rebecka Peebles report that the lifetime prevalence of eating disorders is about 5%. Although most children and adolescents with eating disorders are female, males account for between 10% and 25% of cases and younger patients are more likely to be boys, with a female-to-male ratio of 6 to 1, compared with a 10 to 1 ratio in adults.

Which Variables Are Associated with Dieting, Overweight, and Eating Disorders?

Dianne Neumark-Sztainer and Peter J. Hannan of the University of Minnesota, Minneapolis, analyzed a representative sample of 6,728 adolescents in grades five through 12 who completed Commonwealth Fund surveys about health. The results of the research were detailed in the landmark study "Weight-Related Behaviors among Adolescent Girls and Boys: Results from a National Survey" (*Archives of Pediatrics and Adolescent Medicine*, vol. 154, no. 6, June 2000). The research aimed to assess the prevalence of dieting and disordered eating among adolescents; the sociodemographic, psychosocial, and behavioral variables that were associated with dieting and disordered eating; and whether adolescents report having discussed weight-related issues with their health care providers. (Neumark-Sztainer and Hannan defined disordered eating as weight-related behaviors such as anorexia and bulimia, self-induced vomiting, binge eating, inappropriate or extreme dieting, and obesity.)

Subjects were assessed by calculating their BMI and eliciting weight-related attitudes and behaviors. For example, dieting was assessed by asking questions such as "Have you ever been on a diet?" and "Why were you dieting?" Behaviors were assessed by posing a question such as "Have you ever binged and purged (which is when you eat a lot of food and then make yourself throw up, vomit, or take something that makes you have diarrhea) or not?" Subjects were also asked, "Right now, how would you describe yourself?" to gain an understanding of their perceptions of their weight. Psychosocial and behavioral variables including self-esteem, stress, depression, substance use (of tobacco, alcohol, or illegal drugs), and level of physical activity were also measured and scored using standardized questionnaires and inventories.

Alcohol and drug use were directly associated with dieting and disordered eating among girls and boys; however, the association between substance use and disordered eating was stronger than the association between substance use and dieting. Tobacco use was associated with dieting and disordered eating among girls, but not among boys.

Campbell and Peebles confirm that dieting is a risk factor for developing an eating disorder. One survey found that about 50% of girls and 25% of boys said they had dieted within the past year. The same study found that 30% of girls and 15% of boys had problematic eating behaviors serious enough to call for medical evaluation, and that 9% of girls and 4% of boys said they made themselves vomit daily.

In "Psychosocial Risk Factors for Eating Disorders" (*International Journal of Eating Disorders*, vol. 46, no. 5, July 2013), Pamela K. Keel and K. Jean Forney seek to identify risk factors for eating disorders in adolescents. Like other investigators, Keel and Forney find that an excessive drive for thinness, body dissatisfaction, negative self-evaluation, low self-esteem, and perfectionism are risk factors. These characteristics also influence the selection of peer groups, which in the case of adolescents who are at risk for eating disorders means choosing peers who share their traits and views, which in turn can magnify and reinforce insecurity about weight and body dissatisfaction.

CHAPTER 5
DIETARY TREATMENT FOR OVERWEIGHT AND OBESITY

We rarely repent of having eaten too little.

—Thomas Jefferson

Americans have long been consumed with losing weight, seemingly willing to suffer deprivation and to embrace each new diet that debuts, even if the "new diet" is simply a twist on a previous weight-loss plan. The fixation with weight loss is so long-standing that even the word *diet* has assumed a new meaning. As a verb, diet means to eat and drink a prescribed selection of foods; however, since the latter part of the 20th century dieting became synonymous with an effort to lose weight.

During the 19th century fashionable body shapes and sizes varied from decade to decade, but most periods celebrated plumpness as a sign of health and prosperity and considered being thin a sign of poverty and ill health. At the start of the 20th century rising interest in dieting seemingly coincided with some of the social and cultural changes that would make it necessary: food became increasingly plentiful, and sedentary work and public transportation reduced Americans' level of physical activity. In *Fat History: Bodies and Beauty in the Modern West* (1997), Peter N. Stearns explains how fat became "a turn-of-the-century target" with anti-fat sentiments intensifying from the 1920s to the 21st century.

Stearns asserts that the contemporary obsession with fat arose in tandem with the dramatic growth in consumer culture, women's increasing equality, and changes in women's sexual and maternal roles. Dieting, with its emphasis on deprivation, self-control, and moral discipline, seemed the perfect antidote to the indulgence of consumer culture, and Stearns contends that "weight morality bore disproportionately on women precisely because of their growing independence, or seeming independence, from other standards."

Fashion trends fueled anti-fat sentiments as women shed the corsets that had created the illusion of narrow waists and aspired to duplicate the wasp-waisted silhouettes by becoming slimmer. The shorter, close-fitting "flapper" dresses of the 1920s revealed women's legs and rekindled their desire to be slender. The emergence of the first actuarial tables (data compiled to assess insurance risk and formulate life insurance premiums), which showed the relationship between overweight and premature mortality (death), reinforced the growing sentiment that thinness was the key to health and longevity. Capitalizing on the increasing interest in monitoring and reducing body weight, the new Detecto and Health-o-Meter bathroom scales enabled people to weigh themselves regularly in the privacy of their own home, as opposed to relying on periodic visits to the physician's office or the pharmacy to use the balance scale.

SELECTED MILESTONES IN THE HISTORY OF DIETING

Not unlike fashion trends, the history of dieting reveals the emergence and popularity of specific diets, which over time are cast aside in favor of different approaches but then are recycled and resurface as "new and miraculous." The first low-carbohydrate diet to earn popular acclaim was described by William Banting (1797–1878) during the 1860s. In *Letter on Corpulence, Addressed to the Public* (1863), Banting, then 66 years old, claimed that by adhering to his low-carbohydrate regimen he was never hungry and had lost 46 pounds (20.9 kg) of his initial 202 pounds (91.6 kg) in one year.

The Early to Mid-20th Century

The early 1900s marked the beginning of diets that restricted calories. *Diet and Health, with Key to the Calories* (1918) by Lulu Hunt Peters (1873–1930) advised readers to think in terms of consuming calories rather than food items and remained in print for 20 years. The 1920s saw the rise of very-low-calorie diets to promote weight loss. For example, the Hollywood 18-day diet advised just 585 calories per day, which required the dieter to eat mostly citrus fruit.

Throughout the 1920s and 1930s the low-calorie diet remained a popular weight-loss strategy. Other approaches, however, such as food-limiting plans that restricted dieters to just one or two foods (e.g., lamb chops, pineapples, grapefruits, or cabbage), were introduced, as were diets that prescribed combinations of certain foods and forbid others. For example, some diets prohibited eating protein and carbohydrates together; others were more specific, advising which vegetables could be served together. The 1930s also saw the first condemnations of carbohydrates as causes of overweight. A high-fat, low-fiber diet consisting primarily of milk and meat was thought to be protective against disease. The Italian poet Filippo Tommaso Marinetti (1876–1944) exhorted Italians to forgo their pasta because he claimed it made them sluggish, pessimistic, and fat.

In 1943 the U.S. Department of Agriculture (USDA) released the "Basic Seven" food guide in the *National Wartime Nutrition Guide*. It emphasized a patriotic wartime austerity diet that included between two and four servings of protein-rich meat and milk products, three servings of fruits or vegetables, and the rather vague recommendation of "bread, flour, and cereals every day and butter, fortified margarine—some daily."

In 1948 Esther Manz (1908–1996), a 208-pound (94.3-kg) homemaker, established Take Off Pounds Sensibly (TOPS; http://www.tops.org/), the first support-group program for weight loss. Manz was inspired to start the program after she attended childbirth preparation classes, where women benefited from mutual support and encouragement. As of February 2016, the annual membership of $33.50 supported the international nonprofit organization, which is based in Milwaukee, Wisconsin. Along with weekly meetings and private weigh-ins, TOPS participants are encouraged to adhere to a calorie-counting meal plan that is based on a program developed by the Academy of Nutrition and Dietetics. In "TOPS Quick Facts" (December 2014, http://www.tops .org/TOPS/PublicDocs/Wellness/PI-009B-TOPSQuickFacts .pdf), TOPS indicates that in 2014 it had more than 125,000 members in North America. Members who achieve their weight goals become KOPS (Keep Off Pounds Sensibly) and often keep attending meetings to maintain their weight and serve as role models for others.

In 1950 the physician and biophysicist John W. Gofman (1918–2007) hypothesized that blood cholesterol was involved in the rise in coronary heart disease. Gofman found not only that heart attacks correlated with elevated levels of cholesterol but also that the cholesterol was contained in one lipoprotein particle: low-density lipoprotein (LDL). Early reports of the connection between overweight and elevated blood cholesterol intensified interest in weight loss, which was now promoted as a strategy for preventing heart disease. During the late 1950s injections of human chorionic gonadotropin, which was derived from the urine of pregnant women or animals, enjoyed fleeting popularity as a weight-loss agent; however, it was quickly proven entirely ineffective. Fad diets, such as a diet advocating the consumption of several bananas to satisfy sugar cravings and another that involved ingesting a blend of oils to boost metabolism, continued to lure Americans seeking quick weight loss. In 1959 the American Medical Association called dieting a "national neurosis."

In 1960 Metrecal, the first high-protein beverage, was widely advertised by the Mead Johnson Company as a weight-reducing aid. It was originally sold as a powder, which when mixed with 1 quart (0.9 L) of water yielded four 8-ounce (237-mL) glasses intended to serve as four meals per day, totaling 900 calories. The powder was made from milk, soy flour, starch, corn oil, yeast, vitamins, coconut oil, and vanilla, chocolate, or butterscotch flavoring. The low-calorie regimen enabled dieters to lose 10 pounds (4.5 kg) in a few weeks, without the trouble of meal preparation or counting calories. Later, Metrecal was sold in a premixed, liquid form that could be consumed right from the can. It was the forerunner of liquid diet products such as Slim-Fast.

Support Groups and Diet Books during the 1960s

The 1960s also witnessed the birth of Overeaters Anonymous (OA) and Weight Watchers. OA began as a support group modeled on the 12-step emotional, physical, and spiritual recovery program used by Alcoholics Anonymous. In *About OA* (2012, http://www.oa.org/pdfs/ oafinalmediamaterials.pdf), the OA notes that about 7,000 OA groups meet each week in more than 80 countries. In 1961 Jean Nidetch (1923–2015), an overweight housewife in New York City, invited a few friends to her home to gain support for her efforts to diet and overcome an "obsession for cookies." From this first meeting, the friends gathered weekly, offering one another encouragement and sharing advice and ideas. The weekly support meetings proved successful, providing motivation and encouragement for long-term weight loss. In 1963 Nidetch incorporated Weight Watchers, and hundreds of people turned out for its first meeting. Weight Watchers grew in both size and popularity by developing nutritious and convenient eating plans and promoting exercise, cookbooks, healthful prepared food, and a magazine. The company became so successful that it was acquired by the H.J. Heinz Company in 1978 and then by Artal Luxembourg S.A. in 1999. In 2015 Weight Watchers was ranked by *U.S. News and World Report* (http://health .usnews.com/best-diet) as the best weight-loss diet. In October of that year Oprah Winfrey (1954–) bought a 10% stake in the company and joined its board, boosting the company's stock prices.

Two best-selling diet books also debuted during the 1960s. The first was Herman Taller's *Calories Don't Count* (1961), which told dieters to avoid carbohydrates and refined sugars and to eat a high-protein diet that included large quantities of unsaturated fat. The second was Irwin Maxwell Stillman and Samm Sinclair Baker's *The Doctor's Quick Weight Loss Diet* (1967), which instructed dieters to avoid carbohydrates altogether and to consume just meat, poultry, fish, cheese, eggs, and water. Although Taller and Stillman and Baker were not the first to tout low-carbohydrate diets, they introduced the first modern high-protein weight-loss diets. Taller's career as a diet guru ended abruptly in 1967, when he was convicted of mail fraud for the sale of safflower capsules as weight-loss aids. Stillman and Baker, however, followed up their wildly successful first book with several other additional weight-loss titles, including *The Doctor's Quick Teenage Diet* (1971), one of the first diet books to address the needs of overweight adolescents. High-protein, low-carbohydrate diets washed down by liberal amounts of alcohol were also advocated by other books from the 1960s, including Gardner Jameson's *The Drinking Man's Diet* (1965) and Sidney Petrie's *Martinis and Whipped Cream: The New Carbo-Cal Way to Lose Weight and Stay Slim* (1966) and *The Lazy Lady's Easy Diet: A Fast-Action Plan to Lose Weight Quickly for Sustained Slenderness and Youthful Attractiveness* (1969).

Development of Nonnutritive Sweeteners

During this same decade chemically processed, nonnutritive sweeteners were marketed as calorie- and guilt-free substitutes that enabled dieters to enjoy many of their favorite sweet treats. Saccharin, which is 300 times sweeter than sugar, was the first artificial sweetener to be widely used in diet foods and beverages. Other chemically processed, artificial, and nonnutritive sweeteners followed, including cyclamate, which was withdrawn from the U.S. market in 1969 because research findings in animals suggested that it might increase the risk of bladder cancer in humans. According to the National Cancer Institute, in "Artificial Sweeteners and Cancer" (August 5, 2009, http://www.cancer.gov/cancertopics/factsheet/Risk/artificial-sweeteners), animal studies have failed to demonstrate that cyclamate is a carcinogen (a substance known to cause cancer) or a cocarcinogen (a substance that enhances the effect of a cancer-causing substance); regardless, cyclamate is not approved for commercial use as a food additive in the United States.

Aspartame and acesulfame potassium were approved by the U.S. Food and Drug Administration (FDA) in 1981 and 1988, respectively. In 1999 the FDA approved the noncaloric sweetener sucralose for general use. Sucralose has gained popularity because it is derived from and tastes like sugar, has no aftertaste, does not promote tooth decay, and is deemed safe for use by pregnant women and diabetics, as well as by those in the general population who are trying to cut down on their sugar intake.

In 2002 the FDA approved neotame, another nonnutritive sweetener, for use as a general-purpose sweetener. Neotame is approximately 7,000 to 13,000 times sweeter than sugar and has been approved for use in food products including baked goods, nonalcoholic beverages (including soft drinks), chewing gum, confections and frostings, frozen desserts, gelatins and puddings, jams and jellies, processed fruits and fruit juices, toppings, and syrups.

In 2008 the FDA approved the sale of stevia, a naturally occurring, zero-calorie sweetener, as a sugar substitute. Stevia is sold in various forms: in combination with other naturally occurring flavors and sweeteners, such as the sugar alcohol erythritol, as well as on its own. Because it has a negligible effect on blood glucose, it is an attractive sugar alternative for people on low-carbohydrate diets.

However, some researchers think sugar substitutes may sabotage dieters by interfering with the body's own innate ability to monitor calorie consumption based on a food's flavor: sweet or savory. Susan E. Swithers of Purdue University reports in "Artificial Sweeteners Produce the Counterintuitive Effect of Inducing Metabolic Derangements" (*Trends in Endocrinology and Metabolism*, vol. 24, no. 9, September 2013) that research confirms that nonnutritive sweeteners promote weight gain and increase risk for metabolic disorders. Swithers suggests that the consumption of nonnutritive sweeteners may result in sweet tastes no longer serving as consistent predictors of energy consumption and physiological consequences. This disconnect between the sweet taste cues and the caloric consequences may lead to a decrease in the ability of sweet tastes to stimulate the bodily responses that regulate energy balance.

The Atkins Diet

In 1972 the cardiologist Robert Atkins (1930–2003) published *Dr. Atkins' Diet Revolution: The High Calorie Way to Stay Thin Forever*, which provided a new explanation about how an extremely low-carbohydrate diet targets insulin to promote weight loss. Atkins called insulin, the hormone that regulates blood sugar levels, a "fat-producing hormone." He asserted that most overeaters are continually in a state of hyperinsulinism, in that they are primed and ever-ready to convert excess carbohydrates to fat. As a result, they have excess circulating insulin, which primes the body to store fat. Atkins contended that when people with hyperinsulinism dieted to lose weight—especially when they reduced their fat intake and increased carbohydrate consumption—their efforts were doomed to fail. He claimed that dieters could alter their metabolism and burn fat by inducing a state of ketosis (the accumulation of ketones from partly digested fats due to inadequate carbohydrate intake) that they monitored by testing their urine for the presence of ketones. Tired of limiting portion size, weighing and measuring their foods, counting calories, and assiduously avoiding fatty foods such as steak, bacon, butter, cheese, and heavy cream, dieters embraced the low-carbohydrate diet with religious fervor.

The high-protein, low-carbohydrate diet was not only satisfying but also produced the immediate benefit of weight loss through water loss because the body flushes the waste products of protein digestion in the form of urine. Especially during the early weeks of dieting this additional weight loss delivered a psychological boost to dieters and provided the motivation to continue. Many researchers and health professionals agreed with Atkins's premise that sharply limiting carbohydrate intake can help curb the appetite by maintaining even levels of insulin and preventing the insulin surges and blood sugar drops that may trigger hunger. For example, in "A High-Protein Diet Induces Sustained Reductions in Appetite, ad Libitum Caloric Intake, and Body Weight Despite Compensatory Changes in Diurnal Plasma Leptin and Ghrelin Concentrations" (*American Journal of Clinical Nutrition*, vol. 82, no. 1, July 2005), David S. Weigle et al. observe that there is considerable evidence that high-protein diets, such as the Atkins regimen, increase satiety (the feeling of fullness or satisfaction after eating). The researchers posit that the increased satiety produced by high-protein diets may help explain the weight loss produced by low-carbohydrate diets.

Critics of the low-carbohydrate regimen were concerned about the long-term health consequences of the high-fat diet and wondered if it might elevate cholesterol and triglyceride levels in people who by virtue of being overweight were already at increased risk for heart disease. There were also concerns that high-protein diets might cause kidney damage or bone loss over time. Rigorous research to compare the effectiveness and assess the health outcomes of low-carbohydrate and low-fat diets was not conducted until the late 1990s. Although Atkins enjoyed tremendous popularity, published weight-loss books, and oversaw the sale of food products bearing his name, his contributions to the scientific understanding of nutrition and weight loss were not fully appreciated until the year preceding his death in 2003.

Pritikin and Other Diets of the 1970s

The 1970s also witnessed several fad diets. Robert Linn's *The Last Chance Diet—When Everything Else Has Failed* (1976) advised a protein-sparing fast, which was so dangerously deficient in essential nutrients that several deaths were attributed to it. In *The Complete Scarsdale Medical Diet Plus Dr. Tarnower's Lifetime Keep-Slim Program* (1978), Herman Tarnower (1910–1980) advocated a fat-free, high-protein diet that allowed 700 calories per day.

At the close of the 1970s Nathan Pritikin's (1915–1985) *The Pritikin Program for Diet and Exercise* (1979) championed a nearly fat-free diet that consisted of fresh and cooked fruits and vegetables, whole grains, breads and pasta, and small amounts of lean meat, fish, and poultry, in concert with daily aerobic exercise. Advocating heart health and fitness, Pritikin opened in 1975 the Pritikin Longevity Center, where people could learn to modify not only their diet but also their lifestyle. Although Pritikin's plan, which essentially eliminated fat from the diet, was considered by many health professionals too extreme to gain long-term adherents, Pritikin enjoyed as loyal a following as did Atkins.

Jenny Craig, the Zone, and Other Diets of the Late 20th Century

During the 1980s Judy Mazel (1943–2007) resurrected the notion of specific food combinations as central to weight loss in *The Beverly Hills Diet* (1981). Mazel asserted that eating foods together, such as protein and carbohydrates, destroyed digestive enzymes and caused weight gain and poor digestion. Her diet featured an abundance of fruit, and some observers speculated that weight loss attributable to the diet resulted from the combined effects of caloric restriction and fluid loss resulting from diarrhea. Celebrity endorsements and Mazel's frequent media interviews stimulated interest in the diet.

In 1983 Jenny Craig (1932–) launched a weight-loss program that would become one of the world's two-largest diet companies (the other being Weight Watchers). With more than 600 centers in Australia, Canada, New Zealand, Puerto Rico, and the United States, the company (2016, http://www.jennycraig.com/corporate/company-profile/) that bears her name sells prepared foods, along with other weight-loss materials. The company offers telephone and online support and home delivery of food and support materials. In 2002 the company founders Jenny Craig and Sid Craig (1932–2008) sold their majority stake in the company to ACI Capital Co. and MidOcean Capital Partners Inc. Four years later, in 2006, the company was acquired by the Swiss food giant Nestlé S.A. North Castle Partners, a private-equity firm that owns Curves International, purchased Jenny Craig from Nestlé in 2013.

The 1990s served up so-called new and revised versions of high-protein, high-fat, and low-carbohydrate diets and the low-fat diet. The cardiologist Dean Ornish (1953–) rekindled enthusiasm for low-fat eating with *Eat More, Weigh Less: Dr. Dean Ornish's Life Choice Program for*

Losing Weight Safely while Eating Abundantly (1993). Atkins's 1999 update of *Dr. Atkins' New Diet Revolution*, which offered advice about how to achieve total wellness and weight loss, spent more than four years on the *New York Times* best-seller list and won over a new generation of dieters. Ornish's approach was directly opposed to Atkins's: he espoused the health benefits of vegetarianism and limiting dietary fat to just 10% of the total daily calories. However, both physicians encouraged readers to engage in moderate exercise, foster social support, and reconnect with themselves to support their physical and emotional well-being.

The diet that generated the most fanfare during the 1990s was by the biochemist Barry Sears (1947–), who published *The Zone: A Dietary Road Map* (1995). Sears's high-protein, low-carbohydrate plan promised that by eating the correct ratio of protein, fat, and carbohydrates dieters would lose weight permanently, avoid disease, enhance mental productivity, achieve maximum physical performance, balance and control insulin levels, and enter "that mysterious but very real state in which your body and mind work together at their ultimate best."

South Beach, the Glycemic Index, and Other Developments

Since the start of the 21st century the fiery debate about the merits of low-carbohydrate and low-fat diets has intensified, with both sides citing scientific evidence to support the supremacy of one diet as the healthier and more effective weight-loss strategy. The cardiologist Arthur Agatston (1947–) offered a kind of compromise between the two regimens in *The South Beach Diet: The Delicious, Doctor-Designed, Foolproof Plan for Fast and Healthy Weight Loss* (2003). Agatston condemned simple carbohydrates, such as white flour and white sugar, citing them as the source of the continuous cravings that sabotage dieters, but did not eliminate complex carbohydrates from the diet. (Carbohydrates are classified as simple or complex. The classification depends on the chemical structure of the particular food source and reflects how quickly the sugar is digested and absorbed. Simple carbohydrates have one or two sugars, whereas complex carbohydrates have three or more.) Agatston's diet recommended plenty of high-fiber foods, lean proteins, and healthful fats, while cutting back on, but not entirely banishing, bread, rice, pastas, and fruits.

Americans' enthusiasm for low-carbohydrate diets cooled in 2004, and Atkins Nutritionals Inc., the company that catapulted low-carbohydrate diets into a national obsession, filed for bankruptcy court protection in 2005. Many dieters abandoned low-carbohydrate diets in favor of regimens that focused on the glycemic index—a ranking system for carbohydrates according to their immediate effect on blood glucose levels, in which a numerical value is assigned to a carbohydrate-rich food based on its average increase in blood glucose.

Diet books that extolled the virtues of the low glycemic index diet—including Michel Montignac's *Eat Yourself Slim* (1999), Rick Gallop's *The G.I. Diet: The Easy, Healthy Way to Permanent Weight Loss* (2002), and H. Leighton Steward et al.'s *The New Sugar Busters!: Cut Sugar to Trim Fat* (2003)—gained popularity. Proponents of low glycemic index diets observed that the regimen not only produced weight loss but also improved overall health by reducing the risk for both type 2 diabetes and cardiovascular disease.

In 2006 Stephen Lanzalotta offered *The Diet Code: Revolutionary Weight Loss Secrets from Da Vinci and the Golden Ratio*, which promotes Mediterranean-style eating and emphasizes bread, fish, cheese, vegetables, meat, nuts, and wine. In *Food Rules: An Eater's Manual* (2009) by Michael Pollan, readers are offered advice such as "eat mostly plants, especially leaves," "eat your colors," "limit your snacks to unprocessed plant food," "don't eat anything your great-grandmother wouldn't recognize as food," "avoid food products that contain more than five ingredients," and "avoid foods that contain high-fructose corn syrup." Some contemporary diets provide behavioral insights and strategies rather than food plans. For example, *The Eat This, Not That! No Diet! Diet: The World's Easiest Weight-Loss Plan* (2011) by David Zinczenko describes how to navigate the supermarket to select healthful foods, and *The Amen Solution: The Brain Healthy Way to Lose Weight and Keep It Off* (2011) by Daniel G. Amen describes how to determine an individual's type of overeating, such as compulsive overeater or emotional eater, and then tailor weight-loss and nutritional strategies for each type of overeater.

Recent Weight-Loss Plans

Although diet industry observers cannot predict the next craze, they are certain that new diets will emerge. By 2014 several popular weight-loss plans stressed portion control and organic foods. Some of these programs had been around for many years. For example, Nutrisystem, a diet delivery service, offers subscribers low-calorie, portion-controlled prepared meals, along with online and telephone access to weight management information and counselors. The program, in operation for more than 40 years, offers customers convenience and simplicity by providing home delivery of a variety of shelf-stable foods that are low in fats and carbohydrates and high in fiber.

Other recent diets that have gained popularity include juice fasts, raw-only plans, and the paleo diet, which is outlined by Loren Cordain in *The Paleo Diet Revised: Lose Weight and Get Healthy by Eating the Foods You Were Designed to Eat* (2010). Cordain suggests returning to the diet of hunter-gatherer times when humans consumed primarily animal products and plants. The high-protein, low glycemic index, and high-fiber diet emphasizes lean meats and fish, fresh fruits, snacks, and nonstarchy vegetables. Juice fasts aim to detox the body, improve health, and promote weight loss by restricting dieters to fruit and vegetable juices and water for periods ranging from two to 60 days. Raw food plans are often associated with veganism and consist of foods such as fruits, vegetables, seeds, sprouts, nuts, and legumes that have not been cooked, processed, or heated above 115° F (46° C).

Dave Asprey's *The Bulletproof Diet: Lose up to a Pound a Day, Reclaim Your Energy and Focus, and Upgrade Your Life* (2014) calls for dieters to consume meat from grass-fed animals and organic eggs, vegetables, and oil and to eliminate all sugar, grains, legumes, pasteurized dairy, farmed seafood, and alcohol. Similar to the paleo diet, *The Whole30* (2015), developed by Dallas Hartwig, a personal trainer, and Melissa Hartwig, a sports nutritionist, is an elimination diet that advises dieters to forgo dairy, grains, legumes, alcohol, and most sugars to eat natural foods, including meat, fish, fruits, vegetables, nuts, and seeds. In *The 22-Day Revolution: The Plant-Based Program That Will Transform Your Body, Reset Your Habits, and Change Your Life* (2016), the exercise physiologist Marco Borges proposes that it takes 21 days to make or break a habit. His vegan diet, which excludes all animal products, has been embraced by celebrities, including Beyoncé (1981–), Jay Z (1970–), Jennifer Lopez (1969–), Pharrell Williams (1973–), Gloria Estefan (1957–), and Shakira (1977–) and is endorsed by Ornish.

AMERICANS' DIETS

Evan Cohen et al. observe in "Statistical Review of US Macronutrient Consumption Data, 1965–2011: Americans Have Been following Dietary Guidelines, Coincident with the Rise in Obesity" (*Nutrition*, vol. 31, no. 5, May 2015) that the rise in overweight and obesity from 42% in 1971 to 66% in 2011 is often attributed to Americans' failure to adhere to nutrition guidelines issued by the American Heart Association and the USDA. The researchers analyzed consumption patterns and body mass index (body weight in kilograms divided by height in meters squared) during this period and find that "Americans in general have been following the nutrition advice that the American Heart Association and the US Departments of Agriculture and Health and Human Services have been issuing for more than 40 years." Between 1971 and 2011 consumption of fats decreased from 45% to 34%, while carbohydrate consumption increased from 39% to 51% of total caloric intake. Cohen et al. conclude, "General adherence to government dietary recommendations to decrease fat share of total dietary intake has been accompanied by a rapid increase in obesity rates. The

results from this study compel a full analysis of the potential causal relationship between Americans seeming adherence to the government's nutrition recommendations and obesity."

Dietary Guidelines for Americans

Every five years the *Dietary Guidelines for Americans* are updated and revised to translate the most current scientific knowledge about individual nutrients and food components into dietary recommendations that may be adopted by the public. The recommendations are based on the preponderance of scientific evidence for reducing the risk of chronic disease and promoting health.

According to the U.S. Department of Health and Human Services and the USDA, in *Scientific Report of the 2015 Dietary Guidelines Advisory Committee* (February 2015, http://health.gov/dietaryguidelines/2015-scientific-report/PDFs/Scientific-Report-of-the-2015-Dietary-Guidelines-Advisory-Committee.pdf), the dietary patterns of Americans are not as good as they could be and are linked to higher chronic disease rates. Consumers' food choices have not improved much in recent decades; they remain low in fruit, vegetables, and whole grains and high in saturated fat, sodium, refined grains, and added sugars.

The *Scientific Report of the 2015 Dietary Guidelines Advisory Committee* identifies a healthful diet as one that is high in fruits, vegetables, whole grains, fat-free or low-fat dairy, seafood, legumes, and nuts. A healthful diet is moderate in alcohol (among adults) and low in red and processed meat, sugar-sweetened food and drinks, and refined grains. The report states that the dietary characteristics recommended by the 2015 guidelines reaffirm those recommended by the 2010 guidelines.

Table 5.1 shows the recommended proportions of carbohydrate, protein, and fat for children, adolescents, and adults. Specific recommendations stipulate that fewer than 10% of calories should come from saturated fatty acids, and trans fatty acids, which are considered to be the most harmful to health, should be avoided.

TABLE 5.1

Recommended proportions of carbohydrate, protein, and fat, by age group, 2010

	Carbohydrate	Protein	Fat
Young children (1–3 years)	45–65%	5–20%	30–40%
Older children and adolescents (4–18 years)	45–65%	10–30%	25–35%
Adults (19 years and older)	45–65%	10–35%	20–35%

SOURCE: "Table 2-4. Recommended Macronutrient Proportions by Age," in *Dietary Guidelines for Americans, 2010*, 7th ed., U.S. Department of Health and Human Services and U.S. Department of Agriculture, December 2010, http://health.gov/dietaryguidelines/dga2010/dietaryguidelines2010.pdf (accessed October 14, 2015)

Cholesterol intake should be less than 300 milligrams per day. Total fat intake should not exceed 20% to 35% of calories. Preferred fat sources are fish, nuts, and vegetable oils that contain polyunsaturated and mono-unsaturated fatty acids. Lean, low-fat, or fat-free meats, poultry, dry beans, and milk or milk products are preferable to full-fat foods. Daily sodium intake should be 2,300 milligrams or less for people to age 51 and 1,500 milligrams or less for older adults, African Americans, and people with diabetes, hypertension, or chronic kidney disease.

In general, the guidelines encourage most Americans to eat fewer calories, increase their physical activity, and choose nutrient-dense foods. They advocate increased consumption of fruits, vegetables, whole grains, and fat-free or low-fat milk and milk products. For example, two cups of fruit and two and a half cups of vegetables per day are recommended for a 2,000-calorie diet, along with three or more servings of whole-grain products per day and three cups per day of fat-free or low-fat milk or equivalent milk products. The guidelines also advise consuming at least half of all grains as whole grains and increasing seafood consumption by replacing some meat and poultry with seafood. Figure 5.1 shows three ways to ensure that at least half of all grains consumed are whole grains.

The *Scientific Report of the 2015 Dietary Guidelines Advisory Committee* observes that a variety of eating patterns adhere to the dietary guidelines. For example, Table 5.2 compares three eating patterns at the 2,000-calories-per-day level: a healthy American adult diet, a healthy vegetarian diet, and a healthy Mediterranean diet. Compared with the typical American adult diet, these eating patterns contain greater quantities of vegetables, fruits, beans and peas, whole grains, fat-free and low-fat dairy, and oils and smaller amounts of solid fats, added sugars, and sodium. Table 5.3 shows the limits for added sugars for the three diets at calorie levels ranging from 1,000 to 3,200.

Both the 2010 and 2015 guidelines specifically address weight management by advising Americans to "[maintain] calorie balance over time to achieve and sustain a healthy weight" and to focus on "consuming nutrient-dense foods and beverages." For people who are overweight, the guidelines advise gradual, steady weight loss by decreasing caloric consumption while maintaining sufficient nutrients and increasing physical activity. Parents of overweight children are counseled to reduce the rate of weight gain while children grow and develop and to consult a health care provider before placing children on weight-reduction diets. Women are encouraged to achieve and maintain a healthy weight before becoming pregnant.

FIGURE 5.1

Three ways to make at least half of total grain intake whole grains

1. 3 ounces of 100% whole grains and 3 ounces of refined-grain products

100% 100% 100% 0% 0% 0%

2. 2 ounces of 100% whole grains, 2 ounces of partly whole-grain products,* and 2 ounces of refined-grain products

100% 100% ≥51% ≥51% 0% 0%

3. 6 ounces of partly whole-grain products

≥51% ≥51% ≥51% ≥51% ≥51% ≥51%

Notes: Each one-ounce slice of bread represents a 1 ounce-equivalent of grains: 1 one-ounce slice bread; 1 ounce uncooked pasta or rice; 1/2 cup cooked rice, pasta, or cereal; 1 tortilla (6" diameter); 1 pancake (5" diameter); 1 ounce ready-to-eat cereal (about 1 cup cereal flakes). The figure uses an example for a person whose recommendation is 6 ounces of total grains with at least 3 ounces from whole grains per day.
*Partly whole-grain products depicted are those that contribute substantially to whole-grain intake. For example, products that contain at least 51% of total weight as whole grains or those that provide at least 8 grams of whole grains per ounce-equivalent.

SOURCE: "Figure 4-1. Three Ways to Make At Least Half of Total Grains Whole Grains," in *Dietary Guidelines for Americans, 2010*, 7th ed., U.S. Department of Health and Human Services and U.S. Department of Agriculture, December 2010, http://health.gov/dietaryguidelines/dga2010/dietaryguidelines2010.pdf (accessed October 14, 2015)

TABLE 5.2

Comparison of a healthy American adult diet, a healthy vegetarian diet and a healthy Mediterranean diet at the 2000 calorie level

Food group	Healthy US-style pattern	Healthy vegetarian pattern	Healthy Med-style pattern
Fruit	2 c per day	2 c per day	2 ½ c per day
Vegetables	2 ½ c per day	2 ½ c per day	2 ½ c per day
Legumes	1 ½ c per wk	3 c per wk	1 ½ c per wk
Whole grains	3 oz eq per day	3 oz eq per day	3 oz eq per day
Dairy	3 c per day	3 c per day	2 c per day
Protein foods	5 ½ oz eq per day	3 ½ oz eq per day	6 ½ oz eq per day
Meat	12 ½ oz eq/wk	—	12 ½ oz eq/wk
Poultry	10 ½ oz eq/wk	—	10 ½ oz eq/wk
Seafood	8 oz eq/wk	—	15 oz eq/wk
Eggs	3 oz eq/wk	3 oz eq/wk	3 oz eq/wk
Nuts/seeds	4 oz eq/wk	7 oz eq/wk	4 oz eq/wk
Processed soy	½ oz eq/wk	8 oz eq/wk	½ oz eq/wk
Oils	27 g per day	27 g per day	27 g per day

SOURCE: "Table D1.32. Composition of Three USDA Food Patterns (Healthy U.S.-Style, Healthy Vegetarian, and Healthy Mediterranean-Style) at the 2000 Calorie Level Daily or Weekly Amounts from Selected Food Groups, Subgroups, and Components," in *Scientific Report of the 2015 Dietary Guidelines Advisory Committee*, U.S. Department of Agriculture and U.S. Department of Health & Human Services, Dietary Guidelines Advisory Committee, February 2015, http://health.gov/dietaryguidelines/2015-scientific-report/PDFs/Scientific-Report-of-the-2015-Dietary-Guidelines-Advisory-Committee.pdf (October 19, 2015)

TABLE 5.3

Limits for added sugars in a healthy American adult diet, a healthy vegetarian diet, and a healthy Mediterranean diet at 1,000–3,200 calorie levels

Calorie level	1,000	1,200	1,400	1,600	1,800	2,000	2,200	2,400	2,600	2,800	3,000	3,200
Empty calorie limits available for **added sugars** (assuming 45% empty calories from added sugars and 55% from solid fat)												
Healthy U.S.-style	68	50	50	54	77	122	126	158	171	180	212	275
Healthy Med-style	63	50	50	81	72	117	126	135	149	158	194	257
Healthy vegetarian	77	77	81	81	81	131	131	158	158	158	185	234
Average	69	59	60	72	77	123	128	150	159	165	197	255
Average (tsp)	4.3	3.7	3.8	4.5	4.8	7.7	8.0	9.4	9.9	10.3	12.3	15.9
Healthy U.S.-style	7%	4%	4%	3%	4%	6%	6%	7%	7%	6%	7%	9%
Healthy Med-style	6%	4%	4%	5%	4%	6%	6%	6%	6%	6%	6%	8%
Healthy vegetarian	8%	6%	6%	5%	5%	7%	6%	7%	6%	6%	6%	7%
Average	7%	5%	4%	5%	4%	6%	6%	6%	6%	6%	7%	8%

SOURCE: "Table D6.1. Added Sugars Available in the USDA Food Patterns (Healthy U.S.-Style, Healthy Mediterranean-Style, and Healthy Vegetarian Patterns) in Calories, Teaspoons, and Percent of Total Calories per Day," in *Scientific Report of the 2015 Dietary Guidelines Advisory Committee*, U.S. Department of Agriculture and U.S. Department of Health & Human Services, Dietary Guidelines Advisory Committee, February 2015, http://health.gov/dietaryguidelines/2015-scientific-report/PDFs/Scientific-Report-of-the-2015-Dietary-Guidelines-Advisory-Committee.pdf (October 19, 2015)

In an effort to expand on the guidelines and improve their utility, the USDA debuted in 2011 a new, simple graphic food icon called MyPlate to offer Americans a simple representation of how to construct a healthful meal and diet. (See Figure 5.2.) There is a full discussion of MyPlate in Chapter 10.

HOW WEIGHT-LOSS DIETS WORK

Research demonstrates that weight loss is associated with the length of the diet, the pre-diet weight (people who are more overweight tend to lose more weight, more quickly than those who are only mildly overweight), and the number of calories consumed. Any diet that restricts caloric intake such that calories consumed are less than those expended will promote short-term weight loss. The key to weight loss through diet is adherence—if people do not stick to their diet, then they will not lose weight.

The successes achieved using regimens that restrict dieters to a single food or food group such as grapefruit, pineapple, or cabbage are probably in part attributable to the human hankering for variety. When limited to just one food, most dieters experience boredom: there is just no appeal to eating the same food at every meal, for days on end, so naturally less food is consumed. In addition, these diets generally rely on low-calorie foods, so that even if dieters were inspired to consume 15 grapefruits per day, their total daily caloric consumption would be about 1,200 calories, which is sufficient to produce weight loss for most overweight people. Similarly, diets that involve stringent portion control effectively reduce calories to produce weight loss.

FIGURE 5.2

MyPlate aims to help consumers plan healthful meals

SOURCE: "MyPlate," in *News and Media* U.S. Department of Agriculture, September 19, 2011, http://www.choosemyplate.gov/sites/default/files/printablematerials/myplate_grayscale.pdf (accessed October 19, 2015)

Low-Calorie Diets

Traditional dietary therapy for weight loss generally seeks to create a deficit of 500 to 1,000 calories per day with the intent of promoting weight loss of between 1 to 2 pounds (0.5 to 0.9 kg) per week. Low-calorie diets for men usually range from 1,200 to 1,600 calories per day; for women, low-calorie diets contain between 1,000 and 1,200 calories per day. (See Table 5.4 for examples of the recommended percentages of nutrients in low-calorie diets.)

The most successful low-calorie diets take individual food preferences into account to custom-tailor the diet. Table 5.5 and Table 5.6 show examples of how traditional American cuisine may be used to create a low-calorie diet containing 1,200 and 1,600 calories per day, respectively. Table 5.7 incorporates regional southern cuisine into a reduced-calorie diet. Table 5.8 illustrates how Asian American cuisine may be adapted to 1,200- and 1,600-calorie-per-day diets, and Table 5.9 shows how Mexican American cuisine may be adapted for low-calorie diets. Table 5.10 is a sample of a reduced-calorie diet that vegetarians who eat milk and eggs but no meat or fish can use to lose weight. Food exchanges, such as those shown in Table 5.11, enable dieters to enjoy a variety of foods in their reduced-calorie meals, which can prevent boredom and the tendency to abandon the diet.

Research reveals that reducing fat in the diet is an effective way to reduce calories and that when low-calorie diets are combined with low-fat diets, better weight loss is achieved than through calorie reduction alone. Furthermore, although very-low-calorie diets that provide about 500 calories per day have been demonstrated to produce greater initial weight loss than low-calorie diets, the long-term weight loss is not different between the two regimens.

Low-Carbohydrate Diets

During the first decade of the 21st century several rigorous research studies reported that low-carbohydrate diets were as effective, or even more effective, in producing short-term weight loss than low-fat diets. The low-carbohydrate diets owed much of their success to adherence—dieters were better able to stick with their diets, and as a result achieved better results. Another hypothesis about the success of low-carbohydrate regimens is that dieters do not feel as hungry as they do on other diets because protein is the most satisfying of the three macronutrients: carbohydrates, fats, and proteins.

The scientific premise of low-carbohydrate diets is that consuming certain carbohydrates can cause surges in blood sugar and insulin that not only stimulate appetite and weight gain but may also increase the risk for diabetes and heart disease. At first, low-carbohydrate diets viewed all carbohydrates as equally harmful. Increasingly, however, low-carbohydrate diets distinguished between simple and complex carbohydrates, which contain simple (single or double) or complex (three or more) sugars.

Examples of single sugars from foods include fructose, which is found in fruits, and galactose, which is found in milk products. Double sugars include lactose in dairy products; maltose, which is found in certain vegetables and in beer; and sucrose (table sugar). Examples of complex carbohydrates, which are often referred to as starches, include breads, cereals, legumes, brown rice, and pastas. Simple carbohydrates occur naturally in fruits, milk products, and vegetables and, like complex carbohydrates, contain vitamins and minerals, which distinguishes them from the refined simple sugars many nutritionists advise against (or at least recommend limiting in the diet). The simple carbohydrates most nutritionists call "empty calories" are the processed and refined sugars found in candy, table sugar, and sodas, as well as in foods such as white flour and polished white rice.

Besides distinguishing between simple and complex carbohydrates, low-carbohydrate regimens rely on a measure known as the glycemic index (GI), which ranks foods based on how rapidly their consumption raises blood glucose levels. The GI measures how much blood sugar increases over a period of two or three hours after a meal. Carbohydrate foods that break down quickly during digestion have the highest GI. The GI may be used to determine if a particular food will trigger the problematical "carbohydrate–blood sugar–insulin cascade."

TABLE 5.4

Recommended intake amounts at various calorie levels

For each food group or subgroup[a], recommended average daily intake amounts[b] at all calorie levels. Recommended intakes from vegetable and protein foods subgroups are per week.

Calorie level of pattern[c]	1,000	1,200	1,400	1,600	1,800	2,000	2,200	2,400	2,600	2,800	3,000	3,200
Fruits	1 c	1 c	1 1/2 c	1 1/2 c	1 1/2 c	2 c	2 c	2 c	2 c	2 1/2 c	2 1/2 c	2 1/2 c
Vegetables[d]	1 c	1 1/2 c	1 1/2 c	2 c	2 1/2 c	2 1/2 c	3 c	3 c	31/2 c	31/2 c	4 c	4 c
Dark-green vegetables	1/2 c/wk	1 c/wk	1 c/wk	1 1/2 c/wk	1 1/2 c/wk	1 1/2 c/wk	2 c/wk	2 c/wk	2 1/2 c/wk	2 1/2 c/wk	2 1/2 c/wk	2 1/2 c/wk
Red and orange vegetables	2 1/2 c/wk	3 c/wk	3 c/wk	4 c/wk	5 1/2 c/wk	5 1/2 c/wk	6 c/wk	6 c/wk	7 c/wk	7 c/wk	7 1/2 c/wk	7 1/2 c/wk
Beans and peas (legumes)	1/2 c/wk	1/2 c/wk	1/2 c/wk	1 c/wk	1 1/2 c/wk	1 1/2 c/wk	2 c/wk	2 c/wk	2 1/2 c/wk	2 1/2 c/wk	3 c/wk	3 c/wk
Starchy vegetables	2 c/wk	3 1/2 c/wk	3 1/2 c/wk	4 c/wk	5 c/wk	5 c/wk	6 c/wk	6 c/wk	7 c/wk	7 c/wk	8 c/wk	8 c/wk
Other vegetables	1 1/2 c/wk	2 1/2 c/wk	2 1/2 c/wk	3 1/2 c/wk	4 c/wk	4 c/wk	5 c/wk	5 c/wk	5 1/2 c/wk	5 1/2 c/wk	7 c/wk	7 c/wk
Grains[e]	3 oz-eq	4 oz-eq	5 oz-eq	5 oz-eq	6 oz-eq	6 oz-eq	7 oz-eq	8 oz-eq	9 oz-eq	10 oz-eq	10 oz-eq	10 oz-eq
Whole grains	1 1/2 oz-eq	2 oz-eq	2 1/2 oz-eq	3 oz-eq	3 oz-eq	3 oz-eq	3 1/2 oz-eq	4 oz-eq	4 1/2 oz-eq	5 oz-eq	5 oz-eq	5 oz-eq
Enriched grains	1 1/2 oz-eq	2 oz-eq	2 1/2 oz-eq	2 oz-eq	3 oz-eq	3 oz-eq	3 1/2 oz-eq	4 oz-eq	4 1/2 oz-eq	5 oz-eq	5 oz-eq	5 oz-eq
Protein foods[d]	2 oz-eq	3 oz-eq	4 oz-eq	5 oz-eq	5 oz-eq	5 1/2 oz-eq	6 oz-eq	6 1/2 oz-eq	6 1/2 oz-eq	7 oz-eq	7 oz-eq	7 oz-eq
Seafood	3 oz/wk	5 oz/wk	6 oz/wk	8 oz/wk	8 oz/wk	8 oz/wk	9 oz/wk	10 oz/wk	10 oz/wk	11 oz/wk	11 oz/wk	11 oz/wk
Meat, poultry, eggs	10 oz/wk	14 oz/wk	19 oz/wk	24 oz/wk	24 oz/wk	26 oz/wk	29 oz/wk	31 oz/wk	31 oz/wk	34 oz/wk	34 oz/wk	34 oz/wk
Nuts, seeds, soy products	1 oz/wk	2 oz/wk	3 oz/wk	4 oz/wk	4 oz/wk	4 oz/wk	4 oz/wk	5 oz/wk	5 oz/wk	5 oz/wk	5 oz/wk	5 oz/wk
Dairy[f]	2 c	2 1/2 c	2 1/2 c	3 c	3 c	3 c	3 c	3 c	3 c	3 c	3 c	3 c
Oils[g]	15 g	17 g	17 g	22 g	24 g	27 g	29 g	31 g	34 g	36 g	44 g	51 g
Maximum SoFAS[h] limit, Calories (% of calories)	137 (14%)	121 (10%)	121 (9%)	121 (8%)	161 (9%)	258 (13%)	266 (12%)	330 (14%)	362 (14%)	395 (14%)	459 (15%)	596 (19%)

[a] All foods are assumed to be in nutrient-dense forms, lean or low-fat and prepared without added fats, sugars, or salt. Solid fats and added sugars may be included up to the daily maximum limit identified in the table. Food items in each group and subgroup are:

Fruits — All fresh, frozen, canned, and dried fruits and fruit juices: for example, oranges and orange juice, apples and apple juice, bananas, grapes, melons, berries, raisins.

Vegetables

• Dark-green vegetables — All fresh, frozen, and canned dark-green leafy vegetables and broccoli, cooked or raw: for example, broccoli; spinach; romaine; collard, turnip, and mustard greens.

• Red and orange vegetables — All fresh, frozen, and canned red and orange vegetables, cooked or raw: for example, tomatoes, red peppers, carrots, sweet potatoes, winter squash, and pumpkin.

• Beans and peas (legumes) — All cooked beans and peas: for example, kidney beans, lentils, chickpeas, and pinto beans. Does not include green beans or green peas. (See additional comment under protein foods group.)

• Starchy vegetables — All fresh, frozen, and canned starchy vegetables: for example, white potatoes, corn, green peas.

• Other vegetables — All fresh, frozen, and canned other vegetables, cooked or raw: for example, iceberg lettuce, green beans, and onions.

Grains

• Whole grains — All whole-grain products and whole grains used as ingredients: for example, whole-wheat bread, whole-grain cereals and crackers, oatmeal, and brown rice.

• Enriched grains — All enriched refined-grain products and enriched refined grains used as ingredients: for example, white breads, enriched grain cereals and crackers, enriched pasta, white rice.

Protein foods — All meat, poultry, seafood, eggs, nuts, seeds, and processed soy products. Meat and poultry should be lean or low-fat and nuts should be unsalted. Beans and peas are considered part of this group as well as the vegetable group, but should be counted in one group only.

Dairy — All milks, including lactose-free and lactose-reduced products and fortified soy beverages, yogurts, frozen yogurts, dairy desserts, and cheeses. Most choices should be fat-free or low-fat. Cream, sour cream, and cream cheese are not included due to their low calcium content.

[b] Food group amounts are shown in cup (c) or ounce-equivalents (oz-eq). Oils are shown in grams (g). Quantity equivalents for each food group are:
• Grains, 1 ounce-equivalent is: 1 one-ounce slice bread; 1 ounce uncooked pasta or rice 1/2 cup cooked rice, pasta, or cereal; 1 tortilla (6" diameter); 1 pancake (5" diameter); 1 ounce ready-to-eat cereal (about 1 cup cereal flakes).
• Vegetables and fruits, 1 cup equivalent is: 1 cup raw or cooked vegetable or fruit 1/2 cup dried vegetable or fruit; 1 cup vegetable or fruit juice; 2 cups leafy salad greens.
• Protein foods, 1 ounce-equivalent is: 1 ounce lean meat, poultry, seafood; 1 egg; 1 Tbsp peanut butter 1/2 ounce nuts or seeds. Also, 1/4 cup cooked beans or peas may also be counted as 1 ounce-equivalent.
• Dairy, 1 cup equivalent is: 1 cup milk, fortified soy beverage, or yogurt; 1/2 ounces natural cheese (e.g., cheddar); 2 ounces of processed cheese (e.g., American).
[c] Food intake patterns at 1,000, 1,200, and 1,400 calories meet the nutritional needs of children ages 2 to 8 years. Patterns from 1,600 to 3,200 calories meet the nutritional needs of children ages 9 years and older and adults. If a child ages 4 to 8 years needs more calories and, therefore, is following a pattern at 1,600 calories or more, the recommended amount from the dairy group can be 2 1/2 cups per day. Children ages 9 years and older and adults should not use the 1,000, 1,200, or 1,400 calorie patterns.
[d] Vegetable and protein foods subgroup amounts are shown in this table as weekly amounts, because it would be difficult for consumers to select foods from all subgroups daily.
[e] Whole-grain subgroup amounts shown in this table are minimums. More whole grains up to all of the grains recommended may be selected, with offsetting decreases in the amounts of enriched refined grains.
[f] The amount of dairy foods in the 1,200 and 1,400 calorie patterns have increased to reflect new RDAs for calcium that are higher than previous recommendations for children ages 4 to 8 years.
[g] Oils and soft margarines include vegetable, nut, and fish oils and soft vegetable oil table spreads that have notrans fats.
[h] SoFAS are calories from solid fats and added sugars. The limit for SoFAS is the remaining amount of calories in each food pattern after selecting the specified amounts in each food group in nutrient-dense forms (forms that are fat-free or low-fat and with no added sugars). The number of SoFAS is lower in the 1,200, 1,400, and 1,600 calorie patterns than in the 1,000 calorie pattern. The nutrient goals for the 1,200 to 1,600 calorie patterns are higher and require that more calories be used for nutrient-dense foods from the food groups.

SOURCE: "Appendix 7. USDA Food Patterns," in *Dietary Guidelines for Americans, 2010*, 7th ed., U.S. Department of Health and Human Services and U.S. Department of Agriculture, December 2010, http://health.gov/dietaryguidelines/dga2010/dietaryguidelines2010.pdf (accessed October 19, 2015)

High-GI foods are those that are rapidly digested and absorbed or transformed metabolically into glucose.

Examples of foods with GI scores of 70 or above are cake, cookies, doughnuts, honey, french fries, rice, baked

TABLE 5.5

Sample reduced calorie menus, traditional American cuisine—1,200 calories

	Calories	Fat (grams)	% Fat	Exchange for
Breakfast				
• Whole wheat bread, 1 medium slice	70	1.2	15	(1 bread/starch)
• Jelly, regular, 2 tsp	30	0	0	(1/2 fruit)
• Cereal, shredded wheat, 1/2 cup	104	1	4	(1 bread/starch)
• Milk, 1%, 1 cup	102	3	23	(1 milk)
• Orange juice, 3/4 cup	78	0	0	(1 1/2 fruit)
• Coffee, regular, 1 cup	5	0	0	(free)
Breakfast total	**389**	**5.2**	**10**	
Lunch				
• Roast beef sandwich:				
Whole wheat bread, 2 medium slices	139	2.4	15	(2 bread/starch)
Lean roast beef, unseasoned, 2 oz	60	1.5	23	(2 lean protein)
Lettuce, 1 leaf	1	0	0	(1 vegetable)
Tomato, 3 medium slices	10	0	0	
Mayonnaise, low calorie, 1 tsp	15	1.7	96	(1/3 fat)
• Apple, 1 medium	80	0	0	(1 fruit)
• Water, 1 cup	0	0	0	(free)
Lunch total	**305**	**5.6**	**16**	
Dinner				
• Salmon, 2 ounces edible	103	5	44	(2 lean protein)
• Vegetable oil, 1 1/2 tsp	60	7	100	(1 1/2 fat)
• Baked potato, 3/4 medium	100	0	0	(1 bread/starch)
• Margarine, 1 tsp	34	4	100	(1 fat)
• Green beans, seasoned, with margarine, 1/2 cup	52	2	4	(1 vegetable) (1/2 fat)
• Carrots, seasoned	35	0	0	(1 vegetable)
• White dinner roll, 1 small	70	2	28	(1 bread/starch)
• Iced tea, unsweetened, 1 cup	0	0	0	(free)
• Water, 2 cups	0	0	0	(free)
Dinner total	**454**	**20**	**39**	
Snack				
• Popcorn, 2 1/2 cups	69	0	0	(1 bread/starch)
• Margarine, 3/4 tsp	30	3	100	(3/4 fat)
Total	**1,247**	**34–36**	**24–26**	

Calories	1,247	Saturated fat, % kcals	7	
Total carbohydrate, % kcals	58	Cholesterol, mg	96	
Total fat, % kcals	26	Protein, % kcals	19	
*Sodium, mg	1,043			

Note: Calories have been rounded. Kcal = kilo calorie.
1,200: 100% RDA met for all nutrients except vitamin E 80%, vitamin B$_2$ 96%, vitamin B$_6$ 94%, calcium 68%, iron 63%, and zinc 73%.
*No salt added in recipe preparation or as seasoning. Consume at least 32 ounces of water.

SOURCE: "Appendix D. Sample Reduced Calorie Menus: Traditional American Cuisine—1,200 Calories," in *The Practical Guide: Identification, Evaluation, and Treatment of Overweight and Obesity in Adults*, National Institutes of Health, National Heart, Lung, and Blood Institute, North American Association for the Study of Obesity, October 2000, http://www.nhlbi.nih.gov/guidelines/obesity/prctgd_b.pdf (accessed October 15, 2015)

potato, and white bread. In contrast, lentils have a GI of 29, whereas broccoli, peanuts, and spinach have GIs of less than 15. Carbohydrates that break down slowly, such as whole-grain breads and cereals, beans, leafy greens, or cruciferous vegetables (which include mustard greens, cabbage, broccoli, cauliflower, kale, and brussels sprouts), generate slower glucose release into the bloodstream and lower GI scores—50 or less. Eating low-GI foods supports weight loss by enhancing satiety and thereby decreasing total food consumption.

The measurement of GI began during the 1990s, following the discovery that specific carbohydrates such as potatoes and cornflakes raised blood sugar faster than others such as brown rice and oatmeal. Harvard University School of Public Health researchers used GI to calculate glycemic load—a measure that considers the food's GI and the amount of carbohydrates contained in a single serving. For example, many whole fruits, vegetables, and grains have low glycemic loads, which when consumed prompt a moderate rise in blood glucose and insulin. When the same fruits, vegetables, and grains are squeezed or pulverized into juice or flour, their glycemic load increases—effectively rendering them with the same high glycemic load of sugar water.

After consuming a meal with a high glycemic load, blood sugar rises higher and faster than it does after eating a meal with a low glycemic load. In an effort to recover from the resulting peaks and plummets, the brain transmits a hunger signal long before the next meal is due. Wildly fluctuating blood sugar and insulin may result in overeating,

TABLE 5.6

Sample reduced calorie menus, traditional American cuisine—1,600 calories

	Calories	Fat (grams)	% Fat	Exchange for
Breakfast				
• Whole wheat bread, 1 medium slice	70	1.2	15.4	(1 bread/starch)
• Jelly, regular, 2 tsp	30	0	0	(1/2 fruit)
• Cereal, shredded wheat, 1 cup	207	2	8	(2 bread/starch)
• Milk, 1%, 1 cup	102	3	23	(1 milk)
• Orange juice, 3/4 cup	18	0	0	(1 1/2 fruit)
• Coffee, regular, 1 cup	5	0	0	(free)
• Milk, 1%, 1 oz	10	0.3	27	(1/8 milk)
Breakfast total	**502**	**6.5**	**10**	
Lunch				
• Roast beef sandwich:				
Whole wheat bread, 2 medium slices	139	2.4	15	(2 bread/starch)
Lean roast beef, unseasoned, 2 oz	60	1.5	23	(2 lean protein)
American cheese, low fat and low sodium, 1 slice, 3/4 oz	46	1.8	36	(1 lean protein)
Lettuce, 1 leaf	1	1	0	
Tomato, 3 medium slices	10	0	0	(1 vegetable)
Mayonnaise, low calorie, 2 tsp	30	3.3	99	(2/3 fat)
• Apple, 1 medium	8	0	0	(1 fruit)
• Water, 1 cup	0	0	0	(free)
Lunch total	**366**	**9**	**22**	
Dinner				
• Salmon, 3 ounces edible	155	7	40	(3 lean protein)
• Vegetable oil, 1 1/2 tsp	60	7	100	(1 1/2 fat)
• Baked potato, 3/4 medium	100	0	0	(1 bread/starch)
• Margarine, 1 tsp	34	4	100	(1 fat)
• Green beans, seasoned, with margarine, 1/2 cup	52	2	4	(1 vegetable) (1/2 fat)
• Carrots, seasoned, with margarine, 1/2 cup	52	2	4	(1 vegetable) (1/2 fat)
• White dinner roll, 1 medium	80	3	33	(1 bread/starch)
• Ice milk, 1/2 cup	92	3	28	(1 bread/starch) (1/2 fat)
• Iced tea, unsweetened, 1 cup	0	0	0	(free)
• Water, 2 cups	0	0	0	(free)
Dinner total	**625**	**28**	**38**	
Snack				
• Popcorn, 2 1/2 cups	69	0	0	(1 bread/starch)
• Margarine, 1/2 tsp	58	6.5	100	(1 1/2 fat)
Total	**1,613**	**50**	**28**	

Calories	1,613	Saturated fat, % kcals	8	
Total carbohydrate, % kcals	55	Cholesterol, mg	142	
Total fat, % kcals	29	Protein, % kcals	19	
*Sodium, mg	1,341			

Note: Calories have been rounded. Kcal = kilo calorie.
1,600: 100% RDA met for all nutrients except vitamin E 99%, iron 73%, and zinc 91%.
*No salt added in recipe preparation or as seasoning. Consume at least 32 ounces of water.

SOURCE: "Appendix D. Sample Reduced Calorie Menus: Traditional American Cuisine—1,600 Calories," in *The Practical Guide: Identification, Evaluation, and Treatment of Overweight and Obesity in Adults*, National Institutes of Health, National Heart, Lung, and Blood Institute, North American Association for the Study of Obesity, October 2000, http://www.nhlbi.nih.gov/guidelines/obesity/prctgd_b.pdf (accessed October 19, 2015)

which in turn causes overweight. For people who are overweight or physically inactive, another potential danger of consuming foods with high glycemic loads is that they may already be insulin resistant, and the overexertion of insulin-producing cells in the pancreas that is required to metabolize the high glycemic loads may ultimately exhaust their insulin-producing cells, leading to diabetes.

Weight-loss diets based on the GI sharply restrict high-index foods in favor of low-index foods. Proponents of low-carbohydrate, low-GI food diets observe that consuming foods with low glycemic loads stabilizes blood sugar and insulin to prevent the fluctuations that can cause overeating and may increase the risk for diabetes. They also assert that reliance on low-fat diets inadvertently led to diets that

were high in simple carbohydrates and indirectly promoted overweight and diabetes in the United States.

Low-Fat Diets

Low-fat diets reduce caloric intake by reducing fat consumption. Fat has 9 calories per gram, whereas protein and carbohydrates have 4 calories per gram. These diets rely on the high-fiber content of complex carbohydrates to satisfy dieters. High-fiber foods also slow the absorption of carbohydrates, so they do not provoke a rapid rise in blood sugar and insulin.

Table 5.12 shows some food substitutions that may be made to reduce dietary fat content. Besides making

TABLE 5.7

Sample reduced calorie menus, southern cuisine

	1,600 calories	1,200 calories
Breakfast		
• Oatmeal, prepared with 1% milk, low fat	1/2 cup	1/2 cup
• Milk, 1%, low fat	1/2 cup	1/2 cup
• English muffin	1 medium	—
• Cream cheese, light, 18% fat	1 T	—
• Orange juice	3/4 cup	1/2 cup
• Coffee	1 cup	1 cup
• Milk, 1%, low fat	1 oz	1 oz
Lunch		
• Baked chicken, without skin	2 oz	2 oz
• Vegetable oil	1 tsp	1/2 tsp
• Salad:		
Lettuce	1/2 cup	1/2 cup
Tomato	1/2 cup	1/2 cup
Cucumber	1/2 cup	1/2 cup
• Oil and vinegar dressing	2 tsp	1 tsp
• White rice	1/2 cup	1/4 cup
• Margarine, diet	1/2 tsp	1/2 tsp
• Baking powder biscuit, prepared with vegetable oil	1 small	1/2 small
• Margarine	1 tsp	1 tsp
• Water	1 cup	1 cup
Dinner		
• Lean roast beef	3 oz	2 oz
• Onion	1/4 cup	1/4 cup
• Beef gravy, water-based	1 T	1 T
• Turnip greens	1/2 cup	1/2 cup
• Margarine, diet	1/2 tsp	1/2 tsp
• Sweet potato, baked	1 small	1 small
• Margarine, diet	1/2 tsp	1/4 tsp
• Ground cinnamon	1 tsp	1 tsp
• Brown sugar	1 tsp	1 tsp
• Corn bread prepared with margarine, diet	1/2 medium slice	1/2 medium slice
• Honeydew melon	1/4 medium	1/8 medium
• Iced tea, sweetened with sugar	1 cup	1 cup
Snack		
• Saltine crackers, unsalted tops	4 crackers	4 crackers
• Mozzarella cheese, part skim, low sodium	1 oz	1 oz

Calories	1,653	Calories	1,225
Total carbohydrate, % kcals	53	Total carbohydrate, % kcals	50
Total fat, % kcals	28	Total fat, % kcals	31
*Sodium, mg	1,231	*Sodium, mg	867
Saturated fat, % kcals	8	Saturated fat, % kcals	9
Cholesterol, mg	172	Cholesterol, mg	142
Protein, % kcals	20	Protein, % kcals	21

1,600: 100% RDA met for all nutrients except vitamin E 97%, magnesium 98%, iron 78%, and zinc 90%.
1,200: 100% RDA met for all nutrients except vitamin E 82%, vitamin B₁ & B₂ 95%, vitamin B₃ 99%, vitamin B₆ 88%, magnesium 83%, iron 56%, and zinc 70%.
*No salt added in recipe preparation or as seasoning. Consume at least 32 ounces of water.
Kcal = kilo calorie.

SOURCE: "Appendix D. Sample Reduced Calorie Menus: Southern Cuisine—Reduced Calorie," in *The Practical Guide: Identification, Evaluation, and Treatment of Overweight and Obesity in Adults*, National Institutes of Health, National Heart, Lung, and Blood Institute, North American Association for the Study of Obesity, October 2000, http://www.nhlbi.nih.gov/guidelines/obesity/prctgd_b.pdf (accessed October 19, 2015)

TABLE 5.8

Sample reduced calorie menus, Asian American cuisine

	1,600 calories	1,200 calories
Breakfast		
• Banana	1 small	1 small
• Whole wheat bread	2 slices	1 slice
• Margarine	1 tsp	1 tsp
• Orange juice	3/4 tsp	3/4 tsp
• Milk 1%, low fat	3/4 cup	3/4 cup
Lunch		
• Beef noodle soup, canned, low sodium	1/2 cup	1/2 cup
• Chinese noodle and beef salad:		
Roast beef	3 oz	2 oz
Peanut oil	1 1/2 tsp	1 tsp
Soya sauce, low sodium	tsp	1 tsp
Carrots	1/2 cup	1/2 cup
Zucchini	1/2 cup	1/2 cup
Onion	1/4 cup	1/4 cup
Chinese noodles, soft type	1/4 cup	1/4 cup
• Apple	1 medium	1 medium
• Tea, unsweetened	1 cup	1 cup
Dinner		
• Pork stir-fry with vegetables:		
Pork cutlet	2 oz	2 oz
Peanut oil	1 tsp	1 tsp
Soya sauce, low sodium	1 tsp	1 tsp
Broccoli	1/2 cup	1/2 cup
Carrots	1 cup	1 cup
Mushrooms	1/4 cup	1/2 cup
• Steamed white rice	1 cup	1/2 cup
• Tea, unsweetened	1 cup	1 cup
Snack		
• Almond, cookies	2 cookies	—
• Milk 1%, low fat	1/2 cup	1/2 cup

Calories	1,609	Calories	1,220
Total carbohydrate, % kcals	56	Total carbohydrate, % kcals	55
Total fat, % kcals	27	Total fat, % kcals	27
*Sodium, mg	1,296	*Sodium, mg	1,043
Saturated fat, % kcals	8	Saturated fat, % kcals	8
Cholesterol, mg	148	Cholesterol, mg	117
Protein, % kcals	20	Protein, % kcals	21

1,600: 100% RDA net for all nutrients except zinc 95%, iron 87%, and calcium 93%.
1,200: 100% RDA net for all nutrients except vitamin E 75%, calcium 84%, magnesium 98%, iron 66%, and zinc 77%.
*No salt added in recipe preparation or as seasoning. Consume at least 32 ounces of water.
Kcal = kilo calorie.

SOURCE: "Appendix D. Sample Reduced Calorie Menus: Asian American Cuisine—Reduced Calorie," in *The Practical Guide: Identification, Evaluation, and Treatment of Overweight and Obesity in Adults*, National Institutes of Health, National Heart, Lung, and Blood Institute, North American Association for the Study of Obesity, October 2000, http://www.nhlbi.nih.gov/guidelines/obesity/prctgd_b.pdf (accessed October 19, 2015)

substitutions, many fat-free or low-fat food products are available—from fat-free frozen desserts to reduced-fat peanut butter. Dieters, however, are cautioned that fat-free or reduced-fat foods are not calorie-free and that their consumption will not result in weight loss when more of the reduced-fat foods are consumed than would be eaten of the full-fat versions. For example, eating twice as many baked tortilla chips would actually result in higher caloric intake than a single serving of regular tortilla chips. (See Table 5.13.)

Low-Fat versus Low-Carbohydrate Diets

In the absence of rigorous scientific research and studies demonstrating the long-term safety and effectiveness of low-carbohydrate and low-fat diets, many investigators and health professionals hesitate to proclaim one

TABLE 5.9

Sample reduced calorie menus, Mexican American cuisine

	1,600 calories	1,200 calories
Breakfast		
• Cantaloupe	1 cup	1/2 cup
• Farina, prepared with 1% low fat milk	1/2 cup	1/2 cup
• White bread	1 slice	1 slice
• Margarine	1 tsp	1 tsp
• Jelly	1 tsp	1 tsp
• Orange juice	1 1/2 cup	3/4 cup
• Milk, 1%, low fat	1/2 cup	1/2 cup
Lunch		
• Beef enchilada:		
Tortilla, corn	2 tortillas	2 tortillas
Lean roast beef	2 1/2 oz	2 oz
Vegetable oil	2/3 tsp	2/3 tsp
Onion	1 T	1 T
Tomato	4 T	4 T
Lettuce	1/2 cup	1/2 cup
Chili peppers	2 tsp	2 tsp
Refried beans, prepared with vegetable oil	1/4 cup	1/4 cup
• Carrots	5 sticks	5 sticks
• Celery	6 sticks	6 sticks
• Milk, 1%, low fat	1/2 cup	—
• Water	—	1 cup
Dinner		
• Chicken taco:		
Tortilla, corn	1 tortilla	1 tortilla
Chicken breast, without skin	2 oz	1 oz
Vegetable oil	2/3 tsp	2/3 tsp
Cheddar cheese, low fat and low sodium	1 oz	1/2 oz
Guacamole	2 T	2 T
Salsa	1 T	1 T
• Corn, seasoned with	1/2 cup	1/2 cup
margarine	1/2 tsp	—
• Spanish rice without meat	1/2 cup	1/2 cup
• Banana	1 large	1/2 large
• Coffee	1 cup	1/2 cup
• Milk, 1%	1 oz	1 oz

Calories	1,638	Calories	1,239
Total carbohydrate, % kcals	56	Total carbohydrate, % kcals	58
Total fat, % kcals	27	Total fat, % kcals	26
*Sodium, mg	1,616	*Sodium, mg	1,364
Saturated fat, % kcals	9	Saturated fat, % kcals	8
Cholesterol, mg	153	Cholesterol, mg	91
Protein, % kcals	20	Protein, % kcals	19

1,600: 100% RDA met for all nutrients except vitamin in E 97% and zinc 84%.
1,200: 100% RDNA met for all nutrients except vitamin E 71%, vitamin B₁ & B₃ 91%, vitamin B₂ & iron 90%, and calcium 92%.
*No salt in recipe preparation or as seasoning. Consume at least 32 ounces of water.
Kcal = kilo calorie.

SOURCE: "Appendix D. Sample Reduced Calorie Menus: Mexican American Cuisine—Reduced Calorie," in *The Practical Guide: Identification, Evaluation, and Treatment of Overweight and Obesity in Adults*, National Institutes of Health, National Heart, Lung, and Blood Institute, North American Association for the Study of Obesity, October 2000, http://www.nhlbi.nih.gov/guidelines/obesity/prctgd_b.pdf (accessed October 19, 2015)

TABLE 5.10

Sample reduced calorie menus, lacto-ovo vegetarian cuisine

	1,600 calories	1,200 calories
Breakfast		
• Orange	1 medium	1 medium
• Pancakes, made with 1% lowfat milk and egg whites	3 4" circles	2 4" circles
• Pancake syrup	2 T	1 T
• Margarine, diet	1 1/2 tsp	1 1/2 tsp
• Milk, 1%, lowfat	1 cup	1/2 cup
• Coffee	1 cup	1 cup
• Milk, 1%, lowfat	1 oz	1 oz
Lunch		
• Vegetable soup, canned, low sodium	1 cup	1/2 cup
• Bagel	1 medium	1/2 medium
• Processed American cheese, lowfat	3/4 oz	—
• Spinach salad:		
Spinach	1 cup	1 cup
Mushrooms	1/2 cup	1/2 cup
• Salad dressing, regular calorie	2 tsp	2 tsp
• Apple	1 medium	1 medium
• Iced tea, unsweetened	1 cup	1 cup
Dinner		
• Omelette:		
Egg whites	4 large eggs	4 large eggs
Green pepper	2 T	2 T
Onion	2 T	2 T
Mozzarella cheese, made from part skim milk, low sodium	1 oz	1/2 oz
Vegetable oil	1 T	1/2 T
• Brown rice, seasoned with	1/2 cup	1/2 cup
margarine, diet	1/2 tsp	1/2 tsp
• Carrots, seasoned with	1/2 cup	1/2 cup
Margarine, diet	1/2 tsp	1/2 tsp
• Whole wheat bread	1 slice	1 slice
• Margarine, diet	1 tsp	1 tsp
• Fig bar cookie	1 bar	1 bar
• Tea	1 cup	1 cup
• Honey	1 tsp	1 tsp
• Milk, 1%, lowfat	3/4 cup	3/4 cup

Calories	1,650	Calories	1,205
Total carbohydrate, % kcals	56	Total carbohydrate, % kcals	60
Total fat, % kcals	27	Total fat, % kcals	25
*Sodium, mg	1,829	*Sodium, mg	1,335
Saturated fat, % kcals	8	Saturated fat, % kcals	7
Cholesterol, mg	82	Cholesterol, mg	44
Protein, % kcals	19	Protein, % kcals	18

1,600: 100% RDA met for all nutrients except vitamin E 92%, vitamin B₃ 97%, vitamin B₆ 67%, iron 73%, and zinc 68%.
1,200: 100% RDA met for all nutrients except vitamin E 75%, vitamin B₁ 92%, vitamin B₃ 69%, vitamin B₆ 59%, iron 54%, and zinc 46%.
*No salt added in recipe preparation or as seasoning. Consume at least 32 ounces of water.
Kcal = kilo calorie.

SOURCE: "Appendix D. Sample Reduced Calorie Menus: Lacto-Ovo Vegetarian Cuisine—Reduced Calorie," in *The Practical Guide: Identification, Evaluation, and Treatment of Overweight and Obesity in Adults*, National Institutes of Health, National Heart, Lung, and Blood Institute, North American Association for the Study of Obesity, October 2000, http://www.nhlbi.nih.gov/guidelines/obesity/prctgd_b.pdf (accessed October 19, 2015)

diet's superiority over all others. Nevertheless, there is consensus that although some diets may produce greater initial weight loss, most perform similarly over time, and that the best predictor of successful weight loss is adherence to a diet.

In "Dietary Intervention for Overweight and Obese Adults: Comparison of Low-Carbohydrate and Low-Fat Diets. A Meta-analysis" (*PLoS One*, vol. 10, no. 10, October 20, 2015), Jonathan Sackner-Bernstein, David Kanter, and Sanjay Kaul present the results of a meta-analysis of 1,797 patients in 17 trials that found that although both diets are effective in reducing weight, low-carbohydrate diets produced more weight loss and less cardiovascular risk than low-fat diets.

TABLE 5.11

Food exchange list

Within each group, these foods can be exchanged for each other. You can use this list to give yourself more choices.

Vegetables contain 25 calories and 5 grams of carbohydrate. One serving equals:
- 1/2 cup   Cooked vegetables (carrots, broccoli, zucchini, cabbage, etc.)
- 1 cup   Raw vegetables or salad greens
- 1/2 cup   Vegetable juice

If you're hungry, eat more fresh or steamed vegetables.

Fat free and very low fat milk contains 90 calories and 12 grams of carbohydrate per serving. One serving equals:
- 8 oz   Milk, fat free or 1% fat
- 1/4 cup   Yogurt, plain nonfat or low fat
- 1 cup   Yogurt, artificially sweetened

Very lean protein choices have 35 calories and 1 gram of fat per serving. One serving equals:
- 1 oz   Turkey breast or chicken breast, skin removed
- 1 oz   Fish fillet (flounder, sole, scrod, cod, haddock, halibut)
- 1 oz   Canned tuna in water
- 1 oz   Shellfish (clams, lobster, scallop, shrimp)
- 3/4 cup   Cottage cheese, nonfat or lowfat
- 2 each   Egg whites
- 1/4 cup   Egg substitute
- 1 oz   Fat free cheese
- 1/2 cup   Beans—cooked (black beans, kidney, chickpeas, or lentils): count as 1 starch/bread and 1 very lean protein

Medium fat proteins have 75 calories and 5 grams of fat per serving. One serving equals:
- 1 oz   Beef (any prime cut), corned beef, ground beef**
- 1 oz   Pork chop
- 1 each   Whole egg (medium)**
- 1 oz   Mozzarella cheese
- 1/4 cup   Ricotta cheese
- 4 oz   Tofu (note that this is a heart-healthy choice)

**Choose these very infrequently.

Fats contain 45 calories and 5 grams of fat per serving. One serving equals:
- 1 tsp   Oil (vegetable, corn, canola, olive, etc.)
- 1 tsp   Butter
- 1 tsp   Stick margarine
- 1 tsp   Mayonnaise
- 1 T   Reduced fat margarine or mayonnaise
- 1 T   Salad dressing
- 1 T   Cream cheese
- 2 T   Lite cream cheese
- 1/8   Avocado
- 8 large   Black olives
- 10 large   Stuffed green olives
- 1 slice   Bacon

Fruits contain 15 grams of carbohydrates and 60 calories. One serving equals:
- 1 small   Apple, banana, orange, nectarine
- 1 medium   Fresh peach
- 1   Kiwi
- 1/2   Grapefruit
- 1/2   Mango
- 1 cup   Fresh berries (strawberries, raspberries, or blueberries)
- 1 cup   Fresh melon cubes
- 1/8   Honeydew melon
- 4 oz   Unsweetened juice
- 4 tsp   Jelly or jam

Lean protein choices have 55 calories and 2 to 3 grams of fat per serving. One serving equals:
- 1 oz   Chicken—dark meat, skin removed
- 1 oz   Turkey—dark meat, skin removed
- 1 oz   Salmon, swordfish, herring, catfish, trout
- 1 oz   Lean beef (flank steak, London broil, tenderloin, roast beef)*
- 1 oz   Veal, roast, or lean chop*
- 1 oz   Lamb, roast, or lean chop*
- 1 oz   Pork, tenderloin, or fresh ham*
- 1 oz   Lowfat luncheon meats (with 3 grams or less of fat per ounce)
- 1/4 cup   4.5% cottage cheese
- 2 medium   Sardines

*Limit to 1 to 2 times per week.

Starches contain 15 grams of carbohydrate and 80 calories per serving. One serving equals:
- 1 slice   Bread (white, pumpernickel, whole wheat, rye)
- 2 slice   Reduced calorie or "lite" bread
- 1/4 (1 oz)   Bagel (varies)
- 1/2   English muffin
- 1/2   Hamburger bun
- 3/4 cup   Cold cereal
- 1/3 cup   Rice, brown or white—cooked
- 1/3 cup   Barley or couscous—cooked
- 1/3 cup   Legumes (dried beans, peas, or lentils)—cooked
- 1/2 cup   Pasta—cooked
- 1/2 cup   Bulgur—cooked
- 1/2 cup   Corn, sweet potato, or green peas
- 3 oz   Baked sweet or white potato
- 3/4 oz   Pretzels
- 3 cups   Popcorn, hot-air popped or microwave (80-percent light)

SOURCE: "Appendix E. Food Exchange List," in *The Practical Guide: Identification, Evaluation, and Treatment of Overweight and Obesity in Adults*, National Institutes of Health, National Heart, Lung, and Blood Institute, North American Association for the Study of Obesity, October 2000, http://www.nhlbi.nih.gov/files/docs/guidelines/prctgd_c.pdf (accessed October 19, 2015)

Although there is no clear winner in the diet wars, research has demonstrated that low-carbohydrate diets are safe and effective in the short term, but long-term outcomes are still unclear. Some results suggest that higher protein and fat intakes lead to lower total caloric intake by producing earlier satiety, but these diets have not been shown to alter fundamental eating behaviors, nor have they demonstrated, as many of their proponents argue, the ability to modify caloric balance such that weight loss persists when more calories are consumed than expended.

Furthermore, some experts are concerned about low-carbohydrate diets because they are often high in animal protein. Ornish explains in "The Myth of High-Protein Diets" (NYTimes.com, March 23, 2015) that animal protein increases chronic inflammation, which has been implicated in many chronic diseases. He asserts that when fat calories are limited, people lose more body fat than when carbohydrates are restricted. He opines, "An optimal diet for preventing disease is a whole-foods, plant-based diet that is naturally low in animal protein, harmful fats and refined carbohydrates. What that means in practice is little or no red meat; mostly vegetables, fruits, whole grains, legumes and soy products in their natural forms; very few simple and refined carbohydrates such as sugar and white

TABLE 5.12

Low-calorie, low-fat food alternatives

Instead of...		Replace with...
• Evaporated whole milk		• Evaporated fat free (skim) or reduced fat (2%) milk
• Whole milk		• Low fat (1%), reduced fat (2%), or fat free (skim) milk
• Ice cream		• Sorbet, sherbet, lowfat or fat free frozen yogurt, or ice milk (check label for calorie content)
• Whipping cream		• Imitation whipped cream (made with fat free [skim] milk) or lowfat vanilla yogurt
• Sour cream		• Plain lowfat yogurt
• Cream cheese	**Dairy**	• Neufchatel or "light" cream cheese or fat free cream cheese
• Cheese (cheddar, Swiss, jack)	**Products**	• Reduced calorie cheese, low calorie processed cheese, etc.
		• Fat free cheese
• American cheese		• Fat free American cheese or other types of fat free cheeses
• Regular (4%) cottage cheese		• Lowfat (1%) or reduced fat (2%) cottage cheese
• Whole milk mozzarella cheese		• Part skim low-moisture mozzarella cheese
• Whole milk ricotta cheese		• Part skim milk ricotta cheese
• Coffee cream (half and half) or nondairy creamer (liquid, power)		• Low fat (1%) or reduced fat (2%) milk or nonfat dry milk power
• Ramen noodles		• Rice or noodles (spaghetti, macaroni, etc.)
• Pasta with white sauce (alfredo)	**Cereals, grains**	• Pasta with red sauce (marinara)
• Pasta with cheese sauce	**and pasta**	• Pasta with vegetables (primavera)
• Granola		• Bran flakes, crispy rice, etc.
		• Cooked grits or oatmeal
		• Whole grains (e.g., couscous, barley, bulgur, etc.)
		• Reduced fat granola
• Cold cuts or lunch meats (bologna, salami, liverwurst, etc.)		• Lowfat cold cuts (95% to 97% fat free lunch meats, lowfat pressed meats)
• Hot dogs (regular)		• Lower fat hot dogs
• Bacon or sausage		• Canadian bacon or lean ham
• Regular ground beef		• Extra lean ground beef such as ground round or ground turkey (read labels)
• Chicken or turkey with skin, duck, or goose		• Chicken or turkey without skin (white meat)
• Oil-packed tuna		• Water-packed tuna (rinse to reduce sodium content)
• Beef (chuck, rib, brisket)	**Meat, fish,**	• Beef (round, loin) (trimmed of external fat) (choose select grades)
• Pork (spareribs, untrimmed loin)	**and poultry**	• Pork tenderloin or trimmed, lean smoked ham
• Frozen breaded fish or fried fish (homemade or commercial)		• Fish or shellfish, unbreaded (fresh, frozen, canned in water)
• Whole eggs		• Egg whites or egg substitutes
• Frozen TV dinners (containing more than 13 gram of fat per serving)		• Frozen TV dinners (containing less than 13 grams of fat per serving and lower in sodium)
• Chorizo sausage		• Turkey sausage, drained well (read label)
		• Vegetarian sausage (made with tofu)
• Croissants, brioches, etc.		• Hard French rolls or soft "brown 'n serve" rolls
• Donuts, sweet rolls, muffins, scones, or pastries		• English muffins, bagels, reduced fat or fat free muffins or scones
• Party crackers		• Lowfat crackers (choose lower in sodium)
• Saltine or soda crackers (choose lower in sodium)	**Baked goods**	
• Cake (pound, chocolate, yellow)		• Cake (angel food, white, gingerbread)
• Cookies		• Reduced fat or fat free cookies (graham crackers, ginger snaps, fig bars) (compare calorie level)
• Nuts	**Snacks and**	• Popcorn (air-popped or light microwave), fruits, vegetables
• Ice cream, e.g., cones or bars	**sweets**	• Frozen yogurt, frozen fruit, or chocolate pudding bars
• Custards or puddings (made with whole milk)		• Puddings (made with skim milk)
• Regular margarine or butter		• Light-spread margarines, diet margarine, or whipped butter, tub or squeeze bottle
• Regular mayonnaise		• Light or diet mayonnaise or mustard
• Regular salad dressings	**Fats, oils, and**	• Reduced calorie or fat free salad dressings, lemon juice, or plain, herb-flavored, or wine vinegar
	salad dressings	
• Butter or margarine on toast or bread		• Jelly, jam, or honey on bread or toast
• Oils, shortening, or lard		• Nonstick cooking spray for stir-frying or sautéing
		• As a substitute for oil or butter, use applesauce or prune puree in baked goods
• Canned cream soups		• Canned broth-based soups
• Canned beans and franks	**Miscellaneous**	• Canned baked beans in tomato sauce
• Gravy (home made with fat and/or milk)		• Gravy mixes made with water or homemade with the fat skimmed off and fat free milk included
• Fudge sauce		• Chocolate syrup
• Avocado on sandwiches		• Cucumber slices or lettuce leaves
• Guacamole dip or refried beans with lard		• Salsa

SOURCE: "Appendix C. Instead of...Replace with...," in *The Practical Guide: Identification, Evaluation, and Treatment of Overweight and Obesity in Adults*, National Institutes of Health, National Heart, Lung, and Blood Institute, North American Association for the Study of Obesity, October 2000, http://www.nhlbi .nih.gov/files/docs/guidelines/prctgd_c.pdf (accessed October 19, 2015)

flour; and sufficient 'good fats' such as fish oil or flax oil, seeds and nuts. A healthful diet should be low in 'bad fats' meaning trans fats, saturated fats and hydrogenated fats. Finally, we need more quality and less quantity."

In "Choosing a Safe and Successful Weight-Loss Program" (December 2012, http://www.niddk.nih.gov/ health-information/health-topics/weight-control/choosing-safe-successful-weight-loss-program/Documents/Choosing program0208.pdf), the National Institute of Diabetes and

TABLE 5.13

Calories in fat-free or reduced-fat and regular food

Fat free or reduced fat	Calories	Regular	Calories
Reduced fat peanut butter, 2 T	187	Regular peanut butter, 2 T	191
Cookies		Cookies	
Reduced fat chocolate chip cookies, 3 cookies (30 g)	118	Regular chocolate chip cookies, 3 cookies (30 g)	142
Fat free fig cookies, 2 cookies (30 g)	102	Regular fig cookies, 2 cookies (30 g)	111
Ice cream		Ice cream	
Nonfat vanilla frozen yogurt (1% fat), 1/2 cup	100	Regular whole milk vanilla frozen yogurt (3–4% fat), 1/2 cup	104
Light vanilla ice cream (7% fat), 1/2 cup	111	Regular vanilla ice cream (11% fat), 1/2 cup	133
Fat free caramel topping, 2 T	103	Caramel topping, homemade with butter, 2 T	103
Low fat granola cereal, approx. 1/2 cup (55 g)	213	Regular granola cereal, approx 1/2 cup (55 g)	257
Low fat blueberry muffin, 1 small (2 1/2 inch)	131	Regular blueberry muffin, 1 small (2 1/2 inch)	138
Baked tortilla chips, 1 oz.	113	Regular tortilla chips, 1 oz.	143
Low fat cereal bar, 1 bar (1.3 oz.)	130	Regular cereal bar, 1 bar (1.3 oz.)	140

SOURCE: "Fat Free or Reduced Fat [versus] Regular," in *The Practical Guide: Identification, Evaluation, and Treatment of Overweight and Obesity in Adults*, National Institutes of Health, National Heart, Lung, and Blood Institute, North American Association for the Study of Obesity, October 2000, http://www.nhlbi .nih.gov/files/docs/guidelines/prctgd_c.pdf (accessed October 19, 2015)

TABLE 5.14

Questions to ask when choosing a weight-loss plan

- Does the program provide counseling to help you change your eating activity and personal habits?
- Is the staff made up of a variety of qualified counselors and health professionals such as nutritionists, registered dietitians, doctors, nurses, psychologists, and exercise physiologists?
- Is training available on how to deal with times when you may feel stressed and slip back to old habits?
- Is attention paid to keeping the weight off? How long is this phase?
- Are food choices flexible and suitable? Are weight goals set by the client and the health professional?
- What percentage of people complete the program?
- What is the average weight loss among people who finish the program?
- What percentage of people have problems or side effects? What are they?
- Are there fees or costs for additional items, such as dietary supplements?

SOURCE: Adapted from "Selecting a Weight-Loss Program—Check It Out: Before You Sign up for Any Weight-Loss Program," in *Aim for a Healthy Weight* National Heart, Lung, and Blood Institute, 2015, https://www.nhlbi .nih.gov/health/educational/lose_wt/wtl_prog.htm (accessed October 19, 2015)

Digestive and Kidney Diseases (NIDDK) offers advice about how to choose a weight-loss program. Besides consulting with a health care provider, the NIDDK recommends considering programs that include ongoing feedback, monitoring, and support as well as a plan for how to maintain weight loss long term. People considering weight-loss programs should also inquire about the credentials of the program and personnel and the costs associated with the program. Table 5.14 lists some of the questions to ask about a weight-loss program.

CHAPTER 6

PHYSICAL ACTIVITY, DRUGS, SURGERY, AND OTHER TREATMENTS FOR OVERWEIGHT AND OBESITY

Lack of activity destroys the good condition of every human being, while movement and methodical physical exercise save it and preserve it.

—Plato

One credible hypothesis about the cause of the epidemic of overweight and obesity in the United States is the progressive decrease in physical activity expended in daily life for work, transportation, and household chores. Some researchers contend that by reducing daily physical activity, the caloric imbalance between calories consumed and expended has shifted to favor weight gain. Although no data conclusively prove this hypothesis, there is some evidence to support it.

Among the studies that support the premise that Americans' sedentary lifestyle has precipitated the obesity epidemic is a landmark study that examined the diets of an Amish community in Ontario, Canada. In "Physical Activity in an Old Order Amish Community" (*Medicine and Science in Sports and Exercise*, vol. 36, no. 1, January 2004), David R. Bassett, Patrick L. Schneider, and Gertrude E. Huntington describe the "Amish paradox"— that despite a diet that is high in fat, calories, and refined sugar, the Amish community had a scant 4% obesity rate, compared with 31% in the general U.S. population. The researchers chose this particular Amish population because it has rejected technological advances such as automobiles and electricity, and its physically demanding lifestyle is comparable to the way Americans lived 150 years ago. (Other Amish communities that have assumed occupations less physically active than farming have obesity rates that are similar to those found in the general U.S. population.) Bassett, Schneider, and Huntington analyzed the daily routines of 98 Amish people and found that the men averaged 18,425 steps per day and the women 14,196 steps per day, compared with the recommended 10,000 steps per day that most Americans do not achieve. The Amish men performed about 10 hours

per week of vigorous exercise, and the women spent 3.4 hours engaged in heavy lifting, shoveling, digging, shoeing horses, or tossing straw bales. The men devoted an additional 42.8 hours per week and the women an average of 39.2 hours to moderate physical activities such as gardening, performing farm-related chores, or doing laundry.

PHYSICAL ACTIVITY

In sharp contrast to the Amish farmers, many Americans are not physically active. In "How Much Physical Activity Do Adults Need?" (June 4, 2015, http://www.cdc.gov/physicalactivity/everyone/guidelines/adults.html), the U.S. Centers for Disease Control and Prevention (CDC) defines the minimum recommended physical activity level for adults as: moderate-intensity aerobic physical activity for 150 minutes every week and muscle-strengthening activities on at least two days per week, or vigorous-intensity physical activity for 75 minutes or more every week and muscle-strengthening activities on at least two days per week. Table 6.1 shows that the percentage of men and women who met the federal guidelines for aerobic and muscle-strengthening exercise increased between 1998 and 2013. In 2013, however, just 21% of Americans obtained the physical activity prescribed by the guidelines. Across all age groups, a lower percentage of women than men met the guidelines.

Table 6.1 shows that the overall percentage of adults who were inactive (meeting neither the aerobic nor the muscle-strengthening activity guidelines) decreased from 56.6% in 1998 to 46.5% in 2013. Inactivity was higher, however, among specific groups. For example, the percentage of inactive adults was higher among non-Hispanic African Americans (54.7%) and Hispanics (53.8%) than among non-Hispanic whites (43.1%). Inactivity declined with increasing education, from 66.6% of people with no high school diploma to 40.6% of those

TABLE 6.1

Participation in leisure-time physical activities that meet federal guidelines for adults, by selected characteristics, selected years 1998–2013

[Data are based on household interviews of a sample of the civilian noninstitutionalized population]

| | 2008 physical activity guidelines for Americans[a] | | | | | | | | | |
| | Met both aerobic activity and muscle-strengthening guidelines | | | | | Met neither aerobic activity nor muscle-strengthening guideline | | | | |
Characteristic	1998	2000	2010	2012	2013	1998	2000	2010	2012	2013
					Percent					
18 years and over, age-adjusted[b, c]	14.3	15.0	20.7	20.8	21.0	56.6	54.7	49.1	46.6	46.5
18 years and over, crude[c]	14.5	15.1	20.4	20.3	20.4	56.3	54.6	49.5	47.1	47.2
Age										
18–44 years	18.9	18.9	25.7	25.7	25.7	50.7	49.1	43.1	41.0	40.3
18–24 years	23.8	23.8	29.6	29.7	30.3	46.5	44.5	39.4	37.9	35.5
25–44 years	17.4	17.3	24.3	24.2	24.0	51.9	50.6	44.4	42.2	42.0
45–64 years	11.4	12.8	17.7	17.2	17.8	58.8	57.6	51.0	49.6	50.2
45–54 years	13.2	14.5	19.2	18.2	20.1	56.9	55.4	48.9	48.3	48.4
55–64 years	8.6	10.1	15.9	16.0	15.3	61.8	61.0	53.7	51.2	52.1
65 years and over	5.5	6.8	10.4	11.9	11.7	71.0	67.0	64.6	58.4	59.4
65–74 years	7.0	8.4	13.6	14.8	14.7	65.6	60.3	59.9	51.7	54.0
75 years and over	3.5	4.9	6.4	7.9	7.6	77.8	75.0	70.3	67.2	66.8
Sex[b]										
Male	17.5	17.9	25.1	24.6	25.0	50.8	49.6	43.8	42.2	42.0
Female	11.4	12.3	16.5	17.1	17.2	61.9	59.4	54.0	50.7	50.7
Sex and age										
Male:										
18–44 years	23.0	23.0	31.8	31.8	31.7	44.3	43.0	37.1	35.9	34.7
45–54 years	16.1	16.0	20.9	18.7	22.3	52.9	52.7	45.2	45.9	46.3
55–64 years	9.4	11.3	19.1	16.8	17.6	58.2	58.7	50.1	49.1	49.6
65–74 years	9.5	9.4	16.6	17.1	15.9	58.9	55.3	55.6	45.9	49.7
75 years and over	4.9	7.1	9.1	10.5	7.8	69.5	66.7	62.8	61.3	60.6
Female:										
18–44 years	14.9	15.0	19.6	19.8	19.8	56.9	55.0	49.0	46.0	45.7
45–54 years	10.5	13.1	17.5	17.7	18.0	60.8	57.9	52.4	50.5	50.5
55–64 years	7.8	9.0	13.1	15.3	13.2	65.0	63.1	57.0	53.2	54.4
65–74 years	5.1	7.7	11.0	12.8	13.6	70.9	64.3	63.6	56.7	57.7
75 years and over	2.6	3.6	4.6	6.2	7.5	83.0	80.0	75.3	71.2	71.0
Race[b, d]										
White only	14.8	15.7	21.4	21.5	21.7	55.2	53.1	47.6	45.4	45.2
Black or African American only	11.7	12.2	17.2	16.8	17.7	65.7	64.6	58.5	55.0	54.7
American Indian or Alaska Native only	16.0	10.6*	12.7*	18.7	16.8	57.6	67.1	54.0	50.8	50.8
Asian only	13.5	14.1	17.8	17.1	18.3	59.1	55.0	51.7	47.8	47.6
Native Hawaiian or other Pacific Islander only	—	*	*	*	*	—	*	*	*	*
2 or more races	—	19.0	25.9	28.7	22.4	—	52.8	45.0	40.5	44.4
Hispanic origin and race[b, d]										
Hispanic or Latino	9.4	9.2	14.4	15.7	16.6	67.7	66.5	60.2	54.5	53.8
Mexican	8.7	8.1	13.2	14.9	15.0	69.5	67.0	60.7	53.8	53.4
Not Hispanic or Latino	14.9	15.8	21.9	21.7	21.9	55.3	53.2	47.2	45.1	45.2
White only	15.5	16.5	22.9	23.0	22.9	53.6	51.4	45.0	43.2	43.1
Black or African American only	11.7	12.2	17.4	16.7	17.8	65.8	64.6	58.4	55.1	54.7
Education[e, f]										
No high school diploma or GED	4.6	4.3	7.7	7.6	8.0	76.3	74.0	69.8	66.3	66.6
High school diploma or GED	8.6	9.5	12.7	12.4	13.8	64.6	61.7	59.0	57.4	57.0
Some college or more	18.2	18.9	25.0	24.9	24.4	48.0	47.1	42.1	39.7	40.6
Percent of poverty level[b, g]										
Below 100%	8.0	9.3	12.0	11.6	12.6	71.3	68.0	63.9	60.5	59.5
100%–199%	9.0	9.0	12.7	14.5	14.3	67.1	65.5	60.6	56.3	56.7
200%–399%	12.6	13.2	19.2	18.8	19.2	58.0	56.8	50.6	47.9	48.0
400% or more	20.2	20.5	29.1	29.4	29.1	46.2	45.0	36.9	35.5	35.6
Hispanic origin and race and percent of poverty level[b, d, g]										
Hispanic or Latino:										
Below 100%	4.6	4.4	8.9	9.6	8.7	78.0	75.2	68.6	64.6	65.1
100%–199%	7.0	5.0	9.3	12.2	12.2	71.2	72.2	66.7	59.3	60.1
200%–399%	11.1	10.2	15.7	17.7	20.6	63.8	63.1	57.6	51.6	48.5
400% or more	17.4	19.6	28.1	29.1	27.6	55.6	52.8	42.5	37.2	39.5

TABLE 6.1

Participation in leisure-time physical activities that meet federal guidelines for adults, by selected characteristics, selected years 1998–2013 [CONTINUED]

[Data are based on household interviews of a sample of the civilian noninstitutionalized population]

	2008 physical activity guidelines for Americans[a]									
	Met both aerobic activity and muscle-strengthening guidelines					Met neither aerobic activity nor muscle-strengthening guideline				
Characteristic	1998	2000	2010	2012	2013	1998	2000	2010	2012	2013
	Percent									
Not Hispanic or Latino:										
White only:										
Below 100%	9.9	11.7	13.7	14.2	14.9	66.9	63.5	60.5	56.9	56.2
100%–199%	9.6	10.3	14.1	16.5	15.7	65.1	62.6	56.4	53.7	53.8
200%–399%	13.1	13.9	20.0	19.0	19.0	56.1	54.7	48.6	46.7	46.8
400% or more	20.2	21.0	29.9	30.2	30.0	45.2	43.7	35.2	34.0	33.9
Black or African American only:										
Below 100%	7.1	9.5	11.3	8.2	11.6	74.6	72.1	66.9	64.6	63.5
100%–199%	8.8	9.5	11.7	12.7	13.8	69.8	69.2	67.0	59.2	62.0
200%–399%	10.6	11.8	20.8	17.9	17.1	64.5	64.3	53.3	53.6	52.7
400% or more	21.2	17.6	26.1	28.8	28.5	54.2	54.9	47.7	43.0	39.4
Disability measure[b, h]										
Any basic actions difficulty or complex activity limitation	10.2	10.3	13.6	14.1	14.1	64.4	62.2	59.1	57.3	56.9
Any basic actions difficulty	9.8	10.3	13.8	14.0	13.8	64.8	62.1	59.2	57.8	57.3
Any complex activity limitation	7.7	7.2	8.9	10.0	10.8	71.9	71.2	67.2	65.4	65.1
No disability	16.0	17.0	24.2	23.9	24.2	52.5	50.6	43.3	40.7	40.2
Geographic region[b]										
Northeast	14.2	17.0	20.2	20.6	22.2	57.0	51.8	49.1	48.7	47.1
Midwest	15.0	16.4	20.7	21.7	21.7	54.9	53.4	49.7	47.0	46.3
South	11.8	12.1	18.8	18.7	18.2	61.4	59.7	51.8	49.9	49.5
West	18.5	16.7	24.0	23.3	23.7	49.5	50.1	44.5	39.3	41.5
Location of residence[b, i]										
Within MSA	14.9	15.7	21.8	22.0	21.9	55.8	54.1	47.8	44.8	45.3
Outside MSA	12.2	12.3	14.5	13.7	15.7	59.7	56.9	56.9	56.2	53.5

—Data not available.

*Estimates are considered unreliable.

[a]Starting with *Health, United States, 2010*, measures of physical activity shown in this table changed to reflect the federal *2008 Physical Activity Guidelines for Americans*. This table presents four measures of physical activity that are of interest to the public health community: the percentage of adults who met the federal 2008 guidelines for both aerobic activity and muscle strengthening; the percentage who met neither the aerobic activity guideline nor the muscle-strengthening guideline; the percentage who met the aerobic activity guideline; and the percentage who met the muscle-strengthening guideline. Persons who met neither the aerobic activity nor the muscle-strengthening guideline were unable to be active, were completely inactive, or had some aerobic or muscle-strengthening activities but amounts were insufficient to meet the guidelines. The percentage of persons who met the aerobic activity guideline includes those who may or may not have also met the muscle-strengthening guideline. Similarly, the percentage of persons who met the muscle-strengthening guideline includes those who may or may not have also met the aerobic activity guideline. The federal 2008 guidelines recommend that for substantial health benefits adults perform at least 150 minutes (2 hours and 30 minutes) a week of moderate-intensity, or 75 minutes (1 hour and 15 minutes) a week of vigorous-intensity aerobic physical activity, or an equivalent combination of moderate- and vigorous-intensity aerobic activity. Aerobic activity should be performed in episodes of at least 10 minutes, and preferably should be spread throughout the week. The 2008 guidelines also recommend that adults perform muscle-strengthening activities that are moderate or high intensity and involve all major muscle groups on 2 or more days a week, because these activities provide additional health benefits.

[b]Estimates are age-adjusted to the year 2000 standard population using five age groups: 18–44 years, 45–54 years, 55–64 years, 65–74 years, and 75 years and over. Age-adjusted estimates in this table may differ from other age-adjusted estimates based on the same data and presented elsewhere if different age groups are used in the adjustment procedure.

[c]Includes all other races not shown separately, unknown education level, and unknown disability status.

[d]The race groups, white, black, American Indian or Alaska Native, Asian, Native Hawaiian or Other Pacific Islander, and 2 or more races, include persons of Hispanic and non-Hispanic origin. Persons of Hispanic origin may be of any race. Starting with 1999 data, race-specific estimates are tabulated according to the 1997 *Revisions to the Standards for the Classification of Federal Data on Race and Ethnicity* and are not strictly comparable with estimates for earlier years. The five single-race categories shown in the table conform to the 1997 Standards. Starting with 1999 data, race-specific estimates are for persons who reported only one racial group; the category 2 or more races includes persons who reported more than one racial group. Prior to 1999, data were tabulated according to the 1977 Standards with four racial groups, and the Asian only category included Native Hawaiian or Other Pacific Islander. Estimates for single-race categories prior to 1999 included persons who reported one race or, if they reported more than one race, identified one race as best representing their race. Starting with 2003 data, race responses of other race and unspecified multiple race were treated as missing, and then race was imputed if these were the only race responses. Almost all persons with a race response of other race were of Hispanic origin.

[e]Estimates are for persons aged 25 and over and are age-adjusted to the year 2000 standard population using five age groups: 25–44 years, 45–54 years, 55–64 years, 65–74 years, and 75 years and over.

[f]GED is General Educational Development high school equivalency diploma.

[g]Percent of poverty level is based on family income and family size and composition using U.S. Census Bureau poverty thresholds. Missing family income data were imputed for 1997 and beyond.

[h]Any basic actions difficulty or complex activity limitation is defined as having one or more of the following limitations or difficulties: movement difficulty, emotional difficulty, sensory (seeing or hearing) difficulty, cognitive difficulty, self-care (activities of daily living or instrumental activities of daily living) limitation, social limitation, or work limitation. Starting with 2007 data, the hearing question, a component of the basic actions difficulty measure, was revised. Consequently, data prior to 2007 are not comparable with data for 2007 and beyond.

[i]MSA is metropolitan statistical area. Starting with 2006 data, MSA status is determined using 2000 census data and the 2000 standards for defining MSAs.

SOURCE: Adapted from "Table 63. Participation in Leisure-Time Aerobic and Muscle-Strengthening Activities That Meet the Federal 2008 *Physical Activity Guidelines for Americans* among Adults Aged 18 Years and over, by Selected Characteristics: United States, Selected Years 1998–2013," in *Health, United States, 2014: With Special Feature on Adults Aged 55–64*, Centers for Disease Control and Prevention, National Center for Health Statistics, May 2015, http://www.cdc.gov/nchs/data/hus/hus14.pdf (accessed October 5, 2015).

with at least some college. Similarly, inactivity declined with increasing income: 59.5% of people at or below poverty level income were inactive, compared with 35.6% of people whose incomes were 400% or more above the poverty level.

Figure 6.1 shows that whereas men were more likely than women to report regularly engaging in leisure-time physical activity across all age groups in early 2015, the difference was relatively small among people aged 25 to 64 years. In early 2015 non-Hispanic white adults (51.3%) were more likely than non-Hispanic African American adults (38.7%) or Hispanic adults (41.3%) to report having participated in sufficient leisure-time physical activity to meet the federal guidelines. (See Figure 6.2.)

Physical Activity and Weight Loss

Increasing physical activity and exercise is an important element of weight-loss regimens, although the addition of exercise to a diet program generally does not produce substantially greater weight loss—most of the weight that is lost is attributable to decreased caloric intake. By favorably affecting blood lipids, increased and sustained physical activity does offer many direct and indirect health benefits, including reducing risks for cardiovascular heart disease and type 2 diabetes beyond the risk reduction possible through diet alone. Physical activity lowers low-density lipoprotein (LDL) cholesterol ("bad cholesterol") and triglycerides, increases high-density lipoprotein (HDL) cholesterol ("good cholesterol"), reduces abdominal fat, and may protect against a decrease in muscle mass during weight loss.

Like those who have been inactive or sedentary, overweight people are advised to initiate physical activity slowly and gradually. Walking and swimming at a slow pace are ideal activities because they are enjoyable, easy to schedule, and less likely than many competitive sports to produce injuries. Table 6.2 presents an example of a walking program that progressively increases physical

FIGURE 6.1

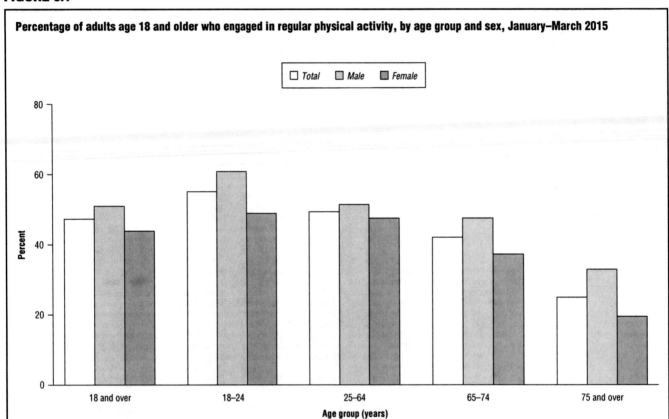

Percentage of adults age 18 and older who engaged in regular physical activity, by age group and sex, January–March 2015

Notes: Data are based on household interviews of a sample of the civilian noninstitutionalized population. Estimates in this figure are limited to leisure-time physical activity only. This measure reflects an estimate of leisure-time aerobic activity motivated by the 2008 federal Physical Activity Guidelines for Americans, which are being used for Healthy People 2020 Objectives (3). The 2008 guidelines refer to any kind of aerobic activity, not just leisure-time aerobic activity, so the leisure-time aerobic activity estimates in this figure may underestimate the percentage of adults who met the 2008 guidelines for aerobic activity. This figure presents the percentage of adults who met the 2008 federal guidelines for aerobic activity. The 2008 federal guidelines recommend that for substantial health benefits, adults perform at least 150 minutes a week of moderate-intensity aerobic physical activity, or 75 minutes a week of vigorous-intensity aerobic physical activity, or an equivalent combination of moderate- and vigorous-intensity aerobic activity. The 2008 guidelines state that aerobic activity should be performed in episodes of at least 10 minutes and preferably should be spread throughout the week. The analyses excluded the 1.5% of persons with unknown physical activity participation.

SOURCE: Tainya C. Clarke et al., "Figure 7.2. Percentage of Adults Aged 18 and over Who Met the 2008 Federal Physical Activity Guidelines for Aerobic Activity through Leisure-Time Aerobic Activity, by Age Group and Sex: United States, January–March 2015," in *Early Release of Selected Estimates Based on Data from the January–March 2015 National Health Interview Survey*, Centers for Disease Control and Prevention, National Center for Health Statistics, September 2015, http://www.cdc.gov/nchs/data/nhis/earlyrelease/earlyrelease201509_07.pdf (accessed October 19, 2015)

FIGURE 6.2

Percentage of adults aged 18 and older who engaged in regular physical activity, by race/ethnicity, January–March 2015

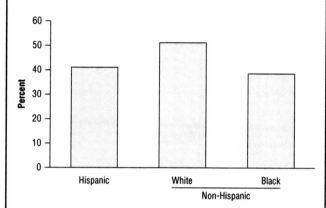

Notes: Data are based on household interviews of a sample of the civilian noninstitutionalized population. Estimates in this figure are limited to leisure-time physical activity only. This measure reflects an estimate of leisure-time aerobic activity motivated by the 2008 federal Physical Activity Guidelines for Americans, which are being used for Healthy People 2020 Objectives (3). The 2008 guidelines refer to any kind of aerobic activity, not just leisure-time aerobic activity, so the leisure-time aerobic activity estimates in this figure may underestimate the percentage of adults who met the 2008 guidelines for aerobic activity. This figure presents the percentage of adults who met the 2008 federal guidelines for aerobic activity. The 2008 federal guidelines recommend that for substantial health benefits, adults perform at least 150 minutes a week of moderate-intensity aerobic physical activity, or 75 minutes a week of vigorous-intensity aerobic physical activity, or an equivalent combination of moderate- and vigorous-intensity aerobic activity. The 2008 guidelines state that aerobic activity should be performed in episodes of at least 10 minutes and preferably should be spread throughout the week. The analyses excluded the 1.5% of persons with unknown physical activity participation. Estimates are age-sex-adjusted using the projected 2000 U.S. population as the standard population and using five age groups: 18–24, 25–34, 35–44, 45–64, and 65 and over.

SOURCE: Tainya C. Clarke et al., "Figure 7.3. Age-Sex-Adjusted Percentage of Adults Aged 18 and over Who Met the 2008 Federal Physical Activity Guidelines for Aerobic Activity through Leisure-Time Aerobic Activity, by Race/Ethnicity: United States, January–March 2015," in *Early Release of Selected Estimates Based on Data from the January–March 2015 National Health Interview Survey*, Centers for Disease Control and Prevention, National Center for Health Statistics, September 2015, http://www.cdc.gov/nchs/data/nhis/earlyrelease/earlyrelease201509_07.pdf (accessed October 19, 2015)

activity. Furthermore, because the amounts of activity and the resulting health benefits are functions of the duration, intensity, and frequency of the activity, the same health benefits can be obtained through long sessions of moderately intense activity, such as brisk walking, as in shorter sessions of more strenuous activity, such as running. Table 6.3 shows how a moderate amount of activity (physical activity that uses about 150 calories of energy per day for a total of about 1,000 calories per week) can be obtained in a variety of ways. The table also indicates how performing common household chores, and even self-care activities such as using a wheelchair, may be used to fulfill requirements for moderate amounts of physical activity. Changing routines to include walking up stairs rather than taking an elevator or parking farther than usual from work or school are ways to increase physical activity incrementally. Even reducing sedentary

TABLE 6.2

A sample walking program

	Warm up	Exercising	Cool down	Total time
Week 1				
Session A	Walk 5 min.	Then walk briskly 5 min.	Then walk more slowly 5 min.	15 min.
Session B	Repeat above pattern			
Session C	Repeat above pattern			

Continue with at least three exercise sessions during each week of the program.

	Warm up	Exercising	Cool down	Total time
Week 2	Walk 5 min.	Walk briskly 7 min.	Walk 5 min.	17 min.
Week 3	Walk 5 min.	Walk briskly 9 min.	Walk 5 min.	19 min.
Week 4	Walk 5 min.	Walk briskly 11 min.	Walk 5 min.	21 min.
Week 5	Walk 5 min.	Walk briskly 13 min.	Walk 5 min.	23 min.
Week 6	Walk 5 min.	Walk briskly 15 min.	Walk 5 min.	25 min.
Week 7	Walk 5 min.	Walk briskly 18 min.	Walk 5 min.	28 min.
Week 8	Walk 5 min.	Walk briskly 20 min.	Walk 5 min.	30 min.
Week 9	Walk 5 min.	Walk briskly 23 min.	Walk 5 min.	33 min.
Week 10	Walk 5 min.	Walk briskly 26 min.	Walk 5 min.	36 min.
Week 11	Walk 5 min.	Walk briskly 28 min.	Walk 5 min.	38 min.
Week 12	Walk 5 min.	Walk briskly 30 min.	Walk 5 min.	40 min.

Week 13 on: Gradually increase your brisk walking time to 30 to 60 minutes, three or four times a week. Remember that your goal is to get the benefits you are seeking and enjoy your activity.

SOURCE: "A Sample Walking Program," in *The Practical Guide: Identification, Evaluation, and Treatment of Overweight and Obesity in Adults*, National Institutes of Health, National Heart, Lung, and Blood Institute, North American Association for the Study of Obesity, October 2000, http://www.nhlbi.nih.gov/files/docs/guidelines/prctgd_c.pdf (accessed October 19, 2015)

time, such as hours spent in front of the television or computer, can serve to increase energy expenditure.

Table 6.3 also shows the relationship between the intensity and duration of physical activities by comparing the amount of time an adult must spend performing each activity to expend 150 calories. It is interesting to note that just five additional minutes of walking at a moderate pace expends the same number of calories as walking at a brisk pace.

In "Weight Loss, Exercise or Both and Cardiometabolic Risk Factors in Obese Older Adults: Results of a Randomized Controlled Trial" (*International Journal of Obesity*, vol. 38, no. 3, March 2014), Matthew F. Bouchonville et al. examine the effects of exercise on weight loss and cardiovascular risk factors. The researchers assigned 107 obese subjects to one of three regimes: diet only, diet and exercise, or a control group. Bouchonville et al. find that body weight decreased similarly in the diet and exercise and the diet alone groups. However, subjects in the diet and exercise group had improved insulin sensitivity and the presence of metabolic syndrome decreased 40% in the diet and exercise group compared with 15% in the diet alone group.

Donal J. O'Gorman and Anna Krook observe in "Exercise and the Treatment of Diabetes and Obesity" (*Medical Clinics of North America*, vol. 95, no. 5, September 2011) that there is a significant dose-response to the effect of exercise and that recommendations such as the minimum

TABLE 6.3

Examples of moderate amounts of physical activity

Common chores	Sporting activities	
Washing and waxing a car for 45–60 minutes	Playing volleyball for 45–60 minutes	**Less vigorous more time***
Washing windows or floors for 45–60 minutes	Playing touch football for 45 minutes	
Gardening for 30–45 minutes	Walking 1 3/4 miles in 35 minutes (20 min/mile)	
Wheeling self in wheelchair for 30–40 minutes	Basketball (shooting baskets) for 30 minutes	
Pushing a stroller 1 1/2 miles in 30 minutes	Bicycling 5 miles in 30 minutes	
Raking leaves for 30 minutes	Dancing fast (social) for 30 minutes	
Walking 2 miles in 30 minutes (15 min/mile)	Water aerobics for 30 minutes	
Shoveling snow for 15 minutes	Swimming laps for 20 minutes	
Stairwalking for 15 minutes	Basketball (playing a game) for 15–20 minutes	
	Jumping rope for 15 minutes	**More vigorous, less time**
	Running 1 1/2 miles in 15 minutes	

Note: A moderate amount of physical activity is roughly equivalent to physical activity that uses approximately 150 calories of energy per day, or 1,000 calories per week.
*Some activities can be performed at various intensities; the suggested durations correspond to expected intensity of effort.

SOURCE: "Appendix H. Examples of Moderate Amounts of Physical Activity," in *The Practical Guide: Identification, Evaluation, and Treatment of Overweight and Obesity in Adults*, National Institutes of Health, National Heart, Lung, and Blood Institute, North American Association for the Study of Obesity, October 2000, http://www.nhlbi.nih.gov/files/docs/guidelines/prctgd_c.pdf (accessed October 19, 2015)

amount of physical activity needed to maintain or improve cardiovascular health are not sufficient to prevent weight gain or promote weight loss. The researchers suggest that exercise recommendations for people seeking to lose weight may have to be revised upward to achieve these objectives. O'Gorman and Krook also reiterate that "exercise by itself exerts clinically beneficial effects in both lean and obese subjects, even in the absence of effects on weight—it exerts an effect on metabolism and changes in gene expression (regulation of the process by which the heritable effects of a gene are displayed)."

O'Gorman and Krook assert that there has been relatively little rigorous research to evaluate the effect of exercise on weight loss. Many studies call for about 150 minutes of exercise per week, or 30 minutes of physical activity on all or most days of the week. O'Gorman and Krook observe that this amount of exercise is only equivalent to a 150- to 200-calorie energy expenditure per day or about 700 to 1,000 calories per week. As such, it is not surprising that this level of exercise does not compare favorably in terms of weight loss with diets that result in a 500-calorie-per-day reduction, or about 3,500 calories per week. O'Gorman and Krook report that there have been just two studies that matched the energy expenditure of exercise with that of a calorie-restricted diet. When exercise and diet both resulted in a deficit of 500 or 700 calories per day, both regimens produced comparable weight loss. O'Gorman and Krook conclude that "exercise is an effective weight-loss strategy but the accumulated energy expenditure required for weight reduction may be greater than the general recommendations."

Although exercise is a key component of weight-loss and weight-maintenance, it cannot offset the effects of an unhealthy diet. In "It Is Time to Bust the Myth of Physical Inactivity and Obesity: You Cannot Outrun a Bad Diet" (*British Journal of Sports Medicine*, vol. 49,

no. 15, August 2015), Aseem Malhotra, Timothy D. Noakes, and Stephen D. Phinney assert that because there has been little change in physical activity levels over the past 30 years and obesity rates have escalated, poor diets must be responsible. Malhotra, Noakes, and Phinney also contend that the message, "all calories count" promoted by the Coca-Cola Company, is misleading because calories from sugar stimulate hunger and promote fat storage, whereas calories from fat induce satiety. The authors conclude, "It is time to wind back the harms caused by the junk food industry's public relations machinery. Let us bust the myth of physical inactivity and obesity. You cannot outrun a bad diet."

EXERCISE MAY COUNTER GENES THAT INCREASE THE RISK OF OBESITY. A gene variant known as FTO (fat mass and obesity associated) is known to increase the risk of obesity by 20% to 30%. In "Influence of Physical Activity on the Association between the FTO Variant rs9939609 and Adiposity in Young Adults" (*American Journal of Human Biology*, vol. 27, no. 5, September 2015), Magdalena Muc, Cristina Padez, and Licino Manco confirm the results of earlier research, finding that physical activity modifies or reduces the risk that is associated with the FTO gene. The researchers find that in more physically active people, there is no significant association of the FTO variant with overweight/obesity. Physical activity may be an effective way of controlling body weight in individuals with a genetic predisposition toward obesity.

MEDICATION

Pharmacotherapy for weight loss involves the use of drugs as one of several strategies including diet, physical activity, behavioral therapy, counseling, and participation in group-support programs that in combination can work to achieve weight loss. Adding weight-loss medications to a comprehensive treatment program consisting of diet, physical activity, and counseling can increase weight loss by 5 to 20 pounds (2.3 to 9.1 kg) during the first six months of treatment. While this is only a modest improvement, demand for weight-loss drugs is high.

The decision to add prescription drugs to a treatment program takes into account the individual's body mass index (BMI; body weight in kilograms divided by height in meters squared), other medical problems, and coexisting risk factors. Table 6.4 shows the therapies that are appropriate for people with differing BMIs and takes into account the presence of comorbidities (the coexistence of two or more diseases) such as diabetes, severe obstructive sleep apnea, or heart disease.

Most drugs used for weight loss are anorexiants (appetite suppressants), which act on neurotransmitters (natural chemical substances that convey impulses from one nerve cell to another) in the brain. Anorexiant drugs vary depending on which neurotransmitters they affect: some affect catecholamines such as dopamine and norepinephrine; others affect serotonin; and a third class of drugs acts on more than one neurotransmitter. The drugs, which include phentermine, diethylpropion, and phendimetrazine, act by increasing the secretion of dopamine, norepinephrine, or serotonin, by inhibiting reuptake of neurotransmitters (causing their effects to last longer), or by inducing a combination of both mechanisms.

Another class of weight-loss drugs blocks the absorption of fat. Orlistat, which was approved by the U.S. Food and Drug Administration (FDA) in 1999, decreases fat absorption in the digestive tract by about one-third. Because it also inhibits absorption of water and vitamins, some users suffer from cramping and diarrhea.

The determination of which type of drug to prescribe is based on individual patient characteristics: anorexiant drugs work best for people who are preoccupied with food and feel constantly hungry, orlistat may be effective for those who are unwilling to reduce fat from their diet, and phentermine may help reduce food cravings.

Several weight-loss drugs that appeared effective and were popular among consumers were withdrawn from the U.S. market due to the number and severity of adverse side effects associated with their use. During the 1990s a combination of two drugs—phentermine and fenfluramine, commonly known as "phen-fen"—was prescribed for long-term use (more than three months). However, rare but unacceptable side effects, including serious damage to the heart valves, prompted the withdrawal of fenfluramine and a similar drug, dexfenfluramine, in 1997. Phentermine is still approved for short-term use.

In 2012 the FDA approved the first new prescription weight-management drug in more than a decade: Belviq (lorcaserin), an anorexiant. As reported by the FDA in "FDA Approves Belviq to Treat Some Overweight or Obese Adults" (June 27, 2012, http://www.fda.gov/News Events/Newsroom/PressAnnouncements/ucm309993.htm), clinical trials showed that obese and overweight individuals who combined Belviq with a program of exercise and a reduced-calorie diet were more likely to lose weight than those who engaged in the same program without using Belviq. After up to a year using Belviq, those in the study had an average weight loss of 3% to 3.7%. Belviq activates serotonin 2C receptors in the brain, which is thought to help people feel full after eating smaller amounts of food.

The FDA also approved Qsymia as a weight-management drug in 2012. Qsymia is a combination of a low dose of phentermine and topiramate (a drug used to prevent seizures and migraine headaches). It acts by increasing satiety, making food taste less appealing and increasing calorie expenditure. When used in combination with a reduced-calorie diet and regular physical activity Qsymia helped obese and overweight adults lose weight. After one year of treatment with Qsymia, nearly two-thirds of patients in the clinical trials had lost 5% or more of their body weight.

TABLE 6.4

A guide to selecting weight-loss treatment by body mass index

| Treatment | BMI category | | | | |
	25–26.9	27–29.9	30–34.9	35–39.9	≥40
Diet, physical activity, and behavior therapy	With comorbidities	With comorbidities	+	+	+
Pharmacotherapy		With comorbidities	+	+	+
Surgery				With comorbidities	

- Prevention of weight gain with lifestyle therapy is indicated in any patient with a BMI ≥25 kg/m², even without comorbidities, while weight loss is not necessarily recommended for those with a BMI of 25–29.9 kg/m² or a high waist circumference, unless they have two or more comorbidities.
- Combined therapy with a low-calorie diet (LCD), increased physical activity, and behavior therapy provide the most successful intervention for weight loss and weight maintenance.
- Consider pharmacotherapy only if a patient has not lost 1 pound per week after 6 months of combined lifestyle therapy.

The + represents the use of indicated treatment regardless of comorbidities.

SOURCE: "Table 3. A Guide to Selecting Treatment," in *The Practical Guide: Identification, Evaluation, and Treatment of Overweight and Obesity in Adults,* National Institutes of Health, National Heart, Lung, and Blood Institute, North American Association for the Study of Obesity, October 2000, http://www.nhlbi .nih.gov/files/docs/guidelines/prctgd_c.pdf (accessed October 19, 2015)

In September 2014 the FDA approved Contrave, a combination of two FDA-approved drugs, naltrexone and bupropion, in an extended-release formulation. Naltrexone is approved to treat alcohol and opioid dependence and bupropion is approved to treat depression and seasonal affective disorder and to help people stop smoking. In one study, 42% of patients treated with Contrave lost at least 5% of their body weight compared with 17% of patients treated with placebo (inactive pill).

In December 2014 the FDA approved Saxenda (liraglutide [rDNA origin] injection), a higher dose of a drug used to treat type 2 diabetes that when injected acts like a hormone, signaling the brain that the stomach is full. In a clinical trial, 62% of patients treated with Saxenda lost at least 5% of their body weight compared with 34% of patients treated with placebo.

Over-the-Counter Use of Orlistat

In 2007 the FDA approved the over-the-counter (nonprescription) sale of orlistat, at doses lower than it had previously approved for prescription sale. In 2008 consumers began buying 60-milligram capsules sold under the brand names Alli and Xenical. The FDA recommended it be used in combination with a reduced-calorie, low-fat diet and an exercise program. The introduction of orlistat as an over-the-counter product made it the only nonprescription FDA-approved product for weight loss, since the FDA had withdrawn phenylpropanolamine in 2005. The FDA notes in "FDA Drug Safety Communication: Completed Safety Review of Xenical/Alli (Orlistat) and Severe Liver Injury" (May 26, 2010, http://www.fda .gov/Drugs/DrugSafety) that in rare cases orlistat can cause severe liver damage. Those taking the drug are advised to be watchful for signs of liver problems, such as itching, yellow eyes or skin, and dark urine.

Promising, New Weight-Loss Drugs in Development

According to Jonathan R. S. Arch of the University of Buckingham, in "Horizons in the Pharmacotherapy of Obesity" (*Current Obesity Reports*, September 8, 2015), effective drug therapy may have to target multiple pathways involved in the regulation of energy balance including the endocrine signals in the brain that govern hunger and satiety. Some new drugs aim to increase metabolic rate, and others are attempting to achieve the same results as produced by bariatric surgery by mimicking or opposing hormones in the gut.

In "Intestinal FXR Agonism Promotes Adipose Tissue Browning and Reduces Obesity and Insulin Resistance" (*Nature Medicine*, vol. 21, no. 2, January 2015), Sungsoon Fang et al. describe one such drug in the early stage of development. Fexaramine stimulates a protein in the brain to induce feelings of satiety. In animal studies, the drug induced reactions involved in digestion, which "tricked" each animal's metabolism into acting as it had consumed a meal.

Another promising drug undergoing clinical trials in 2016 is beloranib, an injected drug that aims to help the body produce less fat and burn off excess fat as fuel. In "Efficacy and Safety of Beloranib for Weight Loss in Obese Adults: A Randomized Controlled Trial" (*Diabetes, Obesity and Metabolism*, vol. 17, no. 6, June 2015), Dennis D. Kim et al. report that in a 12-week study beloranib produced dose-dependent weight loss, with weight loss of more than 10 pounds at the highest dose compared with a loss of less than one pound in subjects treated with placebo.

SURGERY

Bariatric (weight-loss) surgery is considered a good treatment option only for people for whom all other treatment methods have failed and who have a BMI of 30 or greater in the presence of comorbidities, or a BMI of 40 or higher regardless of comorbidities. Two types of surgical procedures have been demonstrated to be effective in producing weight loss maintained for five years: restrictive techniques, which reduce gastric volume, and malabsorptive procedures, which not only limit food intake but also alter digestion. An example of the first type is banded gastroplasty, in which an inflatable band that can be adjusted to different diameters is placed around the stomach, reducing its size and thus the amount of food that it can digest. (See Figure 6.3.) Another

FIGURE 6.3

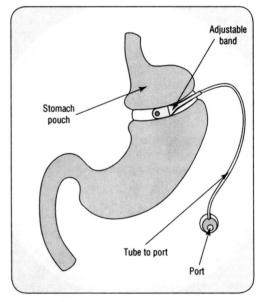

Adjustable gastric band

SOURCE: "Adjustable Gastric Band," in *Weight-Loss Surgery for Adults with Diabetes or Prediabetes Who Are at the Lower Levels of Obesity: A Review of the Research for Adults with a BMI between 30 and 35*, Agency for Healthcare Research and Quality, September 2013, http:// effectivehealthcare.ahrq.gov/ehc/products/227/1693/weight-loss-surgery-130913.pdf (accessed October 19, 2015)

FIGURE 6.4

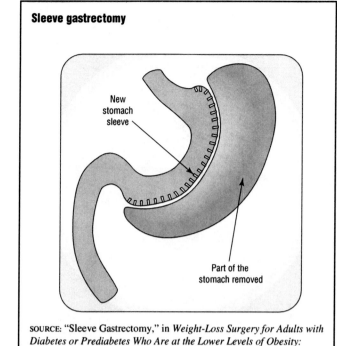

Sleeve gastrectomy

New stomach sleeve

Part of the stomach removed

SOURCE: "Sleeve Gastrectomy," in *Weight-Loss Surgery for Adults with Diabetes or Prediabetes Who Are at the Lower Levels of Obesity: A Review of the Research for Adults with a BMI between 30 and 35,* Agency for Healthcare Research and Quality, September 2013, http:// effectivehealthcare.ahrq.gov/ehc/products/227/1693/weight-loss-surgery-130913.pdf (accessed October 19, 2015)

FIGURE 6.5

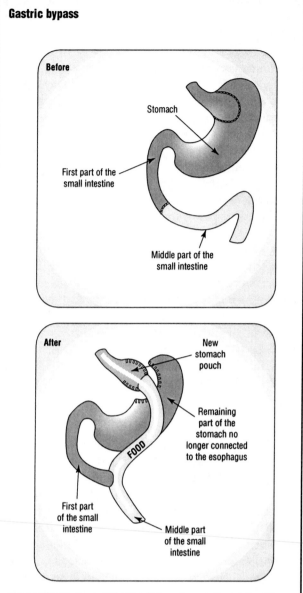

Gastric bypass

Before

Stomach

First part of the small intestine

Middle part of the small intestine

After

New stomach pouch

Remaining part of the stomach no longer connected to the esophagus

FOOD

First part of the small intestine

Middle part of the small intestine

SOURCE: "Gastric Bypass," in *Weight-Loss Surgery for Adults with Diabetes or Prediabetes Who Are at the Lower Levels of Obesity: A Review of the Research for Adults with a BMI between 30 and 35,* Agency for Healthcare Research and Quality, September 2013, http:// effectivehealthcare.ahrq.gov/ehc/products/227/1693/weight-loss-surgery-130913.pdf (accessed October 19, 2015)

restrictive technique is sleeve gastrectomy, in which the stomach is reduced to about 25% of its original size. (See Figure 6.4.) The Roux-en-Y gastric bypass is an example of the second technique. (See Figure 6.5.) On average, patients maintain a weight loss of 25% to 40% of their preoperative body weight after these procedures.

Bariatric surgeries improve patients' quality of life by causing weight loss and the resolution of many weight-related conditions, such as sleep apnea, joint pain, and diabetes. It also significantly improves and frequently eliminates obesity-related diabetes, hypertension, and hyperlipidemia (elevated blood lipids). Furthermore, in "Treatment of Obesity: Bariatric Surgery" (*International Textbook of Diabetes Mellitus*, 4th ed., 2015), Ralph A. DeFronzo et al. report that bariatric surgery is associated with reduced deaths from cardiovascular disease and cancer and increased life span.

Bariatric surgical procedures are generally performed laparoscopically (via a tube inserted through a small incision in the abdomen), as opposed to open surgery. This reduces, but does not eliminate, the risk of complications, which can include death. According to Muhammad Asad Khan et al., in "Perioperative Risk Factors for 30-Day Mortality after Bariatric Surgery: Is Functional Status Important?" (*Surgical Endoscopy*, vol. 27, no. 5, May 2013), people without comorbidities and a BMI equal to or less than 50 have the lowest reported mortality rates and the fewest postsurgical complications. Not

unexpectedly, those with a BMI equal to or greater than 60 with one or more comorbidities have higher mortality rates. The possibility of death or other complications due to bariatric surgery is why it is generally only recommended in cases where other treatments have failed and the risks from the obesity itself are high.

People who undergo weight-loss surgeries require lifelong medical monitoring. After surgery, they are no longer able to eat in the way to which they were accustomed. Those who have undergone gastric bypass experience "dumping syndrome" when they ingest significant amounts of calorie-dense food, with symptoms such as sweating, palpitations, lightheadedness, and nausea. Over time most become conditioned not to eat such foods. Patients who have had gastric restriction surgery can only eat a limited amount of food during a single sitting without vomiting, so they must eat several small meals per day to maintain adequate nutrition. Those who do not adhere to a prescribed regimen of vitamins and minerals may develop vitamin and iron deficiencies. There are also potential postoperative and long-term complications following surgery, such as wound infections, hernias at the incision site, and gallstones. Generally, however, patients fare extremely well, experiencing dramatic improvement and even complete resolution of diabetes, hypertension (high blood pressure), and infertility, as well as improved mobility, self-esteem, and overall quality of life.

The Number of Weight-Loss Surgeries

The American Society for Metabolic and Bariatric Surgery (an organization that advocates for the study and practice of bariatric surgery) reports in the fact sheet "Estimates of Bariatric Surgery Numbers" (July 2015, personal communication with the author) that while approximately 193,000 people had bariatric surgery in 2014, up from 158,000 in 2011, this number represented just 1% of the population that met the guidelines for bariatric surgery.

NEW WEIGHT-LOSS DEVICES

In 2015 the FDA approved two new nonsurgical devices to treat obesity. Both help patients feel full with less food. The ReShape System features two connected, sealed balloons filled with saline, which, when placed in the stomach, take up space that would normally be filled by food. It uses two balloons because earlier single-balloon versions were able to dislodge and move through the digestive tract, blocking the bowels. (See Figure 6.6.) The device is inserted through the mouth in an outpatient setting. The balloons are placed into the stomach empty and then filled with saline once in place. The device remains in the stomach for only six months and the balloons are emptied before it is removed.

The ORBERA Intragastric Balloon System uses a single balloon to take up space in the stomach. Like the ReShape System, it is intended for patients participating in diet and exercise programs under the supervision of a health care provider.

In 2015 the FDA also approved an electrical stimulation system that is surgically implanted in the abdomen and blocks nerve activity between the brain and the stomach. The Maestro Rechargeable System works like a pacemaker, sending electrical pulses to the vagus nerve, which is involved in regulating stomach emptying and signaling to the brain whether the stomach is empty or full. Controllers outside the body permit the patient to charge the device and enable health care professionals to adjust the device's settings. (See Figure 6.7.)

FIGURE 6.6

ReShape system uses two balloons to fill space in the stomach

SOURCE: "ReShape Dual Balloon," in *FDA Approved Obesity Treatment Devices*, U.S. Food and Drug Administration, August 5, 2015, http:// www.fda.gov/MedicalDevices/ProductsandMedicalProcedures/ ObesityDevices/ucm350134.htm (accessed October 19, 2015)

FIGURE 6.7

Maestro Rechargeable System uses electrical stimulation to promote weight loss

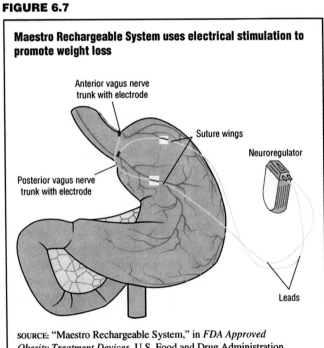

SOURCE: "Maestro Rechargeable System," in *FDA Approved Obesity Treatment Devices*, U.S. Food and Drug Administration, August 5, 2015, http://www.fda.gov/MedicalDevices/ ProductsandMedicalProcedures/ObesityDevices/ucm350134.htm (accessed October 19, 2015)

COUNSELING AND BEHAVIORAL THERAPY

Weight-loss counseling and behavioral therapy aim to assist people to develop the skills needed to identify and modify behaviors and patterns of thinking that undermine weight-control efforts. Behavioral strategies include self-monitoring of weight, food intake, and physical activity; identifying and controlling stimuli that provoke overeating; identifying and solving problems; and using family and social support systems to reinforce weight-control efforts. Counseling and behavioral therapy are perceived as necessary components of comprehensive weight-loss treatment but are also viewed as labor intensive because educating and supporting people seeking to lose weight is time consuming. The effort also requires the active participation of everyone who may be involved in treatment: the affected individuals, their families, physicians, nurses, nutritionists, dieticians, exercise instructors, and mental health professionals. In view of the considerable resources that must be allocated to deliver counseling and behavioral therapy, it is important to know if these approaches promote weight loss effectively.

Jamie Hartmann-Boyce et al. reviewed 37 studies, representing more than 16,000 participants, to determine the efficacy of counseling and behavioral therapy and present their findings in "Effect of Behavioural Techniques and Delivery Mode on Effectiveness of Weight Management: Systematic Review, Meta-analysis and Meta-regression" (*Obesity Reviews*, vol. 15, no. 7, July 2014). The researchers report that most but not all behavioral weight-loss programs effectively promote change in diet, exercise, or both, and behavioral therapy to help patients acquire the skills, motivations, and support to change diet and exercise patterns enabled obese patients to achieve modest but clinically significant and sustained (one to two years) weight loss. However, Hartmann-Boyce et al. find no evidence that more frequent contact with a therapist within a set period led to greater weight loss, nor were programs delivered in-person rather than remotely more effective. Programs that had participants count calories and those that offered some contact with a dietitian promoted greater weight loss as did programs that featured "social comparison," an approach that involves drawing attention to others' performance to draw comparisons.

Assessing the Effectiveness of Weight-Loss Counseling Approaches

In "Changes in Eating, Physical Activity, and Related Behaviors in a Primary-Care-Based Weight Loss Intervention" (*International Journal of Obesity* [London], vol. 37, nos. S12–S18, August 2013), Sheri Volger et al. analyzed changes in eating and physical activity in adults who participated in a two-year behavioral weight-loss intervention conducted in a primary care setting. Study participants were assigned to either:

- Usual care—quarterly visits to a primary care setting that included education about diet and exercise

- Brief lifestyle counseling—quarterly primary care visits plus monthly counseling sessions about weight control

- Enhanced brief lifestyle counseling—quarterly primary care visits, monthly lifestyle counseling, and a choice of meal replacements or weight-loss medication

After two years, participants in the two groups that included lifestyle counseling had significantly more improvement in self-reported measures of appetite control, dietary intake, and physical activity than did the participants receiving only usual care. At month 24, participants in the brief lifestyle counseling had lost an average of 6.4 pounds (2.9 kg), and those in enhanced brief lifestyle counseling had lost an average of 10.1 pounds (4.6 kg). By comparison, those receiving usual care had lost 3.7 pounds (1.7 kg) on average. Volger et al. conclude, "a primary care–based lifestyle intervention delivered by primary care providers, with the assistance of auxiliary health care workers, can result in clinically meaningful weight loss in some patients."

Comparing Behavioral Counseling Delivered by Primary Care Physicians and/or Trained Interventionists

Thomas A. Wadden et al. report an analysis of 12 studies in which behavioral counseling for weight loss was provided by primary care physicians and/or other trained personnel such as registered dietitians, psychologists, exercise specialists, health counselors, and medical assistants and reported their findings in "Behavioral Treatment of Obesity in Patients Encountered in Primary Care Settings: A Systematic Review" (*Journal of the American Medical Association*, vol. 312, no. 17, November 2014). Wadden et al. find limited data to support the supremacy of intensive behavioral weight loss counseling by physicians and other primary care providers such as nurse practitioners and physician assistants over other trained personnel. The researchers acknowledge that primary care providers will "continue to play a critical role in diagnosing obesity, evaluating its causes (including medications associated with weight gain), assessing and treating weight-related co-morbid conditions, and monitoring changes in health that occur with weight loss" but observe that demands on their time will likely require them to refer patients to other trained personnel. For this reason, Wadden et al. call for research to determine the professional qualifications and training needed to provide effective behavioral weight-loss counseling in primary care and other settings.

Comparing Commercial Programs

Kimberly A. Gudzune et al. evaluated 45 studies to determine which commercial program yields better results and reported their findings in "Efficacy of Commercial Weight-Loss Programs: An Updated Systematic Review" (*Annals of Internal Medicine*, vol. 162, no. 7, April 7, 2015). The researchers find that at 12 months Weight Watchers participants lost at least 2.6% more weight and Jenny Craig participants lost at least 4.9% more weight than subjects assigned to education only. Nutrisystem participants lost at least 3.8% more weight at three months than subjects given education and counseling. Atkins resulted in 0.1% to 2.9% greater weight loss at 12 months than counseling. Very-low-calorie programs such as Medifast and OPTIFAST produced at least 4% greater weight loss than counseling at three months, but beyond that time weight loss diminished. Participants in Internet-based programs such as the Biggest Loser Club resulted in 2.7% greater weight loss than those receiving education at three months.

Gudzune et al. report that Weight Watchers participants "consistently have greater weight loss than control/education participants and sustain it beyond 12 months," and also noted that it is one of the least expensive programs. They conclude that overall they "found consistent evidence supporting the long-term efficacy of Weight Watchers and Jenny Craig."

New Approaches

Comprehensive and holistic weight-loss programs that address diet, nutrition, physical activity, stress, and an array of emotional and behavioral issues promise to help people seeking lasting weight loss and better health. Working with individuals, groups, and corporations, many of these programs combine high-tech and high-touch approaches. For example, Retrofit, started by Mark Hyman in 2011, promises to help people lose weight and become healthier over the course of 12 months using team support from a registered dietician, exercise physiologist, behavior coach, and program manager. Clients meet via weekly Skype meetings, and their activity and weight are monitored using wireless activity trackers and scales. As of February 2016 the Retrofit program cost roughly $250 a month.

Weight-Loss Counseling Online

An expanding array of diet plans, counseling programs, and support groups are available on the Internet. However, there is little comparative research available on these approaches, including any studies to determine their efficacy. In the landmark study "A Randomized Trial Comparing Human E-Mail Counseling, Computer-Automated Tailored Counseling, and No Counseling in an Internet Weight Loss Program" (*Archives of Internal Medicine*, vol. 166, no. 15, August 2006), Deborah F. Tate, Elizabeth H. Jackvony, and Rena R. Wing sought to determine whether computer-generated feedback, delivered via the Internet, would be a viable alternative to human counseling via e-mail. They compared the effects of custom-tailored computer-automated interactions with an Internet program that provided weight-loss counseling from a human via e-mail.

Participants were randomly assigned to one of three treatment groups: human e-mail counseling, computer-automated feedback, or no counseling. All subjects received one weight-loss group session, coupons for meal replacements, and access to an interactive website, but the human e-mail counseling and computer-automated feedback groups also had access to an e-diary and a message board. The human e-mail counseling group received weekly e-mail feedback from a counselor, the computer-automated feedback group received automated, custom-tailored messages, and the control group did not receive any counseling. Recommendations included calorie-restricted diets of between 1,200 and 1,500 calories per day, daily exercise equivalent to walking for 30 minutes, and instructions about how to use meal replacement products. All the participants were encouraged to self-monitor their diet and exercise using diaries and calorie books. Both groups accessed the same website, which featured weekly reporting and graphs of weight, weekly e-mail prompts to report weight, weekly weight-loss tips via e-mail, recipes, and a weight-loss e-buddy network system that enabled users to interact with other dieters with similar characteristics via e-mail.

The primary outcome measure used to compare the groups was change in body weight from baseline at three months and six months. Both the human and automated e-counseling groups had greater reductions in weight than the control group at each weigh-in. Tate, Jackvony, and Wing conclude that automated computer feedback was as effective as human e-mail counseling.

Kevin O. Hwang et al. describe in "Website Usage and Weight Loss in a Free Commercial Online Weight Loss Program: Retrospective Cohort Study" (*Journal of Medical Internet Research*, vol. 15, no. 1, January 2013) the association between use of SparkPeople, a free commercial online weight-loss program, and weight loss. Hwang et al. find that active participation—logging in, entering weight, or entering food at least four times per 30 days—was associated with greater weight loss. The researchers posit that in addition to engagement with the program, "weight self-monitoring leads to frequent modification of diet and exercise behavior in response to weights," which in turn spurs weight-loss efforts.

Mobile Apps and Other Self-Directed Weight-Loss Interventions

Smartphones offer dieters a wide range of mobile apps to motivate them and track diet and exercise. In

"Effectiveness of a Smartphone Application for Weight Loss Compared to Usual Care in Overweight Primary Care Patients: A Randomized Controlled Trial" (*Annals of Internal Medicine*, vol. 161, no. 10, November 2014), Brian Yoshio Laing et al. examine the effectiveness of MyFitnessPal, a popular, free app that boasts more than 50 million registered users. The researchers find that while 79% of users said they were satisfied with the app and 92% said they would recommend it to a friend, app users did not lose more weight than the control group, which received usual care from their primary care providers.

Jason Tang et al. reviewed 20 studies of self-directed weight-loss interventions—online programs, mobile phone applications, text messaging, e-mail, electronic and print newsletters, telephone-based communication, print manuals, and booklets—and report in "Self-Directed Interventions to Promote Weight Loss: A Systematic Review of Reviews" (*Journal of Medical Internet Research*, vol. 16, no. 2, February 2014) that some of these interventions appear promising. For example, text-messaging interventions were effective for short-term weight loss, and Internet-based programs that offered individualized feedback or e-mail were more effective than those that did not offer these services. Tang et al. cite the strengths of these interventions as "personal tailoring of information, 24-hour availability, anonymity, online social support, and affordability."

COMPLEMENTARY AND ALTERNATIVE THERAPIES

Many complementary and alternative medicine practices such as yoga, Dahn (a holistic mind-body training method), and mindful eating (which teaches greater awareness of bodily sensations such as hunger and satiety [the feeling of fullness or satisfaction after eating] and helps people to identify "emotional eating") have been used to promote weight loss. However, acupuncture (the Chinese practice of inserting extremely thin, sterile needles into any of 360 specific points on the body) and hypnosis are the only alternative medical practices that have been studied as potential treatments for obesity. Several studies report that acupuncture does not appear to have any benefit greater than a placebo.

Hypnosis is an altered state of consciousness. It is a state of heightened awareness and suggestibility and enables focused concentration that may be used to alter perceptions of hunger and satiety and to modify behavior. Hypnosis is considered a mainstream treatment for addictions and overeating. Regardless, there are conflicting data about its effectiveness. Some studies find that it adds little, if any, benefit beyond that of a placebo, whereas others conclude that hypnosis may have

some initial benefit for people seeking weight loss, but that it has little sustained effect.

In "Does Mindfulness Matter? Everyday Mindfulness, Mindful Eating and Self-Reported Serving Size of Energy Dense Foods among a Sample of South Australian Adults" (*Appetite*, vol. 67, August 2013), Monica Beshara, Amanda D. Hutchinson, and Carlene Wilson report that mindful eating is connected to serving-size moderation, supporting the premise that mindfulness does change eating behaviors.

Although there are few rigorous studies to support their claims, some supplements may enhance weight loss. In "Eight Weeks of Supplementation with a Multi-ingredient Weight Loss Product Enhances Body Composition, Reduces Hip and Waist Girth, and Increases Energy Levels in Overweight Men and Women" (*Journal of the International Society of Sports Nutrition*, vol. 10, no. 1, April 2013), Hector L. Lopez et al. evaluate the effectiveness of a multi-ingredient supplement containing vitamins, raspberry ketone, caffeine, capsaicin, garlic, ginger, and citrus aurantium. One group of subjects followed a calorie-restricted diet, had exercise training, and took the supplement. A second group followed the same diet and exercise plan but did not take the supplement. Lopez et al. find that after eight weeks, subjects taking the supplement lost significantly more weight and body fat and their waist and hip circumference decreased more than subjects who did not take the supplement.

In "Effect of Novel Dietary Supplement on Metabolism In Vitro and In Vivo" (*Journal of Traditional and Complementary Medicine*, May 2015), Roger A. Vaughan et al. analyze and assess the effectiveness of Ripped Freak (RF), a commercially available dietary supplement that claims to increase metabolic rate to help users lose weight. Vaughan et al. find evidence that RF increased metabolic rate in the laboratory and in healthy volunteer subjects, increasing their energy expenditures by about 160 calories per day. The researchers caution, however, that "it is unclear if RF provides any metabolic benefit beyond that previously documented by caffeine or catechin consumption" and call for additional research to determine the effects of RF consumption on metabolism and health.

MIGHT WEIGHT LOSS BE HARMFUL?

Successful weight-loss treatments generally result in improved health: reduced blood pressure, reduced triglycerides, reduced total cholesterol and LDL cholesterol, and increased HDL cholesterol. Weight loss of as little as 5% to 10% of initial weight produces measurable health benefits and may prevent illnesses among people at risk. These findings suggest that treatment should not exclusively focus on the medical consequences of obesity, but that obesity itself should be treated. National Institutes of Health guidelines recommend weight loss for people with a BMI greater than 30 and for people with a BMI greater than 25 with two or more obesity-related risk factors. The guidelines also recommend that for people with a BMI between 25 and 30 without other risk factors, the focus should be on prevention of further weight gain, rather than on weight loss.

There is evidence, however, that weight cycling (repeated cycles of weight gain and loss, a not uncommon occurrence among people trying to lose weight) is associated with metabolic and cardiovascular health problems. In "Weight Cycling Increases T Cell Accumulation in Adipose Tissue and Impairs Systemic Glucose Tolerance" (*Diabetes*, vol. 62, no. 9, September 2013), Emily K. Anderson et al. indicate that weight cycling may contribute to metabolic problems by impairing glucose tolerance and insulin sensitivity. This in turn increases risk for diabetes and cardiovascular disease.

In "Controversies in Obesity Treatment" (*Nutrition and Food Sciences Research*, vol. 2, no. 3, July–September 2015), Majid Karandish and Fatemeh Shirani observe that many weight-loss strategies are ineffective long term and may have unintended consequences including decreasing energy expenditure, complicating appetite control, reinforcing eating disorders, reducing self-esteem, and increasing the plasma and tissue levels of persistent organic pollutants that promote metabolic complications.

Is It Really Dangerous to Be Overweight?

The health risks and consequences of obesity are well understood, but the risk of death associated with overweight remains unclear. In "Association of All-Cause Mortality with Overweight and Obesity Using Standard Body Mass Index Categories" (*Journal of the American Medical Association*, vol. 309, no. 1, January 2, 2013), Katherine M. Flegal et al. estimate the relationship between BMI and risk of death associated with normal weight, overweight, and obesity. The researchers find that compared with normal weight, overweight (BMI 25 to 29.9) was associated with a significantly decreased risk of death. People who were somewhat obese (BMI 30 to 34.9) had roughly the same mortality level as people of normal weight. People with a BMI of 35 or higher had a higher risk of death than people of normal weight.

Karandish and Shirani note that many studies find that obese patients with life-threatening diseases fare better than their healthy-weight peers. Examples of this "obesity paradox" are research findings that overweight and obese patients with cardiovascular disease, stroke, hypertension, type 2 diabetes, chronic kidney disease, and some cancers have better short- and long-term survival than their lean counterparts. Further, people who are fit and obese have no greater risk for cardiovascular disease and death from all causes than their normal-weight and fit counterparts. Karandish and Shirani also explain that about 30% of obese Americans are metabolically healthy, meaning they do not have the six risk factors—high fasting glucose/diabetes, insulin resistance, high triglycerides, low HDL cholesterol, high blood pressure, and high C-reactive protein—associated with cardiovascular disease, and this population is not at greater risk for cardiovascular disease than healthy people who are not obese.

Finally, Karandish and Shirani also point out that some researchers view obesity as a biological adaptation and conclude that "obesity is definitely a major risk factor for a few chronic diseases and premature disability and death," but that given the risks and challenges of losing weight and maintaining weight loss, "scientists and practitioners should search for practical recommendations in order to prevent overweight or obesity among the public (healthy or ill)."

CHAPTER 7
THE ECONOMICS OF OVERWEIGHT AND OBESITY

The economic impact of obesity is considerable. In "The Direct and Indirect Costs of Both Overweight and Obesity: A Systematic Review" (*BMC Research Notes*, vol. 7, April 2014), Anne Dee et al. explain that increasing body mass index (BMI; body weight in kilograms divided by height in meters squared) is associated with increased health care consumption and reduced productivity. Per capita costs increase as BMI increases, but obesity accounts for much higher costs than does overweight. In the United States, people with a BMI greater than 35 represent 37% of all obese people but account for 61% of costs. Dee et al. also note the costs associated with lost productivity are higher than direct health care costs.

In "Economic Costs of Overweight and Obesity" (*Best Practice and Research: Clinical Endocrinology and Metabolism*, vol. 27, no. 2, April 2013), Thomas Lehnert et al. report that about 20% of total annual U.S. health care expenditures, about $190 billion, are spent on obesity-related health care. The researchers assert that the direct health care costs for overweight individuals are about 10% greater than costs for normal-weight individuals. Obese individuals have even higher direct health care costs compared with normal-weight individuals. People with class I obesity (those with a BMI of 30 to 34.9) had annual costs around 23% higher, class II obesity (BMI of 35 to 39.9) was associated with 45% higher annual costs, and class III obesity (BMI 40 or higher) led to 81% higher annual costs. People with class III obesity, despite accounting for a relatively small proportion of the total population of people who are overweight, incur a substantial amount of the total direct health care costs associated with overweight and obesity. Examples of direct health care costs are physician office visits, hospital and nursing home charges, prescription drug costs, and special hospital beds to accommodate obese patients. The indirect costs of overweight and obesity are measured in terms of decreased earnings: lost wages and lower

productivity resulting from the inability to work because of illness or disability, as well as the value of future earnings lost by premature mortality (death). Estimates of indirect costs vary, but several studies suggest that the monetary loss resulting from lost productivity is several times larger than direct health care costs.

According to Y. Claire Wang et al., in "Health and Economic Burden of the Projected Obesity Trends in the USA and the UK" (*Lancet*, vol. 378, no. 9793, August 27, 2011), the economic losses attributable to health care costs and lost productivity are projected to increase. By 2020 three out of four Americans will be overweight or obese and by 2030 there will be an additional 65 million obese adults in the United States. Obesity-related health care costs are attributable not only to increased prevalence of type 2 diabetes, cardiovascular diseases, and several forms of cancer but also to costly, disabling conditions such as osteoarthritis, asthma, infertility, and sleep apnea. Along with health care costs and lost productivity, there are indirect costs as a result of decreased years of disability-free life, increased mortality before retirement, early retirement, and disability benefits.

There are other economic consequences and personal costs of obesity: obese workers may earn less than their lower-weight counterparts because of job discrimination. Also, many insurance companies, particularly in the life insurance sector, charge higher premiums with increasing degrees of overweight. When obesity compromises physical functioning and limits activities of daily living, affected individuals may require assistance from home health aides, durable medical equipment such as walkers or wheelchairs, or other costly adaptations to accommodate disability.

THE HIGH COST OF OVERWEIGHT AND OBESITY

Because overweight and obesity have been linked to an increased risk for many chronic conditions, it may be argued that some percentage of the costs attributed to arthritis, cancer, diabetes, heart disease, and stroke are also attributable to obesity. It is important to remember that estimates of the medical care costs, direct and indirect as well as total cost of overweight and obesity in the United States, vary depending on how the conditions are defined, whether overweight and obesity are considered together or separately, and which costs and obesity-related conditions are included in the estimates and projections.

In "Obesity and Severe Obesity Forecasts through 2030" (*American Journal of Preventive Medicine*, vol. 42, no. 6, June 2012), Eric A. Finkelstein et al. observe that the lifetime costs of overweight and obesity borne by the government are likely to be greater than the lifetime costs imposed by smokers. Furthermore, the results of this study reveal that obese people who live to age 65 have much larger annual Medicare expenditures than their normal-weight peers.

In *Obesity and Its Relation to Mortality and Morbidity Costs* (December 2010, https://www.soa.org/Files/ Research/Projects/research-2011-obesity-relation-mortality .pdf), Donald F. Behan et al. estimate that the economic cost of overweight and obesity in the United States and Canada was $300 billion in 2009, with just $30 billion attributed to Canada. Roughly $220 billion is attributed to obesity, the remaining $80 billion to overweight. Behan et al. attribute $127 billion to health care costs, $49 billion to loss of productivity resulting from early death, $43 billion to disability of active workers, and $72 billion to loss of productivity of totally disabled workers.

Finkelstein et al. predict that between 2010 and 2030 the prevalence of obesity in the United States will increase 33% and clinically severe obesity will increase 130%. The researchers observe that if these increases do not occur, and obesity prevalence remains at about the 2010 levels, then the savings in health care expenditures over the two decades would be $549 billion.

Wang et al. concur with Finkelstein et al. and offer projections for 2030 that are based on current trends of BMI in the U.S. population. The researchers forecast an excess of 8 million cases of diabetes, 6 million to 8 million cases of heart disease and stroke, and more than 1.5 million cases of cancer. This forecast translates into an increase in annual medical costs for obesity-related treatment to $66 billion per year in 2030 from $28 billion per year in 2020.

The Costs of Youth Obesity and Treatment

In "Estimating the Medical Care Costs of Youth Obesity in the Presence of Proxy Reporting Error" (American Economic Association, November 18, 2014), Adam I. Biener, Chad Meyerhoefer, and John Cawley analyzed data from the 2000–10 Medical Expenditure Panel Survey on children and teens aged 11 to 17 years to determine the impact of youth obesity on health care costs. The researchers find that average annual medical expenditures for overweight children are $478.21 higher compared with healthy-weight children and for obese children are $1,098.23 higher compared with healthy-weight children. Health care costs for girls who are overweight are $628.39 more per year than costs for healthy-weight girls, and health care for girls who are obese averages $1,448.94 more than for healthy-weight girls.

In "Payment for Obesity Services: Examples and Recommendations for Stage 3 Comprehensive Multidisciplinary Intervention Programs for Children and Adolescents" (*Pediatrics*, vol. 128, suppl. 2, September 1, 2011), Wendy Slusser et al. explain that "health insurers and hospitals often have to evaluate coverage of obesity care services on a case-by-case basis, which creates a barrier between patients and providers." The researchers interviewed several hospital-based programs and find that most programs fall short of operating expenses. For example, the Duke Children's Health Lifestyles Program is funded by grants and clinic-visit payments, and revenue is about 10% less than operating expenses each year. Approximately 40% of reimbursement is from Medicaid, 30% from private insurance such as Blue-Cross, BlueShield, and Aetna, 20% from managed care plans, and 10% from the Duke employee health plan.

The U.S. Preventive Services Task Force reviewed childhood and adolescent obesity interventions and found that medium- to high-intensity comprehensive behavioral interventions were most effective in the treatment of obesity. Slusser et al. indicate that "no statewide or national efforts are testing models of payment packages for children treated by a multidisciplinary team.... Nevertheless, these efforts are desperately needed, given the near-doubling of hospital admissions and an associated increase in costs from $125.9 million in 1999 (adjusted for inflation) to $237.6 million in 2005 among U.S. children aged two to 19 years with a diagnosis of obesity." They assert that intensive obesity interventions should be reimbursed, consistent with the White House Task Force on Childhood Obesity report *Solving the Problem of Childhood Obesity within a Generation: White House Task Force on Childhood Obesity Report to the President* (May 2010, http://www.letsmove.gov/ white-house-task-force-childhood-obesity-report-president), which states that "federally funded and private insurance plans should cover services necessary to prevent, assess, and provide care to overweight and obese children."

In "Treatment of Childhood and Adolescent Obesity: An Integrative Review of Recent Recommendations from Five Expert Groups" (*Journal of Consulting and Clinical*

Psychology, vol. 81, no. 2, 2013), Daniel S. Kirschenbaum and Kristen Gierut explain that cost-effective treatments are urgently needed, stating, "even if all of the professional counselors in the United States devoted themselves only to treating obesity in children and adults (over 100 million potential clients), they could not keep up with the demand. Even if the numbers could work, consider the cost for such services on such a massive scale. Those numbers do not work either." The researchers consider self-help groups such as Weight Watchers and outpatient cognitive-behavioral therapy, especially when delivered by telephone or via the Internet, as effective for adolescents and relatively low-cost. Costlier treatment such as therapeutic summer camps have produced promising results but are not covered by insurance. Kirschenbaum and Gierut acknowledge that bariatric surgery is effective treatment for limited numbers of extremely overweight young people when all other approaches fail.

Medicare and Medicaid Coverage for Obesity Treatment

Medicare is a program run by the U.S. federal government that provides subsidized health care to Americans aged 65 years and older who paid into the system when they were younger (and certain other individuals). It is the single largest health insurance provider in the country. Medicaid provides subsidized health insurance to people who could not otherwise afford health care. The second-largest health insurance provider in the country, it is operated jointly by the federal government and state governments, with many details of the program varying from state to state.

Although Medicare and Medicaid spend billions of dollars annually to treat obesity-related illnesses, these government programs offer limited coverage for treatment of obesity itself. Medicare covers intensive behavioral therapy for obesity, consisting of obesity screening and dietary assessment, behavioral counseling, and behavioral therapy to promote sustained weight loss through diet and exercise. As of 2015 Medicare covered 15 face-to-face individual behavioral therapy sessions and 30-minute face-to-face group behavioral counseling sessions for people with Medicare Part B (medical insurance) with a BMI of 30 or higher.

Medicare covers some weight-loss surgeries for patients with a BMI of 35 or more who have comorbidities (additional disorders, such as diabetes or heart disease) and who have failed to lose weight in a medical weight-loss program. Medicare Part D is the primary means through which prescription drugs are covered under Medicare. When someone enrolls in Medicare Part D, they choose from different drug coverage plans available in their area. Weight-loss drugs are not included in the list of drugs that Medicare requires all plans to cover, but some plans do include them as an added benefit.

At the state level, government programs may choose to cover obesity treatments for Medicaid patients and state employees, but they are not required to do so. In view of the high prevalence of obesity among the populations covered by Medicaid, and the significant Medicaid expenditures for obesity-related illnesses, many health care industry observers believe it is shortsighted that some states specifically exclude coverage of weight-loss treatments in their Medicaid programs. Some health care analysts and advocacy groups, including the Obesity Society (formerly the American Obesity Association), contend that it is difficult to reconcile limited coverage of obesity in light of Medicaid coverage for inpatient and outpatient alcohol detoxification and rehabilitation, chemical dependency treatment and drug rehabilitation, and services for sexual impotence.

In "Severe Obesity in Adults Cost State Medicaid Programs Nearly $8 Billion in 2013" (*Health Affairs*, vol. 34, no. 11, November 2015), Y. Claire Wang et al. analyzed data from the Medical Expenditure Panel Survey for 2007–12, a sample of more than 117,000 Americans to determine the extent to which obesity predicts higher medical care costs in adults aged 18 years and older, compared with their healthy-weight peers. The researchers find that in 2013, severe obesity (BMI of 35 or higher) cost the United States $69 billion and constituted 60% of the total costs associated with obesity. Medicaid paid nearly 11% of the cost of severe obesity, which translates to about $8 billion per year. Medicare and other federal health programs paid 30% ($20.9 billion), private health plans paid 27% ($18.2 billion), and 30% of costs were paid out-of-pocket. Wang et al. note that state Medicaid costs varied, ranging from $5 million in Wyoming, which covered 58,000 severely obese adults to $1.3 billion in California. Wang et al. predict these costs will grow as Medicaid eligibility is expanded. The researchers advise that in order to slow the rise in obesity-related health care costs, states should focus on identifying effective obesity prevention and treatment services, ensure access for those who are Medicaid-eligible, and include obesity in policy discussions around state Medicaid expansions.

In "Medicaid Coverage for Weight Loss Counseling May Make 'Cents'" (*Journal of Internal Medicine*, vol. 28, no. 1, January 2013), Sara N. Bleich and Bradley J. Herring assert that coverage of screening and behavioral weight-loss programs in the Medicaid program may be crucial for cost containment. Screening for obesity without also covering the cost of weight-loss counseling may not reduce obesity rates because a weekly fee for a program such as Weight Watchers may be unaffordable for people at or near poverty. Bleich and Herring opine, "Coverage of commercial weight-loss programs like Weight Watchers by the Medicaid program may not solve the problem of obesity, but—given the magnitude of the epidemic—even modest reductions in weight can lead to significant health benefits and reduced costs."

Private Insurance

In "The Challenges and Opportunities Associated with Reimbursement for Obesity Pharmacotherapy in the USA" (*PharmacoEconomics*, vol. 33, no. 7, July 2015), Charles Baum et al. note that the Patient Protection and Affordable Care Act (ACA) requires private health insurance providers to help obese patients try to lose weight but that determining which services are covered is up to the individual plans. The ACA stipulates that screening and counseling must be covered with no patient cost-sharing, no deductibles or co-payments; health plans, however, vary in terms of covered services. Some plans offer counseling by telephone, others offer visits with a health coach, a dietician, or group counseling sessions, and some refer patients to programs such as Weight Watchers. The American Medical Association's recognition of obesity as a disease in June 2013 also has motivated some plans to cover weight-loss treatments.

The National Council of State Legislatures reports in "Health Reform and Health Mandates for Obesity" (Richard Cauchi, November 1, 2015, http://www.ncsl .org/research/health/aca-and-health-mandates-for-obesity .aspx) that as of July 2015, 23 states require plans to cover bariatric surgery and 16 states include some coverage and reimbursement for dietary or nutritional screening, weight-loss counseling and/or therapy, and/or weight-loss programs.

George Loewenstein, David A. Asch, and Kevin G. Volpp report in "Behavioral Economics Holds Potential to Deliver Better Results for Patients, Insurers, and Employers" (*Health Affairs*, vol. 32, no. 7, July 2013) that many employers, insurers, and health care providers use incentives to encourage patients to take better care of themselves. Loewenstein, Asch, and Volpp opine that many such programs may not be effective because in their existing forms they require people to have high levels of expertise, motivation and self-control to modify their behaviors. Instead, they propose that incentive programs offer people small and frequent payments for positive health and lifestyle behaviors, under the premise that highly visible rewards such as these will be more effective, and cheaper, than typical incentives such as a reduction in a health care premium.

The Pharmacy Benefit Management Institute (PBMI), an independent organization that is not affiliated with any employee benefits program or pharmaceutical manufacturer, periodically surveys employers to determine the extent, cost, and coverage of their pharmacy benefits. It publishes the survey data and trends in *Prescription Drug Benefit Cost and Plan Design Report*. The PBMI explains in *2014–2015 Prescription Drug Benefit Cost and Plan Design Report* (2014, http://reports.pbmi .com/report.php?id=10) that in 2014 nearly half of employers (48.2%) excluded weight-loss drugs from their coverage. About one in five plans (20.4%) covered the drugs with prior authorization (a cost-containment procedure that requires the prescriber to obtain permission before prescribing specific medications) and just 9.6% of employers surveyed offered complete, unlimited coverage of weight-loss drugs.

OVERWEIGHT WORKERS MAY PAY MORE FOR HEALTH INSURANCE COVERAGE. Stephen Soumerai, professor of population medicine and director of the Drug Policy Research Group at Harvard Medical School and Harvard Pilgrim Health Care Institute, writes in "An Obamacare Fine on Overweight Americans: Discriminatory and Ineffective" (HealthCareBlog.com, May 25, 2014), that the ACA authorizes employer-provided health plans to charge high premiums to people who are overweight or obese (as well as people with certain other conditions or behaviors, such as smoking). The higher premiums are intended to encourage people to take action to become healthier. This approach is closely tied to the rise of workplace wellness plans. The specifics of wellness plans vary from one company to another, but in general they involve rewarding employees for participating in health screenings and activities intended to improve their health, or penalizing them for not doing so.

As Soumerai notes, research reveals that use of premium incentives or penalties to encourage weight loss is not effective, erodes trust between employers and employees and is discriminatory. Soumerai states that these penalties disproportionately affect the poor, who may live in neighborhoods with little access to healthy foods and ready access to junk food, and to people with mobility problems, a group that includes many people who are obese. Furthermore, research demonstrates that increasing health care charges reduces access to essential medical care and increases illness and death among low-income people with chronic diseases. Soumerai exhorts payers and plans to "offer respectful long-term behavioral programs that reduce a few realistic pounds at a time, rather than fining those who fail to achieve what are nearly impossible goals."

FUNDING OBESITY RESEARCH

Table 7.1 shows National Institutes of Health (NIH) funding for research into a variety of diseases and

TABLE 7.1

Estimates of funding for various research, conditions, and disease categories, fiscal years 2011–16

Research/disease areas (Dollars in millions and rounded)	Fiscal year 2011 actual	Fiscal year 2012 actual	Fiscal year 2013 actual	Fiscal year 2014 actual	Fiscal year 2015 estimated	Fiscal year 2016 estimated
Acute respiratory distress syndrome	$96	$98	$95	$85	$86	$88
Adolescent sexual activity	$69	$76	$70	$68	$69	$70
Agent Orange & dioxin	$8	$8	$10	$8	$8	$8
Aging	$2,572	$2,593	$2,429	$2,556	$2,548	$2,585
Alcoholism	$452	$455	$437	$475	$476	$490
Allergic rhinitis (hay fever)	$7	$7	$9	$6	$6	$6
ALS	$44	$44	$39	$48	$48	$50
Alzheimer's disease	$448	$503	$504	$562	$586	$638
American Indians/Alaska Natives	$136	$170	$160	$166	$167	$172
Anorexia	$11	$14	$11	$11	$11	$11
Anthrax	$87	$84	$70	$67	$67	$67
Antimicrobial resistance	$369	$377	$325	$277	$361	$461
Aphasia	$21	$24	$24	$24	$24	$25
Arctic	$28	$23	$19	$16	$16	$16
Arthritis	$231	$258	$231	$239	$240	$245
Assistive technology	$250	$237	$220	$228	$229	$234
Asthma	$221	$229	$207	$241	$242	$246
Ataxia telangiectasia	$13	$11	$11	$8	$8	$8
Atherosclerosis	$475	$477	$374	$375	$376	$385
Attention deficit disorder (ADD)	$55	$60	$49	$44	$45	$46
Autism	$169	$192	$186	$188	$189	$193
Autoimmune disease	$869	$867	$821	$822	$832	$845
Basic behavioral and social science	$1,173	$1,215	$1,172	$1,234	$1,242	$1,272
Batten disease	$4	$4	$5	$5	$5	$5
Behavioral and social science	$3,573	$3,682	$3,535	$3,688	$3,711	$3,797
Biodefense[a]	$1,803	$1,791	$1,692	$1,746	$1,745	$1,848
Bioengineering	$3,303	$3,498	$3,234	$3,329	$3,353	$3,432
Biotechnology	$5,823	$6,089	$5,698	$5,889	$5,925	$6,046
Brain cancer	$280	$281	$280	$289	$290	$299
Brain disorders	$3,864	$3,968	$3,708	$3,894	$3,920	$4,014
Breast cancer	$715	$800	$657	$682	$685	$704
Burden of illness	$40	$84	$72	$73	$74	$76
Cancer	$5,448	$5,621	$5,274	$5,392	$5,414	$5,568
Cardiovascular	$2,049	$2,040	$1,964	$1,950	$1,957	$2,004
Cerebral palsy	$23	$42	$18	$21	$21	$21
Cervical cancer	$119	$112	$98	$116	$116	$119
Charcot-Marie-Tooth disease	$13	$13	$11	$14	$14	$14
Child abuse and neglect research	$30	$32	$30	$30	$30	$31
Childhood leukemia	$59	$77	$67	$105	$105	$108
Chronic fatigue syndrome (ME/CFS)	$6	$5	$5	$5	$5	$6
Chronic liver disease and cirrhosis	$303	$288	$282	$293	$294	$300
Chronic obstructive pulmonary disease	$108	$101	$102	$107	$108	$110
Climate change	$6	$8	$8	$6	$6	$6
Climate-related exposures and conditions[b]	$155	$157	$137	$131	$131	$134
Clinical research	$10,503	$10,951	$10,604	$11,087	$11,132	$11,376
Clinical trials	$3,093	$3,208	$3,155	$3,221	$3,233	$3,298
Colo-rectal cancer	$313	$302	$281	$271	$272	$280
Comparative effectiveness research	$517	$597	$559	$610	$612	$627
Complementary and alternative medicine	$442	$493	$380	$367	$369	$378
Conditions affecting the embryonic and fetal periods[c]	$157	$165	$151	$175	$176	$180
Contraception/reproduction	$415	$448	$408	$394	$397	$405
Cooley's anemia	$20	$20	$15	$18	$18	$18
Cost effectiveness research	$71	$78	$82	$70	$70	$71
Crohn's disease	$67	$76	$61	$65	$66	$67
Cystic fibrosis	$79	$86	$78	$77	$77	$79
Dementia	$0	$0	$650	$704	$731	$789
Dental/oral and craniofacial disease	$501	$516	$480	$483	$484	$495
Depression	$426	$429	$415	$396	$397	$404
Diabetes[d]	$1,076	$1,061	$1,007	$1,011	$1,020	$1,039
Diagnostic radiology	$1,071	$1,090	$1,079	$1,078	$1,085	$1,110
Diethylstilbestrol (DES)	$3	$3	$1	$1	$1	$1
Digestive diseases	$1,698	$1,719	$1,575	$1,607	$1,613	$1,646
Digestive diseases—(gallbladder)	$4	$11	$10	$9	$9	$10
Digestive diseases—(peptic ulcer)	$18	$20	$19	$15	$15	$15
Down syndrome	$20	$20	$18	$18	$18	$19
Drug abuse (NIDA only)[e]	$1,051	$1,052	$993	$1,018	$1,016	$1,047
Duchenne/Becker muscular dystrophy	$32	$34	$33	$32	$32	$33
Dystonia	$13	$14	$13	$12	$12	$13

research areas for fiscal years (FYs) 2011 to 2013, as well as estimates for FYs 2015 and 2016. Baseline funding for obesity increased to a projected $878 million in FY 2016 from $830 million in FY 2011.

TABLE 7.1

Estimates of funding for various research, conditions, and disease categories, fiscal years 2011–16 [CONTINUED]

Research/disease areas (Dollars in millions and rounded)	Fiscal year 2011 actual	Fiscal year 2012 actual	Fiscal year 2013 actual	Fiscal year 2014 actual	Fiscal year 2015 estimated	Fiscal year 2016 estimated
Eating disorders[f]	$27	$34	$31	$30	$30	$30
Emerging infectious diseases	$2,190	$2,153	$1,804	$1,930	$1,933	$1,942
Emphysema	$22	$20	$24	$27	$27	$27
Endometriosis	$14	$9	$7	$7	$7	$7
Epilepsy	$152	$156	$129	$154	$156	$161
Estrogen	$227	$221	$218	$203	$204	$209
Eye disease and disorders of vision	$831	$841	$774	$824	$826	$849
Facioscapulohumeral muscular dystrophy	$6	$5	$5	$7	$7	$7
Fetal alcohol syndrome	$36	$32	$33	$34	$34	$35
Fibroid tumors (uterine)	$12	$14	$10	$9	$9	$9
Fibromyalgia	$11	$13	$11	$10	$10	$11
Food allergies	$33	$31	$36	$35	$35	$35
Food safety	$287	$257	$229	$232	$232	$233
Fragile X syndrome	$29	$27	$30	$36	$37	$37
Frontotemporal dementia (FTD)	$23	$26	$32	$37	$37	$38
Gene therapy	$248	$256	$226	$253	$255	$260
Gene therapy clinical trials	$14	$15	$15	$26	$26	$27
Genetic testing	$270	$255	$272	$231	$231	$237
Genetics	$7,223	$7,632	$7,144	$7,324	$7,364	$7,535
Global warming climate change	$5	$6	$6	$4	$4	$4
Headaches	$21	$24	$25	$24	$24	$25
Health disparities[g]	$2,718	$2,740	$2,722	$2,734	$2,736	$2,750
Health services	$1,172	$1,317	$1,262	$1,342	$1,347	$1,376
Heart disease	$1,236	$1,278	$1,230	$1,224	$1,228	$1,258
Heart disease—coronary heart disease	$437	$468	$404	$421	$423	$433
Hematology	$1,006	$1,091	$1,020	$1,189	$1,194	$1,225
Hepatitis	$208	$210	$195	$251	$252	$256
Hepatitis—A	$4	$2	$2	$3	$3	$3
Hepatitis—B	$58	$51	$48	$48	$48	$49
Hepatitis—C	$114	$112	$101	$111	$111	$112
HIV/AIDS[h]	$3,059	$3,074	$2,898	$2,978	$3,000	$3,100
Hodgkin's disease	$20	$21	$13	$14	$14	$14
Homelessness	$9	$10	$11	$14	$14	$15
Homicide and legal interventions	$1	$1	$0	$0	—	—
HPV and/or cervical cancer vaccines	$24	$26	$25	$38	$38	$39
Human fetal tissue[i]	$66	$71	$67	$76	$76	$77
Human genome	$1,907	$2,271	$2,473	$2,701	$2,717	$2,785
Huntington's disease	$56	$65	$55	$50	$51	$53
Hydrocephalus	+	$7	$6	$5	$5	$6
Hyperbaric oxygen	$2	$2	$1	$2	$2	$2
Hypertension	$240	$215	$222	$216	$217	$222
Immunization	$1,756	$1,733	$1,656	$1,607	$1,610	$1,621
Infant mortality/(LBW)	$286	$287	$253	$268	$269	$275
Infectious diseases	$3,883	$3,867	$4,887	$5,002	$5,015	$5,181
Infertility	$74	$74	$78	$76	$77	$79
Inflammatory bowel disease	$113	$121	$114	$125	$126	$128
Influenza	$272	$251	$304	$262	$263	$284
Injury—childhood injuries	$33	$37	$37	$35	$35	$36
Injury—trauma—(head and spine)	$166	$171	$183	$216	$218	$225
Injury—traumatic brain injury	$81	$79	$88	$87	$88	$91
Injury—unintentional childhood injury	$20	$22	$20	$22	$22	$22
Injury (total) accidents/adverse effects	$356	$366	$367	$404	$407	$418
Intellectual and developmental disabilities (IDD)[c]	$333	$355	$343	$356	$358	$365
Interstitial cystitis	$13	$10	$10	$9	$10	$10
Kidney disease	$557	$556	$551	$549	$551	$563
Lead poisoning	$10	$8	$8	$7	$7	$7
Lewy body dementia	+	+	+	$15	$15	$15
Liver cancer	$74	$73	$71	$74	$74	$76
Liver disease	$623	$632	$594	$605	$607	$619
Lung	$1,278	$1,286	$1,230	$1,329	$1,335	$1,363
Lung cancer	$221	$233	$208	$254	$255	$263
Lupus	$106	$108	$92	$99	$99	$100
Lyme disease	$28	$25	$20	$23	$23	$23
Lymphoma	$199	$213	$233	$251	$252	$259
Macular degeneration	$105	$101	$98	$82	$82	$83
Malaria	$145	$152	$147	$169	$169	$173
Malaria vaccine	$39	$40	$34	$36	$36	$36
Mental health	$2,275	$2,287	$2,174	$2,213	$2,234	$2,299
Methamphetamine	$70	$69	$68	$63	$63	$65
Migraines	$16	$18	$19	$20	$20	$21
Mind and body	$533	$533	$210	$211	$212	$216

TABLE 7.1

Estimates of funding for various research, conditions, and disease categories, fiscal years 2011–16 [CONTINUED]

Research/disease areas (Dollars in millions and rounded)	Fiscal year 2011 actual	Fiscal year 2012 actual	Fiscal year 2013 actual	Fiscal year 2014 actual	Fiscal year 2015 estimated	Fiscal year 2016 estimated
Minority health[g]	$2,504	$2,487	$2,428	$2,514	$2,515	$2,528
Mucopolysaccharidoses (MPS)	$10	$10	$8	$6	$7	$7
Multiple sclerosis	$122	$115	$112	$102	$103	$105
Muscular dystrophy	$75	$75	$76	$78	$79	$81
Myasthenia gravis	$9	$7	$7	$8	$8	$8
Myotonic dystrophy	$9	$10	$10	$9	$9	$9
Nanotechnology[i]	$409	$456	$430	$409	$411	$421
Networking and information technology R&D[i]	$551	$532	$521	$612	$613	$628
Neuroblastoma	$25	$34	$33	$37	$37	$39
Neurodegenerative	$1,622	$1,671	$1,619	$1,743	$1,752	$1,788
Neurofibromatosis	$23	$18	$17	$21	$21	$22
Neuropathy	$146	$145	$151	$156	$157	$161
Neurosciences	$5,548	$5,618	$5,340	$5,580	$5,634	$5,791
Nutrition	$1,411	$1,692	$1,524	$1,555	$1,566	$1,600
Obesity	$830	$836	$812	$857	$857	$878
Organ transplantation	$164	$150	$140	$142	$143	$144
Orphan drug	$749	$809	$764	$809	$813	$830
Osteogenesis imperfecta	$9	$9	$8	$11	$11	$12
Osteoporosis	$179	$181	$164	$141	$142	$144
Otitis media	$15	$17	$14	$16	$16	$16
Ovarian cancer	$138	$147	$133	$131	$131	$135
Paget's disease	$1	$1	$0	$0	—	—
Pain conditions—chronic	$386	$396	$402	$402	$404	$414
Pain research	$0	$479	$475	$499	$501	$514
Pancreatic cancer	$112	$127	$125	$123	$123	$127
Parkinson's disease	$151	$154	$135	$139	$140	$144
Patient safety	$839	$845	$858	$1,008	$1,012	$1,035
Pediatric	$3,277	$3,612	$3,266	$3,486	$3,523	$3,598
Pediatric AIDS[h]	$228	$219	$188	$166	$163	$168
Pediatric cancer	+	+	+	$276	$277	$285
Pediatric research initiative	$362	$379	$258	$343	$346	$353
Pelvic inflammatory disease	$4	$3	$3	$2	$2	$2
Perinatal—birth—preterm (LBW)	$214	$217	$198	$206	$207	$211
Perinatal—neonatal respiratory distress syndrome	$37	$38	$33	$52	$53	$54
Perinatal period—conditions originating in perinatal period	$498	$538	$486	$534	$536	$549
Physical rehabilitation	+	+	+	$113	$113	$116
Pick's disease	$3	$2	$3	$4	$4	$4
Pneumonia	$117	$115	$113	$107	$107	$108
Pneumonia & influenza	$382	$358	$407	$362	$363	$384
Polycystic kidney disease	$42	$42	$40	$36	$36	$37
Post-traumatic stress disorder (PTSD)	$0	$0	$77	$79	$79	$81
Prescription drug abuse	$28	$33	$33	$40	$40	$41
Prevention	$5,929	$5,924	$6,686	$6,858	$6,882	$7,005
Prostate cancer	$284	$257	$286	$254	$255	$262
Psoriasis	$10	$10	$12	$13	$13	$13
Rare diseases	$3,527	$3,623	$3,456	$3,639	$3,654	$3,733
Regenerative medicine	$824	$877	$831	$836	$843	$862
Rehabilitation	$459	$449	$446	$494	$496	$508
Rett syndrome	$12	$13	$13	$12	$12	$12
Reye's syndrome	$0	$0	$0	$0	—	—
Rural health	$211	$231	$187	$197	$198	$203
Schizophrenia	$264	$268	$232	$253	$255	$259
Scleroderma	$25	$24	$21	$24	$24	$25
Screening and brief intervention for substance abuse	$30	$31	$25	$30	$30	$31
Septicemia	$91	$96	$88	$100	$100	$102
Serious mental illness	+	+	+	$407	$409	$415
Sexually transmitted diseases/herpes	$259	$275	$242	$263	$263	$267
Sickle cell disease	$65	$65	$70	$75	$75	$77
Sleep research	$232	$238	$229	$233	$233	$239
Small pox	$41	$40	$30	$24	$24	$24
Smoking and health	$360	$353	$321	$320	$321	$330
Spina bifida	$11	$12	$10	$10	$10	$10
Spinal cord injury	$78	$79	$94	$80	$81	$83
Spinal muscular atrophy	$19	$15	$13	$16	$16	$16
Stem cell research	$1,179	$1,374	$1,273	$1,391	$1,402	$1,436
Stem cell research—embryonic—human	$123	$146	$146	$166	$168	$172
Stem cell research—embryonic—non-human	$165	$164	$154	$150	$152	$155

The Obesity Society, along with myriad medical professional organizations and advocacy groups, contends that public funding for obesity research is inadequate in view of the size and scope of this public health problem.

TABLE 7.1

Estimates of funding for various research, conditions, and disease categories, fiscal years 2011–16 [CONTINUED]

Research/disease areas (Dollars in millions and rounded)	Fiscal year 2011 actual	Fiscal year 2012 actual	Fiscal year 2013 actual	Fiscal year 2014 actual	Fiscal year 2015 estimated	Fiscal year 2016 estimated
Stem cell research—nonembryonic—human	$395	$504	$431	$443	$445	$457
Stem cell research—nonembryonic—non-human	$620	$653	$613	$627	$631	$646
Stem cell research—umbilical cord blood/ placenta	$41	$47	$40	$34	$34	$35
Stem cell research—umbilical cord blood/ placenta—human	$36	$43	$35	$28	$28	$29
Stem cell research—umbilical cord blood/placenta—non-human	$10	$8	$7	$7	$7	$7
Stroke	$317	$310	$282	$300	$302	$311
Substance abuse[k]	$1,623	$1,634	$1,525	$1,564	$1,564	$1,611
Substance abuse prevention	$44	$41	$65	$69	$69	$71
Sudden infant death syndrome	$23	$24	$20	$20	$21	$21
Suicide	$49	$44	$37	$39	$39	$40
Suicide prevention	$25	$22	$21	$22	$22	$22
Teenage pregnancy	$19	$18	$17	$16	$16	$16
Temporomandibular muscle/joint disorder (TMJD)	$18	$21	$19	$18	$18	$18
Tobacco	$362	$355	$322	$321	$322	$331
Topical microbicides	$104	$99	$93	$103	$103	$104
Tourette syndrome	$5	$6	$4	$4	$4	$4
Transmissible spongiform encephalopathy (TSE)	$46	$39	$35	$33	$33	$34
Transplantation	$592	$552	$538	$561	$565	$575
Tuberculosis	$209	$218	$240	$279	$279	$285
Tuberculosis vaccine	$17	$21	$26	$31	$31	$31
Tuberous sclerosis	$20	$23	$20	$24	$24	$25
Underage drinking	$77	$80	$75	$83	$83	$85
Underage drinking and prevention & treatment (NIAAA only)[l]	$57	$62	$62	$59	$60	$61
Urologic diseases	$542	$496	$497	$494	$496	$509
Usher syndrome	+	+	+	$19	$19	$19
Uterine cancer	$40	$42	$39	$57	$57	$59
Vaccine related	$1,717	$1,691	$1,608	$1,573	$1,576	$1,587
Vaccine related (AIDS)[h]	$550	$557	$518	$533	$537	$568
Valley fever	+	+	+	$3	$4	$4
Vascular cognitive impairment/dementia	+	+	+	$45	$45	$46
Vector-borne diseases	$466	$441	$437	$487	$487	$492
Violence against women	$34	$36	$31	$35	$36	$36
Violence research	$156	$154	$137	$130	$130	$134
Vulvodynia	$2	$4	$4	$3	$3	$3
West Nile virus	$65	$29	$40	$48	$48	$48
Women's health[g]	$3,891	$3,833	$3,745	$3,935	$3,936	$3,946
Youth violence	$87	$77	$70	$59	$59	$60
Youth violence prevention	$26	$27	$26	$16	$16	$17

Besides insufficient NIH funding for obesity research, the Obesity Society cites inequities in research grants that are awarded by the NIH.

WEIGHING THE PRICE THAT EMPLOYERS PAY

Obese employees incur substantially higher health care costs than normal-weight employees. Obesity significantly increases health expenditures and absenteeism. James P. Moriarty et al. estimate in "The Effects of Incremental Costs of Smoking and Obesity on Health Care Costs among Adults: A 7-Year Longitudinal Study" (*Journal of Occupational and Environmental Medicine*, vol. 54, no. 3, March 2012) that health care costs are $1,400 more for obese employees compared with their healthy-weight colleagues. Moriarty et al. find that obese workers cost $600 more than smokers.

In "Obesity & the Workplace: Direct, Indirect Costs & the Role of Wellness Education" (American Society of Safety Engineers, November 2012), Thomas A. Sherwood reviews multiple studies estimating the costs of obese workers. Sherwood reports that of the $900 billion that U.S. employers spend on health care annually, $75 billion is attributable to obesity. Absenteeism attributable to overweight and obesity results in a cost of $4.3 billion per year. Obese workers file more medical claims (11.65 claims per 100 full-time equivalents) compared with healthy-weight employees (5.80 claims per 100), and their medical claims costs are higher.

Tatiana Andreyeva, Joerg Luedicke, and Y. Claire Wang explain that obesity imposes a significant burden on the U.S. economy in terms of lost productivity in "State-Level Estimates of Obesity-Attributable Costs of Absenteeism" (*Journal of Occupational and Environmental Medicine*, vol. 56, no. 11, November 2014). Obese workers miss from 1.1 to 1.7 extra days per year compared with healthy-weight workers and cost the United States an estimated $8.65 billion per year.

*The minimum reporting threshold for a specific disease/condition is $500,000. Reporting of $0 does not indicate that no research is being conducted.

'+' Indicates a new category. Funding support data not available prior to the initial year reported.

aReporting for this category does not follow the standard RCDC process. The total amount reported is consistent with reporting requirements for this category to the U.S. Office of Management & Budget (OMB). The project listing does not include non-project or other support costs associated with the annual total for this category.

bPrior to fiscal year 2011, this category's title was "Health Effects of Climate Change." The title was revised to more accurately reflect the content of the research conducted and facilitate reporting spending data in response to requests tracking climate change adaptation.

cName revised in fiscal year 2013 to reflect current scientific terminology.

dIncludes research funded from the Type 1 diabetes appropriation. These are project listings only.

eReporting for this category does not follow the standard RCDC process. Spending for this category is reported consistent with U.S. Office of National Drug Control Policy (ONDCP) requirements. This category includes only projects funded by National Institute on Drug Abuse (NIDA). Fiscal year 2014 actual and fiscal year 2015 estimate reported in RePORT can differ from levels identified in the fiscal year 2016 Drug Control budget submission for those fiscal years where comparable adjustments have been applied.

fReported total for this category encompasses research for anorexia, bulimia nervosa, binge eating disorders, and eating disorders not otherwise specified.

gReporting for this category does not follow the standard RCDC process. This category assigns project funding according to populations tracked by gender or ethnicity. The databases used to track gender/ethnicity are complex are not currently compatible with the RCDC system.

hThe total for acquired immunodeficiency syndrome (AIDS) research includes both extramural and intramural research (including research management and support, Management Fund, and Service & Supply Fund), buildings and facilities, research training, and program evaluation, as well as research on the many human immunodeficiency virus (HIV)-associated co-infections and co-morbidities, including TB, hepatitis C, and HIV-associated cancers. It also includes all of the basic science underlying this research. Other RCDC categories are not reported this way; thus the total for AIDS-related research is not comparable to spending reported for other RCDC diseases.

iReporting for this category does not follow the standard RCDC process. This category uses a non-standard approach involving subject matter expert reviews of manually collected project listings.

jThe data provided reflects funding amounts reported by the NIH RCDC process for this category. Actual and estimate levels presented on this site supersede estimates detailed in OMB MAX DE application tables that may have been based on preliminary funding support information.

kReporting for this category does not follow the standard RCDC process. This category includes all spending reported under the Drug Abuse category as well as projects categorized under the broader area of Substance Abuse. These are project listings only.

lReporting for this category does not follow the standard RCDC process. Spending for this category is reported consistent with U.S. Office of National Drug Control Policy (ONDCP) requirements. This category includes only projects funded or administered by National Institute on Alcohol Abuse and Alcoholism (NIAAA). This category represents a subset of spending reported under the RCDC Underage Drinking category and involves manual review of the project listing by subject matter experts.

Note: HPV = Human papillomavirus; LBW = Low birth weight.

SOURCE: "Estimates of Funding for Various Research, Condition, and Disease Categories (RCDC)," in *NIH Categorical Spending*, U.S. Department of Health and Human Services, National Institutes of Health, February 5, 2015, http://report.nih.gov/categorical_spending.aspx (accessed October 22, 2015)

Andreyeva, Luedicke, and Wang observe that in 2012, an estimated 9.3% of all absenteeism costs among American workers aged 18 years and older were attributable to obesity, and nearly the same proportion of health care spending was obesity-related.

THE HIGH COST OF LOSING WEIGHT

According to the market research firm MarketsandMarkets, the global weight-loss market is expected to grow to $206.4 billion by 2019 from $148.1 billion in 2014. The firm's report, "Weight Loss and Weight Management Market by Equipment (Fitness Equipment [Treadmill, Stair Steppers]), Surgical Equipment (Adjustable Gastric Band, Gastric Bypass), Diet (Weight Loss Meals, Diet Soft Drinks), Weight Loss Services—Forecast to 2019" (February 2015, http://www.marketsandmarkets.com/Market-Reports/weight-loss-obesity-management-market-1152.html) explains that although North America accounts for the majority of this market, the Asian market is anticipated to grow in response to "the rising obese and diabetic population, sedentary lifestyle, rise in disposable incomes, and low cost of bariatric surgeries which in turn promote medical tourism in this region."

The report explains that meals, beverages, and supplements accounted for the largest share of the obesity management market, by diet. Key players in the market, by diet, include Atkins Nutritionals, Inc.; Herbalife Ltd.; the Kellogg Company; and NutriSystem, Inc. The key companies in the surgical and fitness equipment market are Amer Sports; Apollo Endosurgery; Brunswick Corporation; Covidien; Cybex International; Ethicon, Inc.; Johnson Health Technology, Ltd.; Olympus Corporation; and Technogym SpA. In the services market, eDiets.com; Equinox, Inc.; Fitness First Group; Gold's Gym; International Duke Diet & Fitness Center; Jenny Craig; Life Time Fitness, Inc. (U.S.); Town Sports International Holdings, Inc.; 24 Hour Fitness; and Weight Watchers International, Inc., are prominent players.

The market research firm Marketdata Enterprises Inc. in *Medical Weight Loss Programs: A Growth Market* (June 2015) describes the U.S. medical weight-loss market as worth $7.9 billion in 2015 and growing and predicts that its growth will surpass that of commercial companies. Medical programs include bariatric surgery ($5.26 billion), prescription antiobesity drugs ($614 million), bariatricians' (physicians who specialize in weight loss) programs ($488 million), very-low-calorie diets ($445 million), and programs provided by hospitals, clinics, and independent physicians ($1.05 billion).

Marketdata predicts that the medical weight-loss market will rise to $9.6 billion by 2019. This growth is fueled by the ACA, which mandates insurance coverage for obesity screening, counseling, and treatment in about half the states. Insurers must pay for counseling by qualified weight-loss professionals (physicians, physician assistants, registered nurses, and registered dieticians). Marketdata explains that the ACA gives medical weight-loss programs a competitive advantage, "an unprecedented opportunity for medically supervised weight-loss programs to provide a higher level of service than commercial diet centers—essentially free of charge for those with insurance."

For example, CVS Health has entered the medical weight-loss market. The pharmacy chain offers one-on-one coaching assisted by doctors or nurse practitioners (eligible for reimbursement under the ACA) and other weight-loss services at nearly 1,000 MinuteClinic locations.

Along with the growth of medical weight-loss programs, the report observes that there has been a shift from programs centered on diet foods to those that emphasize behavior modification. For the first time, services constitute more than half (50.7%) of the market as opposed to diet foods, soft drinks and commercial weight-loss centers.

Technology also has spurred change in the weight-loss industry, with health and wellness apps that can help people track calorie consumption and expenditures. These low-cost or free apps appeal to younger dieters more than many commercial programs such as Weight Watchers, where the average group leader is 48 years old.

Medical and Behavioral Treatments

Behavioral interventions for weight loss, such as one-on-one counseling, involve considerable expense. Prescription drug treatment is also costly—newer drugs Qsymia (phentermine and topiramate) and Belviq (lorcaserin) cost between $100 and $250 per month.

In "Self-Directed Interventions to Promote Weight Loss: A Systematic Review of Reviews" (*Journal of Medical Internet Research*, vol. 16, no. 2, February 2014), Jason Tang et al. conducted a review of studies examining the effectiveness of interactive websites, smartphone applications, and text messaging. Tang et al. also considered the cost-effectiveness of these self-directed interventions. The researchers find two studies indicating that Internet-based interventions are less costly to deliver and afford additional savings in terms of travel time and travel costs and one meta-analysis (a review of multiple studies) that concluded that eHealth interventions were no more cost-effective than in-person programs. Although the researchers could not draw definitive conclusions about the cost-effectiveness of Internet-based interventions, the characteristics of these interventions—personal tailoring of information, 24-hour availability, anonymity, online social support, and affordability—suggest that they may be effective with specific target audiences such as adolescents and young adults.

In "Internet Programs Targeting Multiple Lifestyle Interventions in Primary and Secondary Care Are Not Superior to Usual Care Alone in Improving Cardiovascular Risk Profile: A Systematic Review" (*European Journal of Internal Medicine*, vol. 25, no. 1, 2014), Irene L. Vegting et al. review a variety of programs targeting lifestyle interventions and find that while they may be able to partially replace face-to-face contact with health care workers, on the whole they are not as effective as one-to-one interventions and suffer from high dropout rates. However, Internet-based interventions may be cost effective when they are applied on a large scale because they have the potential to reduce the number of doctor's visits.

Long-Term Savings

Considerable research indicates that the costs of surgical treatment of obesity are offset by a reduction in future utilization of health care services, especially prescription drug use, and a resultant reduction in health care costs. For example, in "Cost-Effectiveness of Bariatric Surgical Procedures for the Treatment of Severe Obesity" (*European Journal of Health Economics*, vol. 22, no. 4, April 2012), Bruce C. M. Wang et al. compared the three most common bariatric surgical procedures in the United States, laparoscopic gastric bypass, conventional Roux-en-Y gastric bypass, and laparoscopic adjustable gastric banding, to no surgery. They conclude that all three surgical procedures resulted in additional years of life, and the significant long-term reductions in morbidity and mortality caused by obesity render these procedures cost effective.

Oleg Borisenko et al. arrived at similar conclusions in a study of the cost-effectiveness of bariatric surgery from the perspective of the Swedish health care system. In "Bariatric Surgery Can Lead to Net Cost Savings to Health Care Systems: Results from a Comprehensive European Decision Analytic Model" (*Obesity Surgery*, vol. 25, no. 9, September 2015), Borisenko et al. find that bariatric surgery has a cost saving effect on the health care system over the patient's lifetime and demonstrates its cost-effectiveness just two years after the procedure.

Medical and commercial weight-loss programs also have the potential to save money. In "Meta- and Cost-Effectiveness Analysis of Commercial Weight Loss Strategies" (*Obesity*, vol. 22, no. 9, September 2014), Eric A. Finkelstein and Eliza Kruger looked at multiple studies describing the effectiveness of two lifestyle interventions (Weight Watchers and Vtrim), one lifestyle and food-replacement intervention (Jenny Craig), and three pharmaceutical interventions (orlistat, Qsymia, and lorcaserin) and find that of the six interventions Weight Watchers and Qsymia appear to be the two most cost-effective strategies for nonsurgical weight loss.

CATERING TO AN EXPANDING MARKET

Many businesses have discovered that they must literally expand their products and services to meet the needs of overweight and obese consumers. The article

"13 Oversize Products for Overweight People" (Health .com, 2015) presents an array of products that are designed to meet the needs of obese Americans, including heavy-duty weight scales, wider toilet seats that can withstand up to 1,200 pounds (544 kg), seat-belt extenders, jumbo-sized jewelry, and bicycles that can accommodate people weighing up to 550 pounds (259 kg). The article also describes electric bed lifts designed to transfer patients up to 1,000 pounds (454 kg) from bed to wheelchair, and wider wheelchairs to accommodate patients up to 700 pounds (318 kg).

Hospitals and other health care facilities also must meet the needs of obese patients. In "Essential Bariatric Equipment: Making Your Facility More Accommodating to Bariatric Surgical Patients" (*Minimally Invasive Bariatric Surgery*, 2015), Hector Romero-Talamas and Stacy A. Brethauer name the furniture and equipment needed to accommodate obese patients, including wide entrance doors, beds, examination tables, wheelchairs, walkers, stretchers, commodes, and blood pressure cuffs, as well as floor-mounted toilets and elevators with adequate weight capacity.

The Plus-Sized Clothing Market Is Growing

In "Retail's Plus-Size Problem: Designing for Larger Sizes" (CNBC.com, April 8, 2015), Courtney Reagan reports that the plus-size clothing market, which generated $17.5 billion in sales in 2014, up 5% from the previous year, is poised for additional growth as new retailers aim to meet the needs of plus-size consumers. One estimate considers two-thirds of American women as plus-sized, although plus-size apparel constitutes just 17% of sales. Target launched its first plus-size brand in 2015, and H&M, J.C. Penney, and other large retailers also have plus-size brands.

Elizabeth Blair observes, "As Plus-Size Fashion Gains Popularity, Retailers Play Catch-Up" (NPR.org, July 9, 2015) that retailers are acknowledging that the average American woman wears a size 14 and are aiming to meet the needs of plus-size consumers. Actors Melissa McCarthy (1970–) and Rebel Wilson (1980–) are designing clothing lines, which will further increase visibility of plus-size apparel, and Blair notes that retailer Lane Bryant is offering sophisticated fashions designed by Isabel Toledo.

In "Full Figured Fashion Week, Where Waifs Are out of Style" (Fortune.com, June 19, 2015), Susan Price reports that 25 brands and 12 independent designers including the event's principal sponsor, Fruit of the Loom, participated in the 2015 Full Figured Fashion Week in New York. Founded by former plus-size model Gwen DeVoe, the first Full Figured Fashion Week took place in 2009. DeVoe credits vocal consumers, the Internet, and social media for spurring retailers' efforts, noting, "The plus-size consumer has become so vocal about what she wants."

In 2001 Hot Topic, a California-based company that specializes in clothing for teenagers and young women, launched a chain of six stores called Torrid that offer fashion-forward plus-sized clothing for young women. The company notes in the press release "TORRID, the Hottest Name in Plus-Size Fashion, Introduces Real Girls Campaign, #MyStoryMyTorrid" (August 18, 2015, http://www.prnewswire.com/news-releases/torrid-the-hottest-name-in-plus-size-fashion-introduces-real-girls-campaign-mystorymytorrid-300130037.html) that in 2015 there were more than 315 Torrid stores and an online store that offered an array of clothing and lingerie for young women sizes 12 to 28. A fall 2015 advertising campaign tagline, "#MyStoryMyTorrid," showcased real girls and young women who wear plus-size clothing. The Torrid fans featured were discovered on Instagram and following photoshoots in their home towns, were featured in Torrid's catalog and website.

CHAPTER 8
POLITICAL, LEGAL, AND SOCIAL ISSUES
OF OVERWEIGHT AND OBESITY

THE GLOBAL POLITICS OF OBESITY

At the international level, the World Health Organization (WHO) has developed a strategy to combat an escalating epidemic of overweight and obesity throughout the world. In *Obesity and Overweight* (January 2015 http://www.who.int/mediacentre/factsheets/fs311/en/), the WHO exhorts individuals and populations to:

- Limit energy intake from total fats and sugars

- Increase consumption of fruit and vegetables, as well as legumes, whole grains, and nuts

- Engage in regular physical activity (60 minutes a day for children and 150 minutes per week for adults)

- Support individuals in following the recommendations above, through sustained political commitment and the collaboration of many public and private stakeholders

- Make regular physical activity and healthier dietary choices available, affordable, and easily accessible to all—especially the poorest individuals

The WHO asserts that the food industry can play an important role, "reducing the fat, sugar and salt content of processed foods; ensuring that healthy and nutritious choices are available and affordable to all consumers; practicing responsible marketing especially those aimed at children and teenagers; and ensuring the availability of healthy food choices and supporting regular physical activity practice in the workplace." The WHO's *Global Action Plan for the Prevention and Control of Noncommunicable Diseases 2013–2020* (2013, http://apps.who.int/iris/bit stream/10665/94384/1/9789241506236_eng.pdf?ua=1) describes these and other actions as necessary to "halt the rise in diabetes and obesity."

At the 63rd World Health Assembly in May 2013, the WHO endorsed a set of guidelines aimed at reducing noncommunicable (noninfectious and nontransmissible) diseases, which includes obesity. In "Follow-Up to the

Political Declaration of the High-Level Meeting of the General Assembly on the Prevention and Control of Non-communicable Diseases" (http://apps.who.int/gb/ebwha/pdf_files/WHA66/A66_R10-en.pdf), the WHO advises "developing or strengthening national food and nutrition policies and action plans and implementation of related global strategies including the global strategy on diet, physical activity and health, the global strategy for infant and young child feeding, the comprehensive implementation plan on maternal, infant and young child nutrition and WHO's set of recommendations on the marketing of foods and nonalcoholic beverages to children. Member States should also consider implementing other relevant evidence-guided strategies, to promote healthy diets in the entire population while protecting dietary guidance and food policy from undue influence of commercial and other vested interests."

Among the dietary recommendations suggested in "Follow-Up to the Political Declaration of the High-Level Meeting of the General Assembly on the Prevention and Control of Non-communicable Diseases" are reducing the content of free and added sugars (sugar added to food and beverages by manufacturers as well as sugar naturally present in honey, syrup, and fruit juices) in food and beverages, developing policies that engage food retailers to improve the availability, affordability, and acceptability of more healthful food products (plant foods, including fruit and vegetables, and products with reduced content of salt/sodium, saturated fatty acids, trans-fatty acids, and free sugars), and reducing the impact of marketing of unhealthful foods to children.

These guidelines are not, however, favored by some food manufacturers. For example, in "Sugar, Obesity, and the Current Environment" (June 23, 2015, http://www .isosugar.org/Workshop/WS15Guatemala/01-Gaine%20-%20ISO%20June%202015%20-%20final.pdf), P. Courtney

TABLE 8.1

Total estimated deliveries of caloric sweeteners for domestic food and beverage use, by calendar year, 1966–2014

Calendar year	Sugar[a]		Corn sweeteners				Honey	Other edible syrups	Total caloric sweeteners[b]
	Raw value	Refined basis	HFCS	Glucose syrup	Dextrose	Total			
					1,000 short tons, dry basis				
1966	10,235	9,565	0	952	415	1,367	98	69	11,099
1967	10,474	9,789	3	984	428	1,415	89	50	11,342
1968	10,656	9,959	15	1,031	444	1,489	90	70	11,608
1969	10,950	10,234	33	1,061	459	1,553	101	61	11,949
1970	11,163	10,433	56	1,102	471	1,629	103	51	12,216
1971	11,345	10,603	86	1,163	482	1,731	93	52	12,478
1972	11,487	10,736	121	1,257	485	1,863	105	52	12,756
1973	11,429	10,681	218	1,384	489	2,092	95	53	12,922
1974	10,945	10,229	295	1,480	486	2,262	75	43	12,609
1975	10,302	9,628	527	1,515	473	2,515	108	43	12,294
1976	10,893	10,180	782	1,514	452	2,748	100	44	13,072
1977	11,099	10,373	1,057	1,517	429	3,003	100	44	13,519
1978	10,889	10,177	1,198	1,551	410	3,159	120	45	13,501
1979	10,756	10,052	1,660	1,519	399	3,578	117	44	13,791
1980	10,189	9,522	2,158	1,472	393	4,024	94	50	13,690
1981	9,769	9,130	2,626	1,486	390	4,501	96	46	13,773
1982	9,153	8,554	3,090	1,479	392	4,961	104	46	13,665
1983	8,812	8,236	3,655	1,523	398	5,577	116	47	13,975
1984	8,428	7,877	4,399	1,552	408	6,359	108	47	14,391
1985	8,003	7,479	5,386	1,607	418	7,411	104	48	15,043
1986	7,731	7,225	5,498	1,632	430	7,561	121	50	14,957
1987	8,103	7,573	5,792	1,679	441	7,912	104	54	15,643
1988	8,136	7,604	5,998	1,747	452	8,197	100	54	15,954
1989	8,304	7,761	5,960	1,587	438	7,985	82	52	15,881
1990	8,615	8,051	6,202	1,700	455	8,358	86	53	16,548
1991	8,622	8,058	6,376	1,776	463	8,615	92	53	16,818
1992	8,826	8,249	6,727	1,943	461	9,131	95	20	17,494
1993	8,886	8,305	7,173	2,050	481	9,704	103	20	18,131
1994	9,072	8,478	7,481	2,093	502	10,076	126	26	18,706
1995	9,258	8,652	7,718	2,176	528	10,423	120	38	19,233
1996	9,381	8,767	7,986	2,216	537	10,739	131	94	19,731
1997	9,473	8,853	8,458	2,364	511	11,333	129	81	20,397
1998	9,592	8,964	8,823	2,358	502	11,683	130	81	20,857
1999	9,905	9,257	9,127	2,281	488	11,897	147	78	21,379
2000	9,899	9,252	9,058	2,230	476	11,764	157	84	21,257
2001	9,839	9,195	9,083	2,205	469	11,757	134	101	21,187
2002	9,742	9,105	9,230	2,224	473	11,926	153	97	21,282
2003	9,468	8,848	9,067	2,209	449	11,725	146	104	20,822
2004	9,661	9,029	8,995	2,292	487	11,774	130	96	21,029
2005	9,977	9,324	8,995	2,261	481	11,736	156	94	21,310
2006	9,936	9,286	8,978	2,053	463	11,495	174	98	21,054
2007	9,876	9,230	8,702	2,067	448	11,217	141	94	20,682
2008	10,605	9,911	8,295	2,036	419	10,750	151	93	20,905
2009	10,422	9,740	7,965	1,991	417	10,372	141	90	20,343
2010	10,923	10,208	7,823	1,956	450	10,230	160	104	20,702
2011	10,996	10,276	7,573	1,908	446	9,927	169	102	20,474
2012	11,198	10,466	7,483	1,969	420	9,873	169	104	20,611
2013	11,506	10,754	7,244	1,903	415	9,562	178	111	20,604
2014	11,666	10,903	7,268	1,941	472	9,681	194	129	20,907

HFCS = High-fructose corn syrup.
[a]Based on U.S. sugar deliveries for domestic food and beverage use.
[b]Total includes sugar, refined basis.
Notes: Per capita deliveries of sweeteners by U.S. processors and refiners and direct-consumption imports to food manufacturers, retailers, and other end users represent the per capita supply of caloric sweeteners. The data exclude deliveries to manufacturers of alcoholic beverages. Actual human intake of caloric sweeteners is lower because of uneaten food, spoilage, and other losses.

SOURCE: "Table 49. U.S. Total Estimated Deliveries of Caloric Sweeteners for Domestic Food and Beverage Use, by Calendar Year," in *Sugar and Sweeteners Yearbook Tables*, U.S. Department of Agriculture, Economic Research Service, June 4, 2015, http://www.ers.usda.gov/data-products/sugar-and-sweeteners-yearbook-tables.aspx (accessed October 26, 2015)

Gaine of the International Sugar Organization asserts, "There is no correlation between added sugars consumption and rates of obesity globally," and strenuously objects to the recommendation that sugar amount to no more than 5% of food and drink calories consumed per day. Table 8.1 shows that the total U.S. consumption of caloric sweeteners spiked in 1999, 2000, 2002, and 2005, but that the overall use of caloric sweeteners has not varied significantly between 1998 and 2014.

There has historically been U.S. opposition to the WHO strategy, and some WHO scientists and consumer advocacy groups suggest the U.S. objections aim to protect industries that have been under attack rather than to improve public health. The 2015 WHO recommendation to limit sugar consumption to just 5% of daily caloric intake rather than its 2003 recommendation of 10% was endorsed by Walter Willett, head of nutrition at the Harvard School of Public Health, and Marion Nestle, a nutrition researcher at New York University, as well as many health and professional associations but not by growers of cane and beet sugar.

In "Storm Brewing over WHO Proposal" (*Nature News*, March 11, 2014), Brian Owens explains that the WHO 2015 guidelines stating that no more than 5% of an adult's daily calories should come from from free sugars prompted the U.S. Sugar Association to call for the U.S. government to withdraw its funding for the WHO if the WHO did not retract its revised guidelines. Nestle understands the industry backlash, observing, "If people follow this advice, that would be very bad for business." For example, because American young adults consume more than 15% of their calories from sugar, complying with WHO guidelines would cut their consumption by more than two-thirds.

Reducing sugar consumption will be difficult for other countries as well. The WHO notes in a March 4, 2015, press release, "WHO Calls on Countries to Reduce Sugars Intake among Adults and Children" (http://www.who.int/mediacentre/news/releases/2015/sugar-guideline/en/), "that sugar consumption among adults ranges from about 7–8% of total calories consumed in Hungary and Norway to 16–17% in Spain and the United Kingdom. Sugar consumption is even higher among children, ranging from 12% in Denmark, Slovenia, and Sweden to nearly 25% in Portugal."

In 2015 the U.S. Dietary Guidelines Advisory Committee, which convenes every five years to review and update the nation's dietary guidelines, recommended that Americans limit their sugar consumption to no more than 10% of their daily calories, which would be about 12 teaspoons per day for many adults—or about half of their current intake of 22–30 teaspoons per day. In "Nutrition Panel Calls for Less Sugar and Eases Cholesterol and Fat Restrictions" (NYTimes.com, February 19, 2015), Anahad O'Connor reports that many experts who took issue with the committee's advice to limit consumption of salt and saturated fat endorsed its recommendation to limit sugar. Table 8.2 presents the recommendations about consumption of sugar or sugar-sweetened beverages from the WHO; American Academy of Pediatrics; American Diabetes Association; American Heart Association; Centers for Disease Control and Prevention (CDC); and National Heart, Lung, and Blood Institute (one of the National Institutes of Health).

Is Sugar the New Tobacco?

The WHO names sugar as one of the chief culprits in the current epidemic of obesity and obesity-related diseases, diabetes, and cardiovascular heart disease. The

TABLE 8.2

Recommendations about consumption of added sugar or sugar-sweetened beverages from international and national organizations, 2015

Organization	Recommendation/statement related to added sugars and/or sugar-sweetened beverages
World Health Organization (WHO)	• WHO recommends reduced intake of free sugars throughout the life-course (*strong recommendation*). • In both adults and children, WHO recommends that intake of free sugars not to exceed 10% of total energy (*strong recommendation*). • WHO suggests further reduction to below 5% of total energy (*conditional recommendation*).
American Heart Association (AHA)	The AHA recommends reductions in added sugars with an upper limit of half of the discretionary calorie allowance that can be accommodated within the appropriate energy intake level needed for a person to achieve or maintain a healthy weight based on the USDA food intake patterns. Most American women should eat or drink no more than 100 calories per day from added sugars (about 6 teaspoons), and most American men should eat or drink no more than 150 calories per day from added sugars (about 9 teaspoons).
Healthy People 2020	Objective NWS-17.2: Reduce consumption of calories from added sugars (target: 10.8%)
American Academy of Pediatrics (AAP)	Limit consumption of sugar-sweetened beverages (consistent evidence) Pediatricians should work to eliminate sweetened drinks in schools *Note: Due to limited studies in children, the American Academy of Pediatrics (AAP) has no official recommendations regarding the use of non-caloric sweeteners.*
American Diabetes Association (ADA)	**Prevention** Research has shown that drinking sugary drinks is linked to type 2 diabetes, and the American Diabetes Association recommends that people limit their intake of sugar-sweetened beverages to help prevent diabetes. **Diabetes management** People with diabetes should limit or avoid intake of sugar-sweetened beverages (from any caloric sweetener including high fructose corn syrup and sucrose) to reduce risk for weight gain and worsening of cardiometabolic risk profile. (evidence rating B)
NHLBI expert panel guidelines for cardiovascular health and risk reduction in childhood	Reduced intake of sugar-sweetened beverages is associated with decreased obesity measures (Grade B).

NHLBI = National Heart, Lung, and Blood Institute.

SOURCE: "Table D6.2. Recommendations or Statements Related to Added Sugars or Sugar-Sweetened Beverages from International and National Organizations," in *Scientific Report of the 2015 Dietary Guidelines Advisory Committee*, U.S. Department of Agriculture and U.S. Department of Health & Human Services, Dietary Guidelines Advisory Committee, February 2015, http://health.gov/dietaryguidelines/2015-scientific-report/PDFs/Scientific-Report-of-the-2015-Dietary-Guidelines-Advisory-Committee.pdf (accessed October 19, 2015)

WHO approach to food is not, however, comparable to its strategy to combat tobacco use. The food strategy aims to provide member states and other interested stakeholders with a range of recommendations and policy options to promote healthier diets and more physical activity. It is up to member states to decide how these should be further developed and implemented at the national level. Because the strategy was endorsed at the World Health Assembly, member states are responsible for determining which specific policy options are appropriate to their circumstances. The WHO provides technical support for the implementation of programs, as requested by member states.

AMERICANS CRAVE SUGAR

The United States is the world leader in sweetener consumption and is among the top sugar producers and importers. Table 8.3 shows monthly estimates of the U.S. sugar supply and use during fiscal year 2016. Dan Pearson explains in "U.S. Sugar Policy Is Not So Sweet" (USNews.com, February 14, 2015) that the federal government uses import restrictions, production quotas, and loan guarantees, among other measures, to ensure that U.S. sugar producers get good prices for their crops. Pearson notes that in 2013 the U.S. Department of Agriculture (USDA) acquired surplus sugar to keep prices high and "then spent more than $250 million of taxpayer

funds to convert that sugar into relatively lower-value ethanol." Pearson observes that although other countries also have policies that influence sugar production and trade, the U.S. sugar industry would remain workable without subsidies and import restrictions and a USDA report, "Sugar and Sweeteners Outlook" (Stephen Haley, May 15, 2014, http://www.ers.usda.gov/media/1423902/sss_m_309.pdf), confirms this assumption.

Many industry observers believe that farm subsidies such as sugar subsidies undermine efforts to improve Americans' diets. For example, in "Food System Policy, Public Health, and Human Rights in the United States" (*Annual Review of Public Health*, vol. 36, March 18, 2015), Kerry L. Shannon et al. assert that many subsidies favor nutrient-poor, processed foods and beverages rather than production of fruits and vegetables. Karen R. Siegel et al. explain in "The Contribution of Subsidized Food Commodities to Total Energy Intake among U.S. Adults" (*Public Health Nutrition*, September 2015) that more than 50% of the energy in U.S. diets is derived from federally subsidized commodities. Current agricultural policies promote the production of refined grains, dairy, and meat products. Apples were the only fresh fruit or vegetable that received federal support from 1995 to 2010.

Sugar (including sucrose, dextrose, fructose, corn syrup, and maltodextrin) is a key ingredient of many processed food products. Table 8.4 lists the names of

TABLE 8.3

Monthly estimates of fiscal year 2016 sugar supply and use, May–October 2015

	May 2015	June 2015	July 2015	August 2015	September 2015	October 2015
	1,000 short tons, raw value					
Beginning stocks	1,607	1,807	1,729	1,821	1,730	1,697
Total production	**8,450**	**8,720**	**8,765**	**8,800**	**8,734**	**8,760**
Beet sugar	4,770	5,040	4,980	4,980	5,034	5,075
Cane sugar	3,680	3,680	3,785	3,820	3,700	3,685
Florida	1,825	1,825	1,875	1,910	1,940	1,940
Hawaii	190	190	190	190	180	165
Louisiana	1,535	1,535	1,590	1,590	1,450	1,450
Texas	130	130	130	130	130	130
Total imports	**3,810**	**3,216**	**3,364**	**3,369**	**3,394**	**3,398**
Tariff-rate quota imports	1,369	1,369	1,491	1,491	1,524	1,528
Other program imports	315	315	315	315	315	315
Non-program imports	2,126	1,531	1,558	1,563	1,555	1,555
Mexico	2,116	1,521	1,548	1,548	1,540	1,540
Total supply	**13,867**	**13,743**	**13,858**	**13,990**	**13,858**	**13,856**
Exports	200	200	200	200	200	200
Adjustments	0	0	0	0	0	0
Total deliveries	**12,120**	**12,010**	**12,010**	**12,010**	**12,010**	**11,920**
Domestic food and beverage	11,985	11,875	11,875	11,875	11,875	11,785
Other use	135	135	135	135	135	135
Total use	**12,320**	**12,210**	**12,210**	**12,210**	**12,210**	**12,120**
Ending stocks	1,547	1,533	1,648	1,780	1,648	1,736
Stocks/use ratio	12.56	12.55	13.50	14.58	13.50	14.32

SOURCE: "Table 26. Monthly Estimates of Fiscal 2016 U.S. Sugar Supply and Use," in *Sugar and Sweeteners Yearbook Tables*, U.S. Department of Agriculture, Economic Research Service, August 13, 2015, http://www.ers.usda.gov/data-products/sugar-and-sweeteners-yearbook-tables.aspx (accessed October 26, 2015)

TABLE 8.4

Names for added sugars that appear on food labels

A food is likely to be high in sugars if one of these names appears first or second in the ingredient list or if several names are listed.

Brown sugar	Invert sugar
Corn sweetener	Lactose
Corn syrup	Malt syrup
Dextrose	Maltose
Fructose	Molasses
Fruit juice concentrate	Raw sugar
Glucose	Sucrose
High-fructose corn syrup	Syrup
Honey	Table sugar

SOURCE: "Box 21. Names for Added Sugars That Appear on Food Labels," in *Nutrition and Your Health: Dietary Guidelines for Americans*, 5th ed., U.S. Department of Health and Human Services and U.S. Department of Agriculture, 2000, http://www.health.gov/dietaryguidelines/dga2000/document/choose.htm (accessed October 26, 2015)

added sugars that may be found in processed foods. Roberto A. Ferdman reports in "Where People Eat the Most Sugar and Fat" (WashingtonPost.com, February 5, 2015) that the average American consumes more than 4.45 ounces (126 g) of sugar per day (more than the sugar contained in three 12-ounce (355 ml) cans of Coca-Cola). U.S. sugar consumption is twice the average intake of 54 countries. The Netherlands, Germany, and Ireland trail the United States with daily consumption of 3.62 ounces (102.5 g), 3.60 ounces (102 g), and 3.41 ounces (96.7 g), respectively. Italy (2.03 ounces [57.6 g]), Japan (2 ounces [56.7 g]) and Greece (1.99 ounces [56.5 g]) consume less than half the U.S. average, and the lowest reported consumption is in China (0.55 ounces [15.7 g]), Indonesia (0.54 ounces [15.2 g]), Israel (0.51 ounces [14.5 g]) and India (0.18 ounces [5.1 g]).

In "The Relationship of Sugar to Population-Level Diabetes Prevalence: An Econometric Analysis of Repeated Cross-Sectional Data" (*PLoS One*, vol. 8, no, 2, February 2013), Sanjay Basu et al. report that there is a direct correlation between how much sugar is available in countries' food supplies and their rates of type 2 diabetes. Countries with higher amounts of sugar in their food supply had higher rates of type 2 diabetes. Specifically, every additional 150 calories of sugar available per person per day (roughly equivalent to the sugar in a can of soda) is associated with a 1.1% increase in diabetes prevalence.

The health food industry has been warning the public about the perils of the overconsumption of refined sugars for more than 40 years, and mainstream nutritionists and public health professionals have joined the ranks of those calling for reduced sugar consumption. Along with ending sugar subsidies, they want to sharply limit the advertising of sugary products to children, ban the sale of soft drinks in schools, and conduct widespread community public health education programs to inform Americans about the health risks of consuming excessive amounts of refined sugars.

THE U.S. WAR ON OBESITY GAINS MOMENTUM

Besides generating international debate, the issue of obesity is receiving considerable attention from lawmakers, public health officials, and politicians throughout the United States. For example, the Trust for America's Health (TFAH; a nonprofit, nonpartisan organization working to make disease prevention a national priority) calls for a national strategy to combat obesity to address the problem. The TFAH and the Robert Wood Johnson Foundation detail in *The State of Obesity 2015: Better Policies for a Healthier America* (September 2015, http://healthyamericans.org/assets/files/TFAH-2015-Obesity Report-final.22.pdf) state and national obesity rates and policies to prevent and reduce obesity. The report describes policy accomplishments over the preceding decade, including changes to nutrition standards for school foods, farm-to-school programs, improved health screenings for children, changes to improve nutrition and health counseling in the Supplemental Nutrition Assistance Program and the Special Supplemental Nutrition Program for Women, Infants, and Children (WIC) programs, increased understanding about how the built environment affects people's ability to eat healthful foods and be physically active, and a growth in community-based programs targeting obesity. Key recommendations include:

- Preventing overweight and obesity in children by helping children maintain a healthy weight

- Providing children and adults with more opportunities to be physically active

- Continuing to improve school nutrition

- Marketing only food and beverage companies' healthiest products to children

- Investing more in preventing disease to save money spent treating it

- Encouraging walking and biking in transportation plans

- Making healthy, affordable foods available for purchase close to consumers' homes

Recommendations based on in-depth interviews with public health experts in African American and Latino communities include:

- Improving access to affordable healthy foods and opportunities for physical activity by increasing resources for programs and connecting obesity-prevention initiatives with other ongoing community programs

- Providing education and addressing cultural differences to improve knowledge about nutrition and physical activity and make health promotion programs relevant to people's daily lives

- Establishing community input, involvement, and shared leadership as top priorities of obesity-prevention initiatives from the outset

Jennifer L. Pomeranz and Kelly D. Brownell of Yale University assert in "Advancing Public Health Obesity Policy through State Attorneys General" (*American Journal of Public Health*, vol. 101, no. 3, March 2011) that the war on obesity requires "government action at multiple levels and across disciplines." The researchers call on state attorneys general to assume lead roles to champion nutrition policy and to protect consumers, especially children, from misleading marketing and advertising practices. Attorneys general can also reach across state lines to tackle issues including food marketing in schools and the use of web-tracking and analytics that target food marketing to individual Internet users, including children. They can advocate consumer education and can issue formal written opinions about issues such as the legality of taxing sugar-sweetened beverages. Pomeranz and Brownell aver that "there is much room for greater attorney general involvement in formulating and championing solutions to this public health problem. Obesity may not be on the radar of every attorney general as a topic for their attention, so state and local advocates should contact and work with their attorneys general to support public health measures at every level."

Skirmishes in the war on obesity do not center on whether there is a problem, but on how best to address it. Participants on one side characterize the food industry, advertisers, and the media as complicit, in that they entice consumers with seductive advertising and sugary, high-calorie treats. Their opponents believe consumers should exercise personal responsibility and make their own choices about food and exercise.

U.S. GOVERNMENT MOVES TO BAN TRANS FAT

In June 2015 the U.S. Food and Drug Administration (FDA) put forth a plan to eliminate trans fats from the U.S. food supply by 2018. Sabrina Tavernise observes in "F.D.A. Sets 2018 Deadline to Rid Foods of Trans Fats" (NYTimes.com, June 16, 2015) that the agency reclassified partially hydrogenated oils (the source of trans fats in fried and baked goods and margarine) as no longer "generally recognized as safe." This would for all intents and purposes ban them from use in food. The FDA's move came nearly a decade after it first required that added trans fats be listed on food labels in 2006, which caused many companies to reformulate their products to eliminate or greatly reduce them and two years after it announced its plan to eliminate the artificial fats from the food supply. For instance, the FDA estimates that consumption of trans fats fell by 78% between 2005 and 2012 in response to the labeling requirement and reformulation of foods that previously contained trans fats.

Tavernise reports, however, that some nutritionists were concerned that health benefits would not be realized if Americans replaced their consumption of trans fats with saturated fats. Barry M. Popkin, an epidemiologist with expertise in nutrition, explained that saturated fats in baked goods, which also pose a threat to Americans' health, increased from 2005 to 2012, in response to the need to reduce use of trans fats.

JUNK FOOD IS IRRESISTIBLE—IS THE FOOD INDUSTRY TO BLAME?

In "The Extraordinary Science of Addictive Junk Food" (NYTimes.com, February 24, 2013), Michael Moss asserts that the food industry has conditioned Americans to crave unhealthful, sugary, salty, fatty, processed foods. Moss describes food industry efforts aimed at getting consumers "hooked" on convenient, inexpensive foods and their efforts to use science not only to produce highly desirable and potentially addictive foods but also to dismiss health concerns about excessive consumption of salt, sugar, and fat. He refers to the sophisticated scientific and market testing that produces food that looks and tastes good but is not necessarily healthy.

Other research argues against the notion that it is possible to become addicted to junk food or any other food. In "'Eating Addiction,' Rather Than 'Food Addiction' Better Captures Addictive-Like Eating Behavior" (*Neuroscience and Biobehavioral Reviews*, vol. 47, November 2014), Johannes Hebebrand et al. assert that "eating addiction" is a behavioral addiction that may contribute to obesity but is not a substance-based addiction. However, Hebebrand et al. concede, "Undoubtedly, the food industry needs to act responsibly given that easy access to highly palatable and calorie-dense foods promotes overeating and potentially the development of an 'eating addiction' in predisposed individuals."

Does Nutrition Labeling Help Consumers Make Healthier Choices?

According to Joanna Parks of the FDA's Center for Food Safety and Applied Nutrition, food labels do affect what people eat. In *The Effects of Food Labeling and Dietary Guidance on Nutrition in the United States* (August 2013, http://ageconsearch.umn.edu/bitstream/149667/2/AAEA%20Nut-Label-DRAFT-IV-5-23-13.pdf), she reports that people who use the Nutrition Facts Panel (NFP) on food packages to learn about their ingredients and nutrients consume 120 fewer calories per day on average than those who do not use the labels. This may help them to regulate body weight. Parks reports that some groups of people were more likely to report using the NFP than others, including women, people with college degrees, those with food allergies, those who think it is important to consider nutrition when making food choices, individuals who engage in vigorous leisure-time physical activity, and people who follow special diets.

Another study, in which "traffic light" labeling—red for unhealthy items, yellow for less healthy items, and green for healthy items—was used to identify foods in a hospital cafeteria, confirms that labels do influence purchasing behavior. In "A Traffic Light Food Labeling Intervention Increases Consumer Awareness of Health and Healthy Choices at the Point-of-Purchase" (*Preventive Medicine*, vol. 57, no. 4, October 2013), Lillian Sonnenberg et al. find that the traffic light labels "prompt people to consider their health at point-of-purchase" and help them make healthier food choices.

Catherine E. Cioffi et al. looked at whether the introduction of nutrition labels in university dining halls influenced food purchases and reported their findings in "A Nudge in a Healthy Direction: The Effect of Nutrition Labels on Food Purchasing Behaviors in University Dining Facilities" (*Appetite*, vol. 92, September 2015). Cioffi et al. analyzed weekly sales data for a sample of packaged food items three semesters before and three semesters after nutrition labels were introduced and find that the labels prompted a small reduction of high-calorie and high-fat foods purchased and an increase in purchases of low-calorie, low-fat foods.

FDA Proposes Changes to the Nutrition Facts Label

In July 2015 the FDA issued proposed changes to the nutrition facts label. The "Factsheet on the New Proposed Nutrition Facts Label" (July 24, 2015, http://www.fda.gov/Food/GuidanceRegulation/GuidanceDocumentsRegulatory Information/LabelingNutrition/ucm387533.htm) explains that the changes are in response to new information about nutrition, obesity, and chronic disease. For example, serving sizes would be updated to reflect the amounts of food and beverages people actually consume in 2015 rather than the amounts consumed 20 years ago when the nutrition facts labels debuted. (See Figure 8.1.) The FDA also proposes requiring the label to display the percent daily value (%DV) for added sugars. The percent daily value would be based on the recommendation that the daily intake of calories from added sugars not exceed 10% of total calories. The updated label also would change the footnote to more clearly explain the meaning of the percent daily value and would replace "Calories from Fat" with "Total Fat," "Saturated Fat," and "Trans Fat" since research demonstrates that the type of fat is more important than the amount.

The FDA also proposes to change the format of the label so that calories, serving sizes, and percent daily value are more prominent. Figure 8.2 shows the original label format and the proposed new format.

FIGURE 8.1

Proposed serving size changes, 2015

Serving size changes

What's considered a single serving has changed in the decades since the original nutrition label was created. So now serving sizes will be more realistic to reflect how much people typically eat at one time.

Packaging affects servings

Package size affects how much people eat and drink. So now, for example, both 12 *and* 20 ounce bottles will equal 1 serving, since people typically drink both sizes in one sitting.

1 Serving per bottle for either bottle size

SOURCE: "Proposed Serving Size Changes: Food Serving Sizes Get a Reality Check," in *Proposed Changes to the Nutrition Facts Label*, U.S. Food and Drug Administration, October 23, 2015, http://www.fda.gov/Food/GuidanceRegulation/GuidanceDocuments-Regulatory Information/LabelingNutrition/ucm385663.htm#images (accessed October 26, 2015)

Can and Should Laws Change Americans' Diets?

The American legal professor John F. Banzhaf III (1940–), who campaigned against tobacco, advocates using the legal system to create change in Americans' diets. He exhorts attorneys to bring lawsuits against fast-food purveyors and junk-food manufacturers to increase consumer awareness of the role the food industry plays in promoting obesity. Banzhaf was interviewed in Morgan Spurlock's (1970–) groundbreaking documentary film *Super Size Me* (2004), which focuses on the fast-food industry's promotion of unhealthful eating and the director's experience subsisting on a diet of fast food for 30 days.

The Center for Consumer Freedom is an advocacy group that is supported by restaurants, food companies,

FIGURE 8.2

Proposed changes to Nutrition Facts label, 2015

Nutrition Facts	
Serving Size 2/3 cup (55 g)	
Servings Per Container About 8	

Amount Per Serving	
Calories 230	Calories from Fat 72
	% Daily Value*
Total Fat 8 g	**12%**
Saturated Fat 1 g	**5%**
Trans Fat 0 g	
Cholesterol 0 mg	**0%**
Sodium 160 mg	**7%**
Total Carbohydrate 37 g	**12%**
Dietary Fiber 4 g	**16%**
Sugars 1 g	
Protein 3 g	
Vitamin A	10%
Vitamin C	8%
Calcium	20%
Iron	45%

*Percent Daily Values are based on a 2,000 calorie diet. Your daily value may be higher or lower depending on your calorie needs.

	Calories:	2,000	2,500
Total Fat	Less than	65 g	80 g
Sat Fat	Less than	20 g	25 g
Cholesterol	Less than	300 mg	300 mg
Sodium	Less than	2,400 mg	2,400 mg
Total Carbohydrate		300 g	375 g
Dietary Fiber		25 g	30 g

Nutrition Facts		
8 servings per container		
Serving Size		2/3 cup (55 g)

Amount per 2/3 cup		
Calories 230		**230**
% DV*		
12%	**Total Fat** 8 g	
5%	Saturated Fat 1 g	
	Trans Fat 0 g	
0%	**Cholesterol** 0 mg	
7%	**Sodium** 160 mg	
12%	**Total Carbs** 37 g	
14%	Dietary Fiber 4 g	
	Sugars 1 g	
	Added Sugars 0 g	
	Protein 3 g	
10%	**Vitamin D** 2 mcg	
20%	**Calcium** 260 mg	
45%	**Iron** 8 mg	
5%	**Potassium** 235 mg	

*Footnote on Daily Values (DV) and calories reference to be inserted here.

SOURCE: Adapted from "Label Formats Original vs. Proposed Original," in *Proposed Changes to the Nutrition Facts Label*, U.S. Food and Drug Administration, October 23, 2015, http://www.fda.gov/Food/GuidanceRegulation/GuidanceDocumentsRegulatoryInformation/LabelingNutrition/ucm385663.htm#images (accessed October 26, 2015).

and individual donors. The center marshals lawyers, publicists, and lobbyists to respond to antiobesity crusaders and derides lawsuits and legislation aimed at limiting consumers' rights to choose the foods they want to consume. It also pokes fun at the self-appointed "food police" (legislators, public health officials, and others) that are intent on modifying Americans' diets, and at mandates by the Center for Science in the Public Interest (CSPI; a nonprofit advocacy group for nutrition, food safety, health, and other issues) to offer consumers nutritional data. It is credited with helping defeat a measure that would have required chain restaurants to offer nutritional data about their products. In "Obamacare's Calorie Mandate Takes a Bite Out of Consumers Wallets" (April 6, 2015, https://www.consumerfreedom.com/op-ed/obamacares-calorie-mandate-takes-a-bite-out-of-consumers-wallets/), Will Coggin of the Center for Consumer Freedom staunchly opposes FDA restaurant menu-labeling requirements. He asserts that complying with the regulations is costly and that these costs will be passed along to consumers. He also contends that labeling fast food will not influence consumer purchasing behavior.

The Obesity Society Action Plan

In its position statement (http://www.obesity.org/obesity/publications/position-and-policies/eradicating-epidemic), the Obesity Society provides an ambitious agenda for the government and private sector that enumerates specific funding priorities, programs, and services to prevent, treat, and educate Americans. It calls for:

- Waging a "war on obesity, not the obese." The Obesity Society asserts that this war will not be waged or won by further stigmatizing obese people and calls for efforts to end discrimination and eliminate the social stigma associated with obesity.

- Educating the public to improve awareness of obesity as "a complex disease involving genes, behavior and environment" rather than as a moral weakness.

- Informing the public about obesity, its causes, and consequences, and engaging in "a national debate on obesity, similar to past campaigns on smoking and cholesterol."

- Expanding access to professional treatment of obesity so that its medical, social, and economic consequences can be averted.

- Ensuring reimbursement for medical treatment for obesity, including drugs and surgery.

- Including nutrition education, lifestyle counseling, and obesity diagnosis and management into medical school curricula and other health professionals' training.

- Revising national policies, such as farm policies promoting the production of energy-dense foods with low nutritional value, that exacerbate the problem.

- Preventing excess weight gain in children and adults, teaching healthy behaviors and lifestyles early in life, and providing healthy school lunches.

- Building environments that encourage healthier behaviors such as walking and more physical activity at work.

- Recognizing the economic impact of obesity on medical expenditures and lost wages.

- Supporting research to address the problem by doubling funding from federal agencies including the CDC, the National Institutes of Health, and the USDA.

To advance its agenda, the Obesity Society works with the U.S. Congress, the U.S. surgeon general, and the CDC as well as with health care organizations and providers. For example, because only four states (California, Massachusetts, Michigan, and New Mexico) cover both weight-loss treatment and weight-loss surgery, together with the American Society of Metabolic and Bariatric Surgeons, the Obesity Society is working at the federal and state levels to improve health insurance coverage for weight-loss treatment. The society is also soliciting support for the Treat and Reduce Obesity Act of 2015, legislation introduced in May 2015 by Senators Bill Cassidy (1957–; R-LA) and Tom Carper (1947–; D-DE) and Representatives Eric Paulsen (1965–; R-MN) and Ron Kind (1963–; D-WI). The act would ensure that Medicare recipients have access to obesity screening and counseling services, and new prescription drugs for chronic weight management. As of February 2016, the bill had not been enacted.

The Healthy, Hunger-Free Kids Act

In December 2010 President Barack Obama (1961–) signed the Healthy, Hunger-Free Kids Act into law. Also known as the Child Nutrition Act, it authorizes funding for federal school meal and child nutrition programs and is intended to increase access to healthful food for low-income children. The bill reauthorizes child nutrition programs for five years and includes $4.5 billion in new funding for these programs over 10 years. Furthermore, it:

- Authorizes the USDA to establish nutritional standards for all foods that are sold in schools during the school day, including vending machines, lunch lines, and school stores

- Provides increased reimbursement to schools that meet updated nutritional standards for federally subsidized lunches

- Assists communities to establish local farm-to-school networks, create school gardens, and use more local foods in schools

- Improves access to drinking water in schools

- Establishes standards for school wellness policies, including goals for nutrition promotion and education and physical activity

- Promotes nutrition and wellness in child care settings through the federally subsidized Child and Adult Care Food Program (CACFP)

- Supports breast-feeding through the WIC program

The USDA describes its school nutrition standards in "Smart Snacks in School: USDA's 'All Foods Sold in Schools' Standards" (July 16, 2013, http://www.fns.usda .gov/cnd/governance/legislation/allfoods.htm). The standards aim to ensure that all foods offered in schools are nutritious. The standards establish limits on how many calories food available in schools can contain, as well as how much sodium, fat, and sugar. In addition, any food sold in schools must meet at least one of four requirements: be whole-grain rich; have a fruit, vegetable, dairy product, or protein food as its first ingredient; be a "combination food" containing at least a quarter cup of fruits or vegetables; contain 10% or more of the recommended daily value of calcium, potassium, vitamin D, or dietary fiber. For a comparison of food offered in schools before and after the new standards, see Figure 4.7 in Chapter 4.

In *State of Obesity 2015*, the TFAH and the Robert Wood Johnson Foundation name the act "a key milestone" toward reversing the obesity epidemic. The act helped raise nutrition standards in schools and child care settings, made school meals more accessible through community eligibility programs, and strengthened requirements for local school wellness policies. It directed the USDA to improve the CACFP, which was designed to ensure that children in day care centers and adults in adult day care programs received nutritious meals.

OVERWEIGHT, OBESITY, AND THE LAW

Health care coverage and the availability of services to prevent or treat obesity vary widely. The Patient Protection and Affordable Care Act (ACA), which was signed into law in 2010, significantly strengthens obesity-prevention efforts. The law authorizes new resources and initiatives, including screening for obesity, diet counseling for adults who are at risk for chronic diseases, and referral to intensive behavioral interventions that are intended to reduce obesity.

The ACA also funded the Childhood Obesity Research Demonstration Project (CORD), which was established through the Children's Health Insurance Program Reauthorization Act of 2009. The demonstration project funds programs aimed at improving children's nutrition. It is aimed at children aged 2 to 12 years who are covered by the Children's Health Insurance Program, which provides low-cost health insurance to over 7 million children of working families. The CDC observes in "Childhood Obesity Research Demonstration Project" (March 13, 2015, http://www.cdc.gov/nccdphp/dnpao/division-information/programs/researchproject.html) that the four grantees successfully helped to reduce obesity among low-income children by increasing their physical activity and consumption of fruits and vegetables, decreasing their screen time and consumption of sugar-sweetened beverages, and encouraging children to get sufficient sleep. CORD project funding ended on September 29, 2015, and a summary report of the project findings was anticipated in the summer of 2016.

In addition, the ACA requires chain restaurants and food establishments to disclose calorie counts and other nutritional information (fat, saturated fat, cholesterol, sodium, total carbohydrates, sugars, fiber, and total protein) for standard menu items. Vending machine operators with 20 or more machines must also disclose calorie content for many items.

Sin Taxes on Sodas and Junk Food?

Sin taxes are taxes imposed on goods at least in part because the government wants to discourage their use by forcing their prices higher. Tobacco and alcohol are subject to sin taxes in many areas. Many industry observers believe that taxes on sugary drinks, or on junk food in general, would reduce the amount of these items that Americans consume.

Bridget Hollingsworth reports in "Purchases of Taxed Beverages Decline in Mexico after Excise Tax Takes Effect" (*Global Food Research Program @ UNC*, June 16, 2015, http://uncfoodresearchprogram.web.unc.edu/822/) that a 10% tax on sugar-sweetened beverages that took effect in 2014 decreased their consumption an average of 6%. Reductions were higher among lower socioeconomic households, averaging 9% during 2014 compared to pretax trends and as high as 17% by the close of 2014. During the same period there was a 4% increase in purchases of untaxed beverages, largely driven by an increase in purchased bottled plain water.

In March 2015 the Navajo Nation became the first U.S. community to impose a tax on junk food. In "This Place Just Became the First Part of the U.S. to Impose a Tax on Junk Food" (Time.com, March 30, 2015), Sabrina Toppa reports that effective April 1, 2015, the Healthy Diné Nation Act imposes a 2% tax on junk food and eliminates a 5% sales tax on healthful foods such as fruits and vegetables. The sin tax revenues will be used to support farmers' markets, vegetable gardens, and greenhouses on Navajo reservations.

The same month, Berkeley, California, instituted a one-cent-per-ounce excise tax on sugar-sweetened beverages. In "Higher Retail Prices of Sugar-Sweetened Beverages 3 Months after Implementation of an Excise Tax in Berkeley, California" (*American Journal of Public Health*, vol. 105, no. 11, November 2015), Jennifer Falbe et al. find that three months after the tax began, retail prices of sugar-sweetened beverages (SSBs) increased more in Berkeley than in neighboring cities. Falbe et al. consider this increase "the first step in the causal pathway toward reduced SSB consumption, which could considerably reduce the burden of chronic disease attributed to obesity and other SSB-related health conditions."

Lawsuits Attack Food Service Industry

A number of individuals and advocacy groups have brought lawsuits against the food service industry. Some claim they deserve compensation for the damage that fattening foods have done to their health. Others focus on advertising and marketing that they think is deceptive and misleads people into eating unhealthy products. Many attorneys and public health professionals believe such lawsuits can serve as vehicles that reverse the obesity epidemic, in part because the media attention generated by such lawsuits motivates food companies to produce healthier products and to reconsider marketing and advertising practices.

The first class-action suit was the widely publicized case of Caesar Barber, a 56-year-old New Yorker weighing 270 pounds (122 kg), who claimed that four fast-food restaurants (Burger King, KFC, McDonald's, and Wendy's) jeopardized his health by promoting high-calorie, high-fat, and salty menu items. In "Whopper of a Lawsuit: Fast-Food Chains Blamed for Obesity, Illnesses" (ABCNews.com, July 26, 2002), Geraldine Sealey reports that Barber filed the lawsuit in the New York State Supreme Court "on behalf of an unspecified number of other obese and ill New Yorkers who also feast on fast food." According to Sealey, Barber's suit alleged that the fast-food restaurants, where he ate "four or five times a week even after suffering a heart attack, did not properly disclose the ingredients of their food and the risks of eating too much." Barber's suit was dismissed, so he filed for a second time. His second suit was also dismissed, and he was barred from filing for a third time.

Pelman v. McDonald's Corporation (237 F. Supp. 2d 512, 543 [S.D.N.Y. 2003]) was a similar case, in which two teenagers sought class-action status to sue McDonald's on the grounds that the company had misled them into thinking that its food was healthier than it really was, and as a consequence they had developed obesity and related disorders. The case ended in dismissal in 2010, after nearly 10 years of legal wrangling. In "Where's the Beef?—The Challenges of Obesity Lawsuits" (BloombergLaw.com, 2013), Saul Wilensky and Kerry C. O'Dell explain that the courts sided with McDonald's in *Pelman* for a number of reasons, among them the fact that to prevail the plaintiffs would need to show that McDonald's food was the specific cause of their health problems, not just one factor among many. They opine that similar lawsuits will most likely fail as well.

Legislation Protects Food Industry Interests

The food industry contends that Americans choose what they eat and should not be able to blame the food industry if their personal choices have unhealthy consequences. State and federal legislators who agree with this viewpoint have enacted or attempted to enact so-called Commonsense Consumption Acts (CCAs). In general, CCAs bar civil lawsuits seeking recovery for obesity-related health harms. Some in the media call these laws "cheeseburger bills," and in "Beyond Cheeseburgers: The Impact of Commonsense Consumption Acts on Future Obesity-Related Lawsuits" (*Food and Drug Law Journal*, vol. 68, no. 3, 2013), Cara L. Wilking and Richard A. Daynard report that CCAs were enacted in 25 states between 2004 and 2012. In 16 states the CCAs conferred broad civil immunity for claims stemming from long-term consumption of food.

Wilking and Daynard discuss the rationale for CCAs in their article. As an example, they describe how Colorado's rationale for its CCA states that obesity and other health problems result from "poor choices that are habitually made" by individuals, and that it asserts that "excessive litigation restricts the wide range of choices otherwise available to individuals who consume products responsibly."

Those in favor of CCAs contend that the central issue is "common sense and personal responsibility" and generally subscribe to the opinion that obesity is an individual health issue as opposed to a larger societal and public health problem. Opponents of legislation limiting liability suggest that it is unrealistic to expect consumers to assume personal responsibility when food companies do not disclose relevant information about their products,

such as the number of calories and fat content. Wilking and Daynard argue that CCAs are not truly motivated by a desire to prevent frivolous lawsuits; instead they claim that CCAs aim to "limit legally and factually sound litigation, which might eventually have harmed industry's bottom line and forced it to change its practices."

THE FOOD INDUSTRY RESPONDS TO PUBLIC OUTCRY

Mounting pressure on the food industry to change its marketing practices and offer healthier products has had some success. For example, in the June 25, 2015, press release "McDonald's and Alliance for a Healthier Generation Announce Progress on Commitment to Promote Balanced Food and Beverage Choices" (http://news.mc donalds.com/press-releases/mcdonald-s-and-alliance-for-a-healthier-generation-announce-progress-on-commitme-nyse-mcd-1203234), McDonald's reported progress made on its commitment to "increase customers' access to fruit and vegetables and help families and children make informed choices in keeping with balanced lifestyles." For example, since it removed soda from the Happy Meal menus for children, customers choosing milk and juice rose from 37% to 46%. By February 2015 the majority of restaurants (83%) offered a fruit, vegetable, or salad option as a substitute for french fries in Extra Value Meals. During 2014 all advertisements directed to children and 14 Happy Meal boxes and bags included messages about nutrition or children's well-being.

In "Profits and Pandemics: Prevention of Harmful Effects of Tobacco, Alcohol, and Ultra-processed Food and Drink Industries" (*Lancet*, vol. 381, no. 9867, February 2013), Rob Moodie et al. assessed the effectiveness of self-regulation, public-private partnerships, and public regulation of unhealthy commodities: tobacco, alcohol, and energy-dense ultra-processed food. The researchers assert that:

- Transnational corporations are major drivers of non-communicable disease epidemics and profit from increased consumption of tobacco, alcohol, and ultra-processed food and drink (so-called unhealthy commodities).

- Alcohol and ultra-processed food and drink industries use strategies similar to those of the tobacco industry to undermine effective public health policies and programs.

- Unhealthy commodity industries should have no role in the formation of national or international policy for noncommunicable disease policy.

- Despite the common reliance on industry self-regulation and public-private partnerships to improve public health, there is no evidence to support their effectiveness or safety.

Moodie et al. point out that these three industries have all employed the same tactics—presenting biased research findings, co-opting policy makers and health professionals, and lobbying politicians and public officials to oppose public regulation—to undermine public health interventions. The researchers note that to deflect claims that their products harm health, companies in these industries often point to factors outside their areas of expertise. For example, food and beverage corporations point to physical inactivity as the culprit in the obesity epidemic. Moodie et al. conclude "the only evidence-based mechanisms that effectively prevent harm caused by unhealthy commodity industries are public regulation and market intervention."

FOOD INDUSTRY INITIATIVES

In "Consumers Want Healthy Foods—and Will Pay More for Them" (Forbes.com, February 18, 2015), Nancy Gagliardi reports that food company representatives attending the February 2015 Consumer Analyst Group conference in New York expressed a commitment to healthful food products. For example, the Campbell Soup Co. is debuting soups with USDA-certified organic ingredients and shelf-stable fruit and vegetable juices with no added sugar or artificial ingredients. Gagliardi asserts that consumer demand for foods that promote health and weight loss and their willingness to pay more for them has spurred food manufacturers' new offerings and cites a 2015 Nielsen poll of more than 30,000 consumers that finds 88% of consumers are willing to pay more for healthier foods.

Mehmood Khan, PepsiCo vice chairman and chief scientific officer of global research and development, states in "Fat & Sugar Reduction: PepsiCo R&D: A Catalyst for Change in the Food and Beverage Industry" (New Food, no. 4, 2015) that nutritious products such as dairy, fruits and vegetables, hummus and other fresh dips, and baked grain snacks account for about 20% of the company's revenue. Fifteen years ago, less than 25% of company sales came from zero- or low-calorie beverages and healthful juices, and in 2014 nearly 50% of sales were from these more healthful beverages. Compared with 2006 levels, PepsiCo aims by 2020 to reduce saturated fats per serving by 15% in key food brands, reduce added sugars in key beverages by 25%, and reduce the average amount of sodium in key foods by 25%.

In "Food Industry: Friend or Foe?" (Obesity Reviews, vol. 15, no. 1, January 2014), Derek Yach calls for collaboration between the public and private sectors to address nutrition issues and provide healthy, sustainable food. Yach observes that neither sector fully understands or appreciates the efforts of the other. For example, he cites the tremendous efforts made by companies to reformulate their products to meet standards for salt, sugar, and saturated fat content. He feels that public sector efforts to inform consumers about the dangers of excessive consumption of salt, sugar, and saturated fat would strengthen companies' motivation and ability to supply these healthier food products. Yach notes that inexpensive commodities in the American diet are those that have been heavily subsidized over decades. More expensive foods such as fruits and vegetables have increased in cost over time. Yach favors making healthier choices more affordable rather than imposing taxes on unhealthful foods. He suggests public-private collaboration to improve the taste of foods with reduced sodium and fat and asks that public funds such as those allocated to the National Institutes of Health be used to research cost-effective, sustainable diet and lifestyle solutions rather than drug treatment of diet and weight-related disorders.

Yach notes that corporate innovation and commitment to healthier foods have been rewarded by investors who understand the long-tem importance of improving consumers' health. He points out that companies do not have to sacrifice profits to combat obesity and promote health. They can succeed in selling less volume if they can sell products with similar value. For example, a quality product with a smaller serving size can have a higher profit margin than a bargain-sized product of lesser quality. Yach concludes, "When common interests and outcomes are at stake, private-public engagement is more likely to achieve faster and more sustainable results than relying on governments to act alone."

THE HEALTHY WEIGHT COMMITMENT FOUNDATION AND CHILDHOOD OBESITY

In October 2009 a group of 41 retailers, nongovernmental organizations, and food and beverage manufacturers launched the Healthy Weight Commitment Foundation (HWCF), a national initiative intended to reduce the rate of obesity, especially among children and adolescents. Members of the foundation, which include the Campbell Soup Co., General Mills Inc., Kellogg Co., Nestlé USA, PepsiCo, and Ralston Foods/Post Foods, invested $20 million in the initiative. The initiative targets three key audiences—markets, the workplace, and schools—with a nationwide public education campaign that focuses on ways to help people reach and maintain a healthy weight by balancing calories consumed with calories expended through physical activity.

In its five-year anniversary report, "Working Together to Change the Outlook of a Generation" (2015, http://www.healthyweightcommit.org/images/uploads/HWCF_5_Report_2014/HWCF_5YearAnniversary_FW.pdf), the HWCF reports that the efforts of its members (250 nonprofit organizations, businesses, and retailers) have resulted in elimination of 6.4 trillion calories from the marketplace—400% more than their initial goal—and earned the trust of the government and public health community. The HWCF awarded more than $1 million in grants to schools in need.

WEIGHT-BASED DISCRIMINATION

Nearly everyone who is overweight or obese has experienced some form of bias, from disapproving glances and unsolicited advice about how to lose weight, to the seemingly unending stream of "fat jokes" and the unflattering and even humiliating portrayal of overweight people in the media. The pervasive anti-fat bias in American culture and negative attitudes toward obese individuals have resulted in stigmatization and clear instances of discrimination.

In "A Multinational Examination of Weight Bias: Predictors of Anti-fat Attitudes across Four Countries" (*International Journal of Obesity*, vol. 39, no. 7, March 2015), Rebecca M. Puhl et al. observe that systematic discrimination against obese individuals occurs in interpersonal relationships, education, employment, and health care. Evidence also points to discrimination in adoption proceedings, jury selection, and housing.

Puhl et al. find negative weight-biased attitudes in Canada, the United States, Iceland, and Australia—countries in which more than half of the adult population is overweight or obese. In all four countries the researchers find that bias was predicted by beliefs that "obesity is attributable to lack of willpower and personal responsibility." People who attributed obesity to physiological or environmental causes had lower levels of weight bias than those attributing it to lack of personal control.

Consistent with previous studies, Puhl et al. find women had lower levels of weight bias. The researchers speculate that in view of "women's increased vulnerability to societal scrutiny and judgment based on their physical appearance, it may be that, in general, women are more sensitive to potential biases and stereotypes related to body weight." Puhl et al. also note that having a family member or friend who experienced weight bias, but not participants' own personal experiences of weight bias, predicted lower levels of weight bias. However, Puhl et al. conclude, "Weight bias remains socially acceptable, is rarely challenged, and sanctions to prohibit weight-based prejudice or discrimination are nonexistent."

Angela R. Sutin and Antonio Terracciano find that weight discrimination also increases risk for obesity. In "Perceived Weight Discrimination and Obesity" (*PLOS One*, vol. 8, no. 7, July 24, 2013), Sutin and Terracciano find that rather than motivating people to lose weight, weight discrimination actually increases risk for obesity. The researchers report that among people who were not obese at the beginning of their study, those who experienced weight discrimination were 2.5 times more likely

to be obese at follow-up four years later than those who did not suffer weight discrimination. Among people who were obese at the start of the study, those who experienced discrimination were more than three times as likely to remain obese at follow-up than those who did not experience discrimination.

Overweight and obese job applicants and workers may be subjected to weight-based discrimination in employment. Many studies document discrimination in hiring practices, especially when the positions sought involved public contact, such as sales or direct customer service. Obese workers face inequities in wages, benefits, and promotions, and several studies confirm that the economic penalties are greater for women than for men. Overweight women earn less doing the same work as their normal-weight counterparts and have dimmer prospects for promotion. The courts have considered cases in which workers contended that their job terminations were weight-related. The outcomes of these cases indicate that termination can occur because of employer prejudice and arbitrary weight standards.

In "New Developments in the Law for Obesity Discrimination Protection" (*Obesity*, vol. 21, no. 3, March 2013), Jennifer L. Pomeranz and Rebecca M. Puhl observe that amendments to the Americans with Disabilities Act of 1990 (ADA) that went into effect in 2009 broaden the definition of disability. The courts now consider severe obesity an impairment using the ADA definition of disability. Pomeranz and Puhl believe that additional protections are warranted and suggest legislation comparable to the Age Discrimination in Employment Act, which prohibits employment discrimination based on age.

Weight Bias among Health Professionals

Anti-fat bias among health care professionals may discourage obese people from seeking medical care and compromise the care they receive. Although research indicates that obese patients often delay or cancel medical appointments for a variety of reasons, including fear about being weighed or undressing in front of health professionals, speculation exists that presumed or real prejudice on the part of health professionals may also deter them from seeking medical care.

In "Implicit and Explicit Anti-fat Bias among a Large Sample of Medical Doctors by BMI, Race/Ethnicity and Gender" (*PLoS ONE*, vol. 7, no. 11, November 2012), Janice A. Sabin, Maddalena Marini, and Brian A. Nosek sought to determine the prevalence of negative attitudes about weight among physicians. Bias was assessed using the Implicit Associations Test (IAT), a timed test that analyzes the automatic associations respondents make about particular attributes. For example, the IAT helped identify whether test takers held negative attitudes and stereotypical views about obese people, such as considering them to be lazy, unmotivated, sluggish, or worthless. About two-thirds of the physicians who took the test were in the normal body mass index (BMI; body weight in kilograms divided by height in meters squared) range, and they demonstrated a strong implicit, or unconscious, anti-fat bias. Sabin, Marini, and Nosek explain that implicit bias may predict discriminatory behavior even among people who have no intention of discriminating.

Rebecca M. Puhl, Joerg Luedicke, and Carlos M. Grilo find that students training in the health professions they questioned (including physician associates, clinical psychologists, and physicians in psychiatric residencies) reported significant weight bias. In "Obesity Bias in Training: Attitudes, Beliefs, and Observations among Advanced Trainees in Professional Health Disciplines" (*Obesity*, October 2013), the researchers report that students say obese patients are targets of negative attitudes and insulting humor by peers (63%), health care providers (65%), and instructors (40%).

OBESE AMERICANS RECEIVE FEWER PREVENTIVE HEALTH SERVICES. Ironically, people who are obese and usually receive more medical care for chronic diseases related to obesity may also receive fewer preventive services. Does bias contribute to this disparity in preventive care? In "Preventive Care and Health Behaviors among Overweight/Obese Men in HMOs" (*American Journal of Managed Care*, vol. 18, no. 1, January 2012), Virginia P. Quinn et al. examine the association between BMI and laboratory tests for cholesterol, glucose, and diabetes control, as well as screening exams for colorectal and prostate cancer. Quinn et al. find no weight-related differences in laboratory tests but do find that despite comparable access to care, overweight and obese men were less likely to be screened for colorectal and prostate cancer. This finding is alarming in view of the fact that overweight and obese men are at greater risk for colorectal cancer and may be at greater risk for aggressive forms of prostate cancer.

Quinn et al. suggest that educating health care providers may help to reduce these disparities in care. The researchers observe, "Education also can help clinicians be sensitive to the stigmatizing experiences heavier patients deal with in the medical setting, and the importance of their attitude and choice of words when treating these patients."

Airlines Consider Their Options

In 2002 Southwest Airlines became the center of a fiery debate when the airline decided to strengthen its enforcement of a policy established in 1980 of requesting and requiring passengers who must occupy two airplane seats because of excessive girth to purchase both tickets. The policy allows passengers to be reimbursed for the additional seat if their flight is not full. The National

Association to Advance Fat Acceptance, an advocacy group, and other consumer groups called the move discriminatory. Regardless, Southwest Airlines is not the only airline with this policy; American, United, and other commercial carriers also require large-sized passengers to pay for two seats.

In 2003 the Federal Aviation Administration (FAA) proposed requiring all passengers on small airlines to be weighed in along with their luggage. The FAA asserted that before takeoff the pilot must calculate the weight of the aircraft as well as that of its passengers, luggage, and crew to determine which seats passengers should occupy to ensure proper balance. For this reason, it is vital to know exact passenger and luggage weights on small planes, where several people with a few extra pounds can tilt the plane away from its center of gravity. Although operators of smaller commuter airlines acknowledged the safety issue, they were reluctant to support the FAA recommendation because they feared that weighing people would discourage them from using commuter airlines, many of which were already strapped financially.

In May 2003 the FAA ruled that airlines must assume that passengers weigh between 190 and 195 pounds (86 and 88 kg), depending on the season. At the same time, checked bags on domestic flights were adjusted from an estimated 25 pounds (11 kg) to 30 pounds (14 kg). The requirement followed shortly after the crash of a commuter plane that killed all 21 people aboard. Investigators suspect the propeller plane was slightly above its maximum weight on takeoff, with most of the weight toward the tail. The weight distribution problem was compounded by a maintenance error that made it difficult to lower the nose with the control column. After the 19-seat plane rose above the ground, its nose pointed dangerously skyward; the pilots were unable to level it off, and the plane spun to the ground.

In "How Long until All Airlines Charge More for Fat People?" (BusinessInsider.com, April 5, 2013), Alex Davies reports that Samoa Airlines is the first airline to charge passengers based on how much they and their luggage weigh. The policy helps offset the cost of fuel for heavier passengers and ensures that the airline's small planes, which hold just 12 passengers each, do not exceed their maximum take-off weights. Davies notes that while this policy may work well for a small operation with few flights and passengers, it would be unwieldy for larger carriers to implement. He also asserts that it would be unpopular and might generate protests arguing that the policy is discriminatory.

In "Airline Begins Weighing Passengers for 'Safety'" (CNN.com, August 13, 2015), Karla Cripps reports that Uzbekistan Airways will weigh passengers and their carry-on bags to determine how much weight will be added to the plane. The airline asserts that the record of weights will identify passengers only by sex and child or adult so confidentiality is ensured. Cripps notes that the airline will not institute a "pay-as-you-weigh" fare structure such as the one Samoa Air instituted in 2012 that charges heavier passengers more.

In "Pay-as-You-Weigh Pricing of an Air Ticket: Economics and Major Issues for Discussions and Investigations" (*Journal of Revenue and Pricing Management*, vol. 12, no. 2, March 2013), Bharat P. Bhatta of Sogn of Fjordane University College in Sogndal, Norway, observes that policies that charge heavier passengers more but do not offer discounts to lighter passengers only benefit the airlines while harming passengers and society at large. Instead, Bhatta favors a model with average, high, and low weight fares, based on whether a passenger is of average weight, above a specific weight, or below a specific weight.

Laws against Weight Discrimination

The San Francisco Human Rights Commission reports in "Compliance Guidelines to Prohibit Weight and Height Discrimination" (http://sf-hrc.org/sites/sf-hrc.org/files/migrated/FileCenter/Documents/LBE_EBO/EBO/Height_and_Weight.pdf) that on July 26, 2001, it unanimously approved historic guidelines for implementing a height-weight antidiscrimination law, and the city became the first jurisdiction in the United States to offer guidelines on how to prevent discrimination based on weight or height.

The strength of the ordinance was tested in 2003, when Jennifer Portnick, a 240-pound (109-kg) aerobics instructor, was refused a job at Jazzercise Inc., an international dance-fitness organization based in Carlsbad, California, and brought her case before the San Francisco Human Rights Commission. She eventually reached an agreement with the company to drop a requirement about the appearance of instructors. It was the first case settled under the San Francisco ordinance, which has become known as the "Fat and Short Law."

As of 2015, only one state (Michigan) and several localities (San Francisco and Santa Cruz, California; District of Columbia; Madison, Wisconsin; Urbana, Illinois; and Binghamton, New York) have passed laws to prohibit weight discrimination. In "Support for Laws to Prohibit Weight Discrimination in the United States: Public Attitudes from 2011 to 2013" (*Obesity*, vol. 22, no. 8, August 2014), Young Suh et al. looked at public attitudes about three proposed laws prohibiting weight discrimination between 2011 and 2013. The researchers find that at least 60% of people supported measures to address weight discrimination. Support was highest for laws prohibiting weight discrimination in the workplace (75%), followed by support for adding body weight as a protected category to civil rights statutes, and for measures extending disability protections to people who are obese.

The Origins of Stigma and Bias

Rebecca M. Puhl and Kelly D. Brownell observe in the landmark study "Psychosocial Origins of Obesity Stigma: Toward Changing a Powerful and Pervasive Bias" (*Obesity Reviews*, vol. 4, no. 4, November 2003) that many people intensely dread the possibility of becoming obese. In one survey 24% of women and 17% of men said they would sacrifice three or more years of their life to be thin. Some women choose not to become pregnant because they fear gaining weight and becoming fat. Others smoke cigarettes in an effort to remain thin or reject the advice that they quit smoking because they fear they will gain weight should they quit. This powerful fear of fat, coupled with widespread perceptions that overweight people lack competence, self-control, ambition, intelligence, and attractiveness, create a culture in which it is socially acceptable to hold negative stereotypes about obese individuals and to discriminate against them.

One explanation of the origin of weight stigma is that Americans traditionally believe in self-determination and individualism—people get what they deserve and are responsible for their circumstances. In this context, when overweight is viewed as a consequence of controllable behaviors, it is possible to understand that if an individual believes overweight people are to blame for their weight, then they should be stigmatized. Other research findings—that many Americans view life as predictable, with effort and ability inevitably producing the desired outcomes, and that attractive people are deemed good and believed to embody many positive qualities—support this theory. Interestingly, researchers find that in other countries the best predictors of anti-fat attitudes were cultural values that held both negative views about overweight and the belief that people are responsible for their life outcome.

Several other theories about the origins of weight stigma have been proposed. Conflict theory suggests that prejudice arises from conflicts of interest between groups and struggles to acquire or retain resources or power. Social identity theory posits that groups develop their social identities by comparing themselves to other groups and designating other groups as inferior. Integrated threat theory proposes that stigmatized groups are perceived as a threat. Proponents of this theory suggest that overweight and obese people threaten deeply held cultural values of self-discipline, self-control, moderation, and thinness. Another theory, evolved dispositions theory, proposes that members of a group will be stigmatized if they threaten or undermine group functioning. This evolutionary adaptation may predispose people to shun obese individuals because they are at increased health risk and may not be able to make sufficient contributions to the group's welfare because of weight-related illness or disability.

Reducing Weight Bias and Stigma

In the landmark study "Demonstrations of Implicit Anti-fat Bias: The Impact of Providing Causal Information and Evoking Empathy" (*Health Psychology*, vol. 22, no. 1, January 2003), Bethany A. Teachman et al. wondered if anti-fat bias would be reduced when people were told that an individual's obesity resulted largely from genetic factors rather than from overeating and lack of exercise. The researchers assigned study participants to one of three groups. The first group received no information about the cause of obesity; the second group was given an article asserting that the principal cause of obesity was genetic; and the third group was given an article that attributed most obesity to overeating and lack of physical activity. As the researchers anticipated, the group told that obesity was controllable (resulting from overeating and inactivity) revealed the greatest amount of bias. However, to their surprise, Teachman et al. find that the group informed that obesity was primarily genetic in origin did not have significantly lower levels of bias than either the control group that had received no prior information or the group informed that obesity was caused by overeating and inactivity.

Teachman et al. also wanted to find out whether eliciting empathy for obese people would significantly reduce negative attitudes. The researchers hypothesized that by sharing written stories about weight-based discrimination with study participants they would feel empathy with the subjects in the stories, which they would then generalize to the entire population of obese people. Although some study participants in the group that read the stories displayed lower bias, the majority did not have lower bias than the control group that had not read the stories of discrimination. The researchers speculate that the stories describing negative evaluations of an obese person might actually have served to reinforce rather than diminish bias.

Puhl and Brownell note that the increasing prevalence of obesity has not acted to reduce weight bias. They also refute the notion that stigma is necessary to motivate overweight and obese people to lose weight. They reiterate that dieting is not associated with long-term weight loss, regardless of the individual's motivation. Furthermore, they indicate that stigma can lead to discrimination and exert a harmful influence on health and quality of life. Puhl and Brownell assert that unless stigma is reduced, obese people will continue to contend with prejudice and discrimination.

Although few studies have evaluated the effectiveness of strategies to reduce weight stigma, a variety of initiatives have produced varying degrees of attitudinal change. These approaches include:

- Educating participants about external uncontrollable causes such as the biological and genetic factors that contribute to obesity.

- Teaching and encouraging young children to practice size acceptance.

- Improving attitudes by combining efforts to elicit empathy with education about the uncontrollable causes of obesity.

- Encouraging direct personal contact with overweight and obese individuals to dispel negative stereotypes.

- Changing individuals' beliefs by exposing them to opposing attitudes and values held by a group that they consider important. This approach, which is called social consensus theory, relies on the observation that after learning that a group does not share the individuals' beliefs, they are more likely to modify their beliefs to be similar to those expressed by the group they respect or wish to join.

Puhl and Brownell describe the results of their experiments using social consensus theory to modify attitudes toward obese people. They conducted experiments with university students in which participants reported their attitudes toward obese people before and after the researchers offered them varying consensus opinions of other students. In one experiment, participants who were told that other students held more favorable attitudes about obese people reported significantly fewer negative attitudes and more positive attitudes about obese people than they had before they learned about the opinions of other students. Furthermore, they also changed their ideas about the causes of obesity, favoring the uncontrollable causes after they were told the other students believed obesity was attributable to these causes.

A second experiment confirmed that the power to alter the participants' beliefs depended on whether the source of the opposing beliefs was an in-group or out-group. Not surprisingly, participants' attitudes toward obese people were more likely to change when the information they were given came from a source they valued—an in-group. In a third experiment the researchers compared attitudinal change produced by social consensus with other methods to reduce stigma, including one in which participants were given written material about the controllable or uncontrollable causes of obesity. Puhl and Brownell find that social consensus theory was as effective as or more effective than any of the other methods they applied. They state that social consensus theory also offers an explanation about why obese individuals themselves express negative stereotypes—they want to belong to the valued social group and choose to accept negative stereotypes to align themselves with current culture. Furthermore, by accepting prevailing cultural values and beliefs, they not only resemble the in-group more closely but also distance themselves from the out-group, where identity and membership are defined by being overweight or obese.

Although Puhl and Brownell consider social consensus a promising approach to reducing weight bias and stigma, they caution that there are many unanswered questions about its widespread utility and effectiveness. They conclude that "an ideal and comprehensive theory of obesity stigma would identify the origins of weight bias, explain why stigma is elicited by obese body types, account for the association between certain negative traits and obesity, and suggest methods for reducing bias. Existing theories do not yet meet all these criteria."

Weight Bias in the Media

Rebecca M. Puhl and Chelsea A. Heuer describe in "The Stigma of Obesity: A Review and Update" (*Obesity*, vol. 17, no. 5, May 2009) how the media take a dim view of people who are obese, often casting them as "targets of humor and ridicule." The researchers point out that in recent years news reports have attributed a host of ills to people who are obese, ranging from playing a role in rising fuel prices and global warming to causing weight gain among their friends. Children's entertainment also consistently presents thin characters in a positive light and overweight characters negatively. Because most American adults are overweight or obese, it would be helpful to see overweight and obese people in lead roles and cast in a flattering light, as opposed to being in television reality shows, "where the entire cast is trying desperately to become thin."

In "What It's Like Being a Fat Amy–Sized Actress in Hollywood" (Slate.com, May 14, 2015), Julie Brister lauds actor Rebel Wilson's (1980–) portrayal of "Fat Amy" in the film *Pitch Perfect* (2012), noting "there are still fat jokes, but Amy's fearlessness transcends any bullying that she may encounter." Brister exhorts the entertainment industry to offer more leading and supporting roles for plus-size actors, citing Melissa McCarthy's (1970–) character, Maggie, in *St. Vincent* (2014). McCarthy also starred in the television series *Mike & Molly* and received an Academy Award for her performance in *Bridesmaids* (2011).

Although reality shows such as *The Biggest Loser* chronicle weight-loss efforts, other shows—such as *The Mindy Project*, *Girls*, and *Awkward*—feature characters who are overweight and unapologetic. These characters are not overly concerned with or obsessing about losing weight. Supporters of these shows believe they are realistic and inspiring, because their characters are not defined by their weight.

Advocacy Groups Promote Size and Weight Acceptance

Our vision [is] a society in which people of every size are accepted with dignity and equality in all aspects of life. Our mission [is] to eliminate discrimination based on body size and provide fat people with the tools for self-empowerment through public education, advocacy, and support.

—National Association to Advance Fat Acceptance (2015)

There is a robust social movement that advocates size and weight acceptance with the overarching goal of assisting people to have a positive body image at any weight and to achieve health at any size. Nearly all the organizations that champion size acceptance characterize society's preoccupation with dieting and weight loss as unhealthy and unproductive, citing statistics about diet failures, the dangers of weight cycling (the repeated loss and regain of body weight), and low self-esteem. The size acceptance movement proposes that it is possible to be fit and fat simultaneously and that health and beauty are attainable at all weights. It also works to reduce "fat phobia," anti-fat bias, and weight-based discrimination.

The Council on Size and Weight Discrimination (2016, http://www.cswd.org), a nonprofit advocacy organization working to end "sizism," bigotry, and discrimination against people who are heavier than average, focuses its advocacy efforts on affecting changes in medical treatment, job discrimination, and media images. The council's basic principles were derived from the "Tenets of the Nondiet Approach" (Karin Kratina, Dayle Hayes, and Nancy King, *Moving Away from Diets: Healing Eating Problems and Exercise Resistance*, 2003) and focus on:

- Total health enhancement and well-being, rather than on weight loss or achieving a specific "ideal weight"

- Self-acceptance and respect for the diversity of bodies that come in a wide variety of shapes and sizes, rather than on the pursuit of an idealized weight at all costs

- The pleasure of eating well, based on internal cues of hunger and satiety (the feeling of fullness or satisfaction after eating), rather than on external food plans or diets

- The joy of movement, encouraging all physical activities, rather than on prescribing a specific routine of regimented exercise

The council urges people to free themselves from weight obsession and the effects of negative body image, to learn about issues such as weight discrimination and eating disorders, and to become educated consumers and seek out health care providers who are competent and unbiased. It also advocates interrupting sizism—pointing out instances of weight discrimination of negative stereotypes and expressing the opinion that "fat jokes" and derogatory stereotypes are both wrong and hurtful.

The National Association to Advance Fat Acceptance (NAAFA; 2015, http://www.naafaonline.com/dev2/about/index.html) is a nonprofit, volunteer civil rights organization dedicated to eliminating discrimination based on body size and providing people with the "tools for self-empowerment through advocacy, public education, and support." Founded in 1969, the NAAFA has assumed a proactive role in protesting social prejudice, bias, and discrimination and in working with the Federal Trade Commission to stop diet fraud. The organization also seeks to improve legal protection for people who are overweight and obese by educating lawmakers and serving as a national legal clearinghouse for attorneys challenging size discrimination.

In an ongoing effort to counter discrimination, the organization has issued statements that aim to prevent overweight and obese children from suffering from bullying in school. In October 2011 the NAAFA (http://issuu .com/naafa/docs/) released guidelines for health care providers who treat people who are overweight and obese. The guidelines detail respectful treatment of overweight and obese patients and advise health care providers to:

- Weigh patients in a private setting
- Ensure that patients have access to waiting room seating, examination room facilities, and durable medical equipment that comfortably accommodates them
- Not assume that all the patient's health problems are caused by excess weight
- Not assume that patients want weight-loss counseling or information

In the July 10, 2015, press release "'Fat' Is NOT a Four-Letter Word" (http://www.prlog.org/12474261-fat-is-not-four-letter-word.html), the NAAFA expressed its opposition to the Obesity Action coalition effort to ban the word *fat*. The NAAFA asserts that there is no evidence that higher-weight people prefer the term *obese*, and the organization announced its intention to reclaim the term *fat*, explaining, "We are not ashamed of our fat bodies and oppose anyone that promotes the use of the phrase 'persons with obesity' to describe fat people and being fat as being diseased. The way to eliminate fat-shaming and stigmatization is for society to accept that we come in ALL sizes."

CHAPTER 9
DIET AND WEIGHT-LOSS LORE, MYTHS, AND CONTROVERSIES

One of the challenges facing public health professionals as they seek to combat obesity among Americans is helping consumers to distinguish myths, lore, legends, and outright fraud from accurate, usable information about nutrition, diet, exercise, and weight loss. Some of these inaccuracies are so long-standing and deeply rooted in American culture that even the most educated consumers unquestioningly accept them as facts. Others began with a kernel of truth but have been so wildly distorted or mis-interpreted that they are confusing, misleading, or entirely erroneous. The rapid influx and dissemination of informa-tion about the origins of overweight and obesity and the conflicting accounts of how best to treat these problems compound the challenge. With media reports and advertise-ments trumpeting different diets nearly every week, it is no wonder that Americans are confused about diet, nutrition, and weight loss.

The fiction that people who are overweight or obese are lazy and weak-willed is among the most harmful myths because it serves to promote stigma, bias, and discrimination. Another common misconception is that it is equally easy or difficult for all people to lose weight. There are biological and behavioral factors that affect an individual's body weight, and people vary in terms of genetic propensity to become overweight, basal meta-bolic rate (BMR), and the number of fat cells. BMR, often referred to simply as the metabolic rate, is the number of calories an individual expends at rest to main-tain normal body functions. BMR changes with age, weight, height, diet, and exercise habits (and varies based on gender) and has been found to vary by as much as 1,000 calories per day. Differences in metabolic rate explain, in part, why not all people who adhere to the same diet achieve the same results in terms of pounds lost or rate of weight loss.

Another factor that produces variation in weight loss is the number of fat cells in the dieter's body. Although fat cells do not determine body weight, they are affected by weight gain and act to limit weight loss because their number cannot be decreased. For example, a normal-weight person has about 40 billion fat cells, whereas an individual who weighs 250 pounds (113 kg) with a body mass index (BMI; body weight in kilograms divided by height in meters squared) of 40 may have as many as 100 billion fat cells. Weight loss causes fat cells to shrink in size but does not decrease their number. As a result, individuals with twice as many fat cells as normal-weight people may be able to shrink their fat cells to a normal size, but even when they have attained a healthy weight they will still have twice as many fat cells.

DIET AND WEIGHT-LOSS MYTHS

It is impossible to recount all the fantastic and improbable claims that have been made over the years. This section considers some of the most persistent myths about diet, exercise, and weight loss.

Small Changes in Caloric Intake or Expenditure Produce Large, Long-Term Weight Loss

MYTH. Small changes in energy intake (consuming fewer calories) or expenditure (burning more calories) will, over time, produce large, long-term weight loss.

FACT. According to Krista Casazza et al., in "Myths, Presumptions, and Facts about Obesity" (*New England Journal of Medicine*, vol. 368, no. 5, January 2013), national health guidelines assert that small, sustained changes in daily behavior such as walking for 20 minutes or eating 10 fewer potato chips will continue to promote the same weight loss over long periods. Casazza et al. point out that this myth arose as a result of the premise that a 3,500-calorie deficit always results in a one-pound weight loss. Recent research demonstrates that many factors influence changes in body composition in response to reduced caloric intake or increased expenditure. For example, the

"3,500 fewer calories equals a one-pound weight loss" premise predicts that if people walk one mile per day, burning 100 calories, then over five years they will lose 50 pounds. The truth is, assuming that the participants did not consume more calories to compensate for those expended, their total weight loss would be just 10 pounds, largely because as they lose weight, their calorie requirements also decrease.

Rate of Weight Loss

MYTH. People who lose large amounts of weight quickly do not fare as well as those who have slow, gradual weight loss.

FACT. Casazza et al. observe that this myth likely originated in response to the use of very-low-calorie diets (fewer than 800 calories per day) in the 1960s. The researchers note that in weight-loss studies, large, rapid weight loss is associated with lower weight in the long term. When the results of rapid weight loss that came from very-low-calories diets was compared with weight loss resulting from low-calorie diets, short-term weight loss was greater among those on very-low-calorie diets— 16.1% of body weight lost compared with 9.7% on low-calorie diets. At the follow-up at the end of one year, there was no significant difference in total weight loss between the two groups of dieters. Casazza et al. acknowledge that although it is not yet known why some dieters have larger initial weight loss than others, advising dieters that slow weight loss is preferable has the potential to hamper the success of their weight-loss efforts.

Physical Education in School Is Key to Preventing Childhood Obesity

MYTH. Traditional physical education (PE) classes play a vital role in preventing or reducing childhood obesity.

FACT. According to Casazza et al., conventional PE classes have not demonstrated the ability to prevent or reduce childhood obesity. Even schools in which students attended PE classes more frequently and schools that promoted PE were not found to influence the prevalence of obesity nor did they reduce BMI of students. Although it is likely that there is a frequency, intensity, and duration of PE that would help to prevent or reduce obesity, the necessary formula has not yet been determined, and even if it were known, might not be feasible in conventional schools.

In fact, a more effective way to prevent and combat childhood obesity may be to supply them with a diet rich in fruits and vegetables at school at no charge. Yiwei Qian et al. report in "The Effect of the Fresh Fruit and Vegetable Program on Childhood Obesity" (*Applied Economic Perspectives and Policy*, online June 20, 2015) find that instituting the U.S. Department of Agriculture Fresh Fruit and Vegetable Program, which aims to increase the amount of fruits and vegetables eaten at breakfast and lunch by students in the poorest elementary schools, reduced obesity rates 3% (from 20% to 17%).

Sexual Activity Burns Hundreds of Calories

MYTH. Sexual activity burns between 100 and 300 calories for each participant.

FACT. Casazza et al. report that the average episode of sexual activity has a duration of about six minutes and a man might burn about 21 calories during sexual intercourse. The researchers point out that just by sitting and watching television, the man would have spent about one-third of those calories, which would mean the benefit of energy expenditure attributable to sexual activity is about 14 calories.

Eating at Night

MYTH. Eating after 8:00 p.m. causes weight gain.

FACT. Weight gain or loss does not depend on the time of day food is consumed—excess calories are stored as fat whether they are consumed midmorning or just before bedtime. In general, weight is governed by the amount of food consumed (measured in total calorie count) and the amount of physical activity expended during the day.

Some nutritionists and dieticians view breakfast as the most important meal of the day and advise dieters to eat breakfast regularly, based on the assumption that skipping breakfast will lead to overeating later in the day. Casazza et al. question this advice, noting that two rigorous studies found no difference in weight between people who ate breakfast and those who did not.

Anne de la Hunty, Sigrid Gibson, and Margaret Ashwell reviewed 14 studies about the relationship of breakfast habits to body weight in children and adolescents and reported the results in "Does Regular Breakfast Cereal Consumption Help Children and Adolescents Stay Slimmer? A Systematic Review and Meta-analysis" (*Obesity Facts*, vol. 6, no. 1, 2013). The researchers found that although energy intake was higher among regular breakfast cereal eaters, they had lower BMIs compared with those who ate breakfast cereal infrequently. Nevertheless, the researchers find that the results did not establish a causal relationship, and cited a need for further research to determine whether other factors were in play.

Natural Weight-Loss Products

MYTH. Organic, natural, or herbal weight-loss products are safer than synthetic (produced in the laboratory), over-the-counter (nonprescription), or prescription drugs.

FACT. Simply because products are organic or naturally occurring does not necessarily mean they are effective, risk-free, or safe. For example, in "How Safe Is the Use of Herbal Weight-Loss Products Sold over the Internet?" (*Human and Experimental Toxicology*, vol. 32, no. 1, January 2013), Bora Ozdemir et al. obtained nine herbal weight-loss products sold over the Internet and analyzed their ingredients. Although all of the products were advertised as purely herbal, three contained sibutramine, a weight-loss drug that was withdrawn from the market in 2010 because it was associated with increased risk for heart attack and stroke. Also, three of the products examined contained caffeine and three contained caffeine and temazepam, a drug used to treat anxiety and insomnia. The researchers also found toxic and trace elements in some of the herbal products.

Low-Fat and Low-Carbohydrate Foods

MYTH. Low fat, nonfat, and low carbohydrate mean few or no calories.

FACT. Low-fat or nonfat food is usually lower in calories than the same sized portion (as measured by weight) of the full-fat food. A food product, however, can contain zero grams of fat and still have a high calorie content. Many fat-free foods replace the fat with sugar or other sweeteners and contain just as many or more calories as full-fat versions. Although most fruits and vegetables are naturally low in fat and calories, processed low-fat or nonfat foods may be high in calories because extra sugar (or other sweeteners), flour, or starch thickeners have been added to enhance the low-fat foods' taste or texture.

Similarly, low-carbohydrate foods are often higher in calories than their "regular" counterparts because their fat content is higher. Many foods that are naturally low in carbohydrates such as meat, butter, and cheese are also calorie-dense. Many nutritionists suggest limiting the consumption of low-carbohydrate versions of foods, such as low-carbohydrate frozen desserts, because they not only contain as many or more calories per serving than regular frozen desserts but are also often sweetened with artificial sweeteners that lack any nutrients.

Eliminating Starchy Foods

MYTH. Pasta, potatoes, and bread are fattening foods and should be eliminated or sharply limited when trying to lose weight.

FACT. Potatoes, rice, pasta, bread, beans, and some starchy vegetables such as squash, yams, sweet potatoes, turnips, beets, and carrots are not innately fattening. (They are often fattening because of the "extras" that are served with them, such as butter, sour cream, margarine, or cheese.) These foods are rich in complex carbohydrates,

which are important sources of energy. Furthermore, foods that are high in complex carbohydrates are often low in fat and calories because carbohydrates contain only four calories per gram, compared with the nine calories per gram contained by fats. In "Calorie for Calorie, Dietary Fat Restriction Results in More Body Fat Loss than Carbohydrate Restriction in People with Obesity" (*Cell Metabolism*, vol. 22, no. 3, September 2015), Kevin D. Hall et al. report the results of a study in which dieters consumed either a low-carbohydrate diet or a low-fat diet. Although the low-carbohydrate diet decreased insulin production and increased fat oxidation, the breakdown of fats that can be used for energy, it did not produce more fat loss than the low-fat diet.

A plant-based, low-fat diet that includes extra-virgin olive oil and nuts has benefits beyond weight loss. In "Primary Prevention of Cardiovascular Disease with a Mediterranean Diet" (*New England Journal of Medicine*, vol. 368, no. 14, April 2013), Ramón Estruch et al. report that among people at high risk for cardiovascular disease, a Mediterranean diet supplemented with extra-virgin olive oil or nuts reduced the incidence of major adverse cardiovascular events, such as heart attack and stroke.

Genetic Destiny

MYTH. People from families in which many members are overweight or obese are destined to become overweight.

FACT. It is true that studies of families find similarities in body weight and that immediate relatives of obese people are at an increased risk for overweight and obesity, compared with people with normal-weight family members. Although it is generally accepted that genetic susceptibility or predisposition to overweight or obesity is a factor, researchers believe environmental and behavioral factors make equally strong, if not stronger, contributions to the development of obesity. As a result, people from overweight or obese families may have to make a concerted effort to maintain healthy body weight and prevent weight gain, but they are not destined to become overweight or obese simply by virtue of the genes they inherited.

Exercise Alone

MYTH. Exercise is a better way to lose weight than dieting.

FACT. Although there are many health benefits from exercise, weight loss is not generally considered a direct benefit. Research consistently demonstrates that for weight loss, diet trumps exercise because it is simpler to reduce caloric intake significantly through diet than to increase caloric expenditure significantly through exercise. For example, if a 155-pound (70-kg) person wants to reduce his or her consumption by 400 calories per day, it might be achieved by simply eliminating dessert and reducing portion sizes. In contrast, expending 400 calories per day requires considerable effort. To burn 400 calories a 155-pound person has to spend an hour bicycling 10 miles per hour (16 km/hr), ice skating at 9 miles per hour (14.5 km/hr), or water skiing or walking uphill at about 3.5 miles per hour (5.6 km/hr). Many studies, however, demonstrate that exercise is an important way to prevent overweight and maintain weight loss.

D. Enette Larson-Meyer et al. combined calorie restriction with exercise and reported their findings in "Caloric Restriction with or without Exercise: The Fitness versus Fatness Debate" (*Medicine and Science in Sports and Exercise*, vol. 42, no. 1, January 2010). The researchers randomly assigned 36 otherwise healthy overweight adults to a 25% caloric restricted diet alone or to a 25% energy deficit regime produced equally by calorie restriction and exercise—12.5% by decreasing food intake and 12.5% by increasing energy expended through regular aerobic exercise.

Subjects in both groups lost about the same amount of weight and visceral fat. The calorie restriction and exercise group, however, had improved insulin sensitivity, low-density lipoprotein and cholesterol levels, and diastolic blood pressure. Larson-Meyer et al. conclude that "results of the current study suggest that beyond changes in fatness, combining caloric restriction with exercise is important for increasing aerobic fitness and optimizing improvements in risk factors for diabetes and cardiovascular disease."

Eating Disorders

MYTH. Eating disorders occur exclusively among middle- and upper-class white females.

FACT. Like many myths about diet, weight, and nutrition, this one is based on fact: an estimated 90% of people with anorexia nervosa or bulimia nervosa are female. The National Eating Disorders Association (NEDA; 2015, http://www.nationaleatingdisorders.org/silent-epidemic) estimates that 30 million Americans suffer from eating disorders and that one-third of them are men.

NEDA also notes that reports of eating disorders among racial and ethnic minorities and older adults are on the rise. In "Classification and Correlates of Eating Disorders among Blacks: Findings from the National Survey of American Life" (*Journal of Health Care for the Poor and Underserved*, vol. 24, no. 1, February 2013), Jacquelyn Y. Taylor et al. note that although the rates of anorexia and bulimia are lower than among whites, there are high rates of binge eating among African American adults and adolescents.

Older adults are affected too. Survey results presented by Danielle Gagne et al., in "Eating Disorder Symptoms and Weight and Shape Concerns in a Large Web-Based Convenience Sample of Women Ages 50 and Above: Results of the Gender and Body Image Study" (*International Journal of Eating Disorders*, vol. 45, no. 7, November 2012), indicate that of women over the age of 50 years, 13% have symptoms of eating disorders, 62% feel that their weight or shape has a negative effect on their life, and well over two-thirds (70%) are attempting to lose weight.

Freshmen in College Gain Weight

MYTH. College freshmen gain an average of 15 pounds (6.8 kg) during their first year of school.

FACT. Historically, college students were warned about the "freshman 15," the 15 pounds that students supposedly gain during their first year of college, presumably because freed from the constraints of healthful eating at home, they subsist on a diet of unhealthful food. Jay L. Zagorsky and Patricia K. Smith, however, dispel the myth of freshman weight gain in "The Freshman 15: A Critical Time for Obesity Intervention or Media Myth?" (*Social Science Quarterly*, vol. 92, no. 5, December 2011). The researchers analyze data from 7,418 college freshmen and find that first-year students, both male and female, gained an average of 2.5 to 3.5 pounds (1.1 to 1.6 kg) during their first year in college. Zagorsky and Smith also find that this weight gain is only one-half pound more than that gained by people of the same age who are not attending college.

Jessica A. Boyce and Roeline G. Kuijer note that baseline (precollege) BMI and stress influence college weight gain. In "Perceived Stress and Freshman Weight Change: The Moderating Role of Baseline Body Mass Index" (*Physiology and Behavior*, vol. 139, February 2015), Boyce and Kuijer looked at the interaction of BMI and stress level on weight gain of college freshman and find that students with high levels of stress and high baseline BMIs gained weight and those with high levels of stress and low baseline BMIs lost weight during their first years of college.

WHY DIETS FAIL

Historically, diets have been considered to have "failed" when lost weight is regained. Many nutritionists and obesity researchers believe diets fail because most are not sustainable. The more restrictive the diet, the less likely an individual will be to remain faithful to it because, in general, people cannot endure extended periods of hunger and deprivation. Diets may also fail because they neglect to teach dieters new eating habits to assist them in maintaining their weight loss. Most overweight people gained their excess weight by consuming more calories per day than they needed. Dieting creates a temporary deficit of calories or specific macronutrients such as carbohydrates or fat. Because the weight-loss diet is viewed as a temporary measure with a beginning and an end, at its conclusion most dieters return to their previous eating habits and often regain the lost weight or gain even more weight. Many nutritionists and dieticians who work with people who are overweight or obese assert that diets do not fail; instead, dieters fail to learn how to eat properly to prevent weight regain.

Consumers are not the only ones who believe that diets are doomed to fail. Many health professionals and researchers cite the statistic that 95% of diets fail. This oft-cited statistic has been attributed to Albert James Stunkard (1922–2014), the director emeritus of the Obesity Society (formerly the American Obesity Association). Stunkard put forth the 95% failure rate based on research he performed in 1959, which involved advising 100 overweight patients to diet, with no follow-up or support to increase their adherence to the diet. In "Whether Obesity Should Be Treated" (*Health Psychology*, vol. 12, no. 5, September 1993), Kelly D. Brownell of Yale University observes that this statistic has been widely applied even though it is quite dated, was not confirmed by subsequent studies, and involved only subjects in university-based research programs.

The article "Psychobehavioural Factors Are More Strongly Associated with Successful Weight Management Than Predetermined Satiety Effect or Other Characteristics of Diet" (*Journal of Obesity*, June 2012), Leila Karhunen et al. find that neither foods with higher satiety value nor the type of diet contribute to better weight management. Instead, Karhunen et al. find that dieters' behaviors, such as better self-control of eating behavior and a decrease in binge eating, are associated with success in weight management.

Improving Long-Term Weight Loss

Research demonstrates that dieters find it challenging to maintain weight loss. Nevertheless, research refutes the 95% failure rate. In "Effects of Dietary Composition on Energy Expenditure during Weight-Loss Maintenance" (*Journal of the American Medical Association*, vol. 307, no. 24, June 2012), Cara B. Ebbeling et al. observe that just one in six overweight and obese adults report ever having maintained a 10% weight loss for one year. Although one explanation for this lack of success may be that the motivation to adhere to a restricted diet erodes over time, another is that weight loss provokes biological adaptations—a decline in energy expenditure and an increase in hunger—that encourage weight regain.

Ebbeling et al. compared the effects of three weight-loss maintenance diets—a low-fat diet, a low-glycemic-index (a measure of a food's ability to raise blood glucose) diet, and a very-low-carbohydrate diet—on energy expenditure, hormones, and other health indicators. The researchers find that energy expenditure during weight-loss maintenance differed significantly for the three diets. The low-fat diet produced changes in energy expenditure and leptin (a hormone that signals satiety) that favor weight regain. By contrast, the very-low-carbohydrate diet had the most beneficial effects on energy expenditure but also exerted potentially harmful effects on other health indicators such as inflammation. The low-glycemic-index diet had comparable but smaller benefits than the very-low-carbohydrate diet, while appearing to not increase inflammation, which suggests that it may be a better approach for weight-loss maintenance.

Because there is considerable variation in individuals' responses to dietary interventions and some interventions may benefit individuals or population subgroups more than others, nutrigenetics (using genetic information to custom-tailor a weight-loss diet) may be used to custom-tailor weight-loss diets and weight-maintenance efforts, which in turn may improve their success. In "Genetics of Weight Loss: A Basis for Personalized Obesity Management" (*Trends in Food Science and Technology*, vol. 42, no. 2, April 2015), J. Alfredo Martínez and Fermin I. Milagro indicate that personalized nutrition using genetic data enables individuals to choose the optimal diet for weight loss based on complex interactions between diet, genes, and the environment.

Approaches to enhance motivation focus on two areas: improved social supports and tangible financial incentives. Strategies to improve social supports emphasize including spouses or significant others in the weight-loss process to teach them to provide social support for their partner's weight-loss efforts. Such strategies demonstrate modest success as do contracts in which groups agree to aim for individual or group weight loss.

Alfredo R. Paloyo et al., in "The Causal Link between Financial Incentives and Weight Loss: An Evidence-Based Survey of the Literature" (*Journal of Economic Surveys*, January 2013), review available research to determine whether financial incentives are effective inducements to lose weight. The researchers considered nine studies. Some of the studies used positive monetary incentives, some used negative monetary incentives, and some combined positive and negative incentives for weight loss. Only five of the studies reported that financial incentives improved weight loss, and none determined that weight lost this way was maintained.

Financial incentives may encourage people to lose weight, but such incentives do not appear to prevent weight regain. In "Financial Incentives for Extended Weight Loss: A Randomized, Controlled Trial" (*Journal of General Internal Medicine*, vol. 26, no. 6, June 2011), Leslie K. John et al. analyze data from a 32-week-long weight-loss program—24 weeks of weight loss followed by eight weeks of weight maintenance. Sixty-six program participants were given the goal of losing 1 pound (0.5 kg) per week and received a financial incentive for achieving this weight loss. To assess longer-term maintenance following the 32-week intervention, participants returned for a weigh-in approximately 36 weeks after they completed the 32-week program. The researchers find that the incentive did promote weight loss and maintenance through the 32-week program. After the program ended, however, there was significant weight regain. John et al. conclude that "future research is needed to devise techniques that promote sustained weight loss over longer periods."

Teaching patients skills that are useful for weight maintenance as opposed to weight loss emphasizes that there are two distinctly different sets of strategies: one set focuses on weight loss and the other set focuses on maintaining a stable energy balance around a lower weight. The most commonly used model for teaching maintenance-specific skills is relapse prevention, which involves teaching people to identify situations in which lapses in behavioral adherence are likely to occur, to plan strategies in advance to prevent lapses, and to get back on track should they occur. Relapse prevention is based on the idea that breaking the so-called rules in terms of remaining faithful to diet and exercise programs may often lead to negative psychological reactions that in turn prompt reversion to pre-weight-loss behaviors.

George A. Bray and Thomas A. Wadden describe strategies for weight-loss maintenance in "Improving Long-Term Weight Loss Maintenance: Can We Do It?" (*Obesity*, vol. 23 no. 1, January 2015). The researchers report that monthly or twice-monthly behavioral health counseling delivered in person or via telephone is effective. They also opine that using new technology to monitor weight such as cellular-connected smart scales and encouraging physical activity through the use of low-cost accelerometers may improve weight maintenance, especially if these approaches are coupled with frequent feedback and economic incentives.

WEIGHT-LOSS SCHEMES DEFRAUD CONSUMERS

The marketing of so-called fat-burning pills, potions, and products to Americans seeking effortless weight loss has a long history. Peter N. Stearns, in *Fat History: Bodies and Beauty in the Modern West* (1997), and Laura Fraser, in *Losing It: False Hopes and Fat Profits in the Diet Industry* (1998), offer detailed histories of magical cures and weight-loss fads. At the beginning of the 20th century, products such as obesity belts and chairs that delivered electrical stimulation, as well as corsets, tonics, and mineral waters, claimed to cause weight loss.

Diet pills appeared in 1910 with the introduction of weight-loss tablets that contained arsenic (a poisonous metallic element), strychnine (a plant toxin formerly used as a stimulant), caffeine, and pokeberries (formerly used as a laxative). During the 1920s cigarette makers promoted their product as a diet aid, urging Americans to smoke rather than eat. During the 1930s diet pills containing dinitrophenol, a chemical used to manufacture explosives, dyes, and insecticides, enjoyed brief popularity after it was observed that factory workers making munitions lost weight. Their popularity was short lived as cases of temporary blindness and death became attributed to their use.

The second half of the 20th century saw the proliferation of questionable, and often entirely worthless, weight-loss devices and gimmicks, including inflatable suits to "sweat off pounds," diet drinks and cookies, and slimming creams, patches, shoe inserts, and wraps to reduce fat thighs and abdomens. Although the claims made for many of these products sounded too good to be true, unsuspecting Americans spent billions of dollars in the hope of achieving quick, easy, and permanent weight loss.

The promotion of dubious and potentially dangerous weight-loss products continued during the second decade of the 21st century. In 2013 alone, the U.S. Food and Drug Administration (FDA) issued more than 25 public notifications about products marketed for weight loss that contained drugs or other potentially harmful ingredients. The agency has also issued warning letters, seized products, and criminally prosecuted people responsible for illegal diet products. For example, in "Beware of Products Promising Miracle Weight Loss" (January 5, 2015, http://www.fda.gov/ForConsumers/ConsumerUpdates/ucm246742.htm#tainted), the FDA explains that many dietary supplements marketed as weight-loss aids are actually powerful drugs that may carry significant risks to unsuspecting consumers. The FDA notes that consumers may unknowingly take products "that contain dangerous concoctions of hidden ingredients including active ingredients contained in approved seizure medications, blood pressure medications, and antidepressants."

Use of Over-the-Counter Weight-Loss Products

In "The Effect of Deceptive Advertising on Consumption of the Advertised Good and Its Substitutes: The Case of Over-the-Counter Weight Loss Products" (National Bureau of Economic Research, Working Paper No. 18863, March 2013), John Cawley, Rosemary Avery, and Matthew Eisenberg report that over-the-counter (OTC) weight-loss products have been used by 20% of adult women, 10% of adult men, 14% of adolescent females, and 7% of adult males. About one-third of people who have ever made a serious weight-loss attempt have used an OTC weight-loss product. The researchers observe that about half of Americans mistakenly believe that OTC weight-loss products are evaluated for safety and efficacy before they are marketed.

Cawley, Avery, and Eisenberg analyzed information on Americans' consumption, magazine reading, and television viewing and measured individual exposure to ads for OTC weight-loss products. They also calculated the percentage of the ads that contained at least one deceptive statement and analyzed the impact of exposure to advertising, including deceptive ads, on the likelihood that an OTC weight-loss product was used in the 12 months prior to the study. The researchers find that deceptive television advertising of OTC weight-loss products reduces the probability that better-educated women will purchase these products; deceptive print advertising, however, increases the likelihood that men will buy them. Deceptive advertising that is unbelievable may unintentionally suggest to consumers that the product is questionable, discouraging consumption.

A promising finding from this research is that deception may make consumers suspicious of the advertised product, prompting them to substitute an established approach, such as diet, exercise, or professional counseling, for the advertised product. Deceptive ads for questionable products that make weight loss seem easy may unintentionally make weight loss in general seem simpler. Cawley, Avery, and Eisenberg conclude, "Advertising, and even deceptive advertising, of questionable products apparently has the potential of a beneficial unintended consequence of inspiring people to undertake healthy and responsible approaches to weight loss."

Weighing the Claims

In May 2000 the Partnership for Healthy Weight Management, a coalition of scientific, academic, health care, government, commercial, and public interest representatives, initiated consumer and media education programs that aimed not only to increase public awareness of the obesity epidemic in the United States but also to promote responsible marketing of weight-loss products and programs. The partnership published a consumer guide, *Finding a Weight Loss Plan That Works for You* (December 2009), designed to help overweight and obese consumers find weight-loss solutions to meet their needs. The guide contains a checklist that enables consumers to compare weight-loss plans based on a variety of criteria. (See Table 9.1.) It also advises consumers about how to select weight-loss programs and services based on specific information from potential providers.

A Harvard Medical School publication available online, "Choosing a Weight-Loss Program: Finding the One that Works Best for You" (adapted from "Healthy Solutions to Lose Weight and Keep It Off," 2015, http://www.helpguide.org/harvard/weight-loss-programs.htm), also advises consumers about how to choose a weight-loss program best suited to their needs. It emphasizes that the best diet offers an array of tasty, healthful foods, is one the consumer can adhere to long term, and is one that promotes overall health as well as weight loss.

The Federal Trade Commission (FTC), in *Deception in Weight-Loss Advertising Workshop: Seizing Opportunities and Building Partnerships to Stop Weight-Loss Fraud* (December 2003, http://www.ftc.gov/os/2003/12/031209weightlossrpt.pdf), describes eight broad categories of advertising claims. The following section considers these advertising claims and assessments of them. It also draws on an analysis of the FTC report by Stephen Barrett in "Impossible Weight-Loss Claims: Summary of an FTC Report" (December 16, 2003, http://www.quackwatch.org/01QuackeryRelatedTopics/PhonyAds/weightlossfraud.html), and the "Being Fooled by Empty Diet Promises" (2015, https://www.youtube.com/watch?v=wcdO6dDnUKE) and "Health Fraud Scams—Weight Loss" (September 4, 2015, http://www.fda.gov/ForConsumers/ProtectYourself/HealthFraud/ucm326842.htm) videos prepared by the FDA.

No Diet or Exercise Required

CLAIM. The advertised product causes substantial weight loss without exercise or diet.

EXAMPLES. "U.S. patent reveals weight loss of as much as 28 pounds in 4 weeks.... Eat all your favorite foods and still lose weight. The pill does all the work," and "Lose up to 2 pounds daily without diet or exercise." Table 9.2 contains other examples of comparable claims.

ASSESSMENT. Products purporting to cause weight loss without diet or exercise would either need to cause malabsorption (impair the absorption) of calories or increase metabolism. Because the number of calories that can be malabsorbed is limited to 1,200 to 1,300 calories per week, or about 0.3 of a pound (0.1 kg) per week, malabsorption alone is unlikely to lead to substantial weight loss. Similarly, there is no thermogenic (heat-producing) agent, such as ephedrine combined with caffeine, able to boost metabolism enough to produce weight loss without diet or exercise. In fact, the mechanism by which ephedrine products appear to assist weight loss is by suppressing appetite rather than by speeding metabolism. Furthermore, although green tea extract was found to increase metabolism, it was by a scant 4%.

No Restrictions on Eating

CLAIM. Users can lose weight while still enjoying unlimited amounts of high-calorie foods.

EXAMPLE. "Eat All the Foods You Love and Still Lose Weight (Pill Does All the Work)."

TABLE 9.1

Checklist for evaluating weight-loss products and services

Use this checklist to gather and compare information from all weight loss programs you're considering.

Make several copies of the blank form so you can fill out one for each program. A provider's willingness to give you this information is an important factor in choosing a program. If you need help to evaluate the information you gather, talk with your primary health care provider or a registered dietitian.

Program name _____

Address _____

Phone number _____

In this program, my daily caloric intake will be: _____

My daily caloric intake is determined by: _____

I   will   will not be evaluated initially by program staff.

The evaluation will be made by (check all that apply):
   Physician   Nurse   Registered dietitian   Other company-trained employee

My progress is supervised by (check all that apply):
   Physician   Nurse   Licensed psychologist
   Registered dietitian   Company-trained employee

I will   will not be evaluated by a physician during the course of my treatment.

During the first month, my progress will be monitored:
   Weekly   Biweekly   Monthly   Other _____

After the first month, my progress will be monitored:
   Weekly   Biweekly   Monthly   Other _____

My weight loss plan includes (check all that apply):
   Nutrition information about healthy eating   At least 1,200 calories/day for women or 1,400 calories/day for men
   Suggested menus and recipes   Keeping food diaries or other monitoring activities
   Portion control   Liquid meal replacements
   Prepackaged meals   Dietary supplements (vitamins, minerals, botanicals, herbals)
   Prescription weight loss drugs   Help with weight maintenance and lifestyle changes
   Surgery

My plan includes regular physical activity that is (check both if both apply):
   Supervised (at the program site)   _____ times per week, _____ minutes per session.
   Unsupervised (on my own time)   _____ times per week, _____ minutes per session.

The physical activity includes (check all that apply):
   Walking   Swimming   Stationary cycling
   Strength training   Aerobic dancing   Other _____

The weight loss plan includes (check all that apply):
   Family counseling   Group support   Lifestyle modification advice
   Weight maintenance advice   Weight maintenance counseling
   The staff explained the risks associated with this weight loss progam. They are:

_____
_____

The staff explained the costs of this program. (Check all that apply and fill in the blanks.)
I will be charged a one-time entry fee of $ ___.
I will be charged $ ___ per visit.
Food replacements will cost about $ ___ per month.
Prescription weight loss drugs will cost about $ ___ per month.
Vitamins and other dietary supplements will cost about $ ___ per month.
Diagnostic tests are required and will cost about $ ___ .
Other costs include _____ at $ ___.

Total cost for this program $____

The program gave me information about:
   The health risks of being overweight.   The difficulty many people have maintaining weight loss.
   The health benefits of weight loss.   How to improve my chances at maintaining my weight.

Other information to ask for:
   Participants in this program have lost an average of ___ lbs. over ___ months/years.
   Participants in this program have kept off ___ % of their weight loss for ___ years.

This information is based on the following (check one):
   All participants.
   Participants who completed the program.
   Other _____

Notes: _____

SOURCE: "Checklist for Evaluating Weight Loss Products and Services," in *Finding a Weight Loss Program That Works for You*, Federal Trade Commission, The Partnership for Healthy Weight Management, December 28, 2009, http://www.checkyourhealth.org/pdf/cyh_materials/wgtloss.pdf (accessed November 2, 2015)

ASSESSMENT. This claim was viewed as a variation of the assertion that dieters can lose weight without reducing caloric intake or increasing exercise because this claim states that users not only can lose weight without reducing caloric intake but also may increase caloric intake and still lose weight. The assembled experts concurred that if this claim were true, it would defy the laws of physics.

TABLE 9.2

TABLE 9.3

Examples of claims that promise weight loss without diet or exercise

"Awesome attack on bulging fatty deposits … has virtually eliminated the need to diet." (Konjac root pill)

"They said it was impossible, but tests prove [that] my astounding diet-free discovery melts away. . . 5, 6, even 7 pounds of fat a day." (ingredients not disclosed)

"The most powerful diet pill ever discovered! No diet or workout required. The secret weight-loss pill behind Fitness models, Show Biz and Entertainment professionals! No prescription required to order." (ingredients not disclosed)

"Lose up to 30 lbs . . . No impossible exercise! No missed meals! No boring foods or small portions!" (plant extract fucus vesiculosus)

"Lose up to 8 to 10 pounds per week … [n]o dieting, no strenuous exercise." (elixir purportedly containing 16 plant extracts)

"My 52 lbs of unwanted fat relaxed away without dieting or grueling exercise." (hypnosis seminar)

"No exercise … [a]nd eat as much as you want—the more you eat, the more you lose, we'll show you how." (meal replacement)

SOURCE: Richard L. Cleland et al., "Table 5. Lose Weight without Diet or Exercise Claims," in *Weight-Loss Advertising: An Analysis of Current Trends*, Federal Trade Commission, September 2002, http://www.ftc.gov/sites/default/files/documents/reports/weight-loss-advertisingan-analysis-current-trends/weightloss_0.pdf (accessed November 2, 2015)

Examples of claims that promise fast results

"This combination of plant extracts constitutes a weight-loss plan that facilitates what is probably the fastest weight loss ever observed from an entirely natural treatment." (elixir purportedly containing 16 plant extracts)

"Just fast and easy, effective weight loss!" (fucus vesiculosus)

"Lose 10 lbs. in 8 Days!" (apple cider vinegar)

"Rapid weight loss in 28 days!" (ephedra)

"Knock off your unwanted weight and fat deposits at warp speeds! You can lose 18 pounds in one week!" (ingredients not disclosed)

"Clinically proven to cause rapid loss of excess body fat." (phosphosterine)

"Two clinically proven fat burning formulations that are guaranteed to get you there fast or it costs you absolutely nothing." (ingredients not disclosed)

SOURCE: Richard L. Cleland et al., "Table 4. Representative Claims That Promise Fast Results," in *Weight Loss Advertising: An Analysis of Current Trends*, Federal Trade Commission, September 2002, http://www.ftc.gov/sites/default/files/documents/reports/weight-loss-advertisingan-analysis-current-trends/weightloss_0.pdf (accessed November 2, 2015)

Permanent Weight Loss

CLAIM. The advertised product causes permanent weight loss.

EXAMPLES. "Take it off and keep it off. You won't gain the weight back afterwards because your weight will have reached an equilibrium," and "People who use this product say that even when they stop using the product, their weight does not jump up again."

ASSESSMENT. Even if a product caused weight loss through a reduction of calories, appetite suppression, or malabsorption, weight would be regained once use of the product stopped and calorie consumption returned to previous levels. Researchers and health professionals have repeatedly observed that dieters tend to regain weight lost over time once the diet, intervention, or other treatment ends. According to the Food and Nutrition Board of the National Academy of Sciences, "Many programs and services exist to help individuals achieve weight control. But without continuing vigilance and a strategy for weight maintenance, many dieters who complete weight-loss programs and lose approximately 10% of their body weight regain two-thirds of it back within 1 year and almost all of it back within 5 years." Furthermore, there are no published scientific studies supporting the claim that a nonprescription drug, dietary supplement, cream, wrap, device, or patch can cause permanent weight loss.

Fat Blockers

CLAIM. The advertised product causes substantial weight loss through the blockage or absorption of fat or calories.

EXAMPLES. "[The named ingredient] can ingest up to 900 times its own weight in fat, that's why it's a fantastic fat blocker," and "The Super Fat Fighting Formula inhibits fats, sugars, and starches from being absorbed in the intestines and turning into excess weight, so that you can lose pounds and inches easily."

ASSESSMENT. Science does not support the possibility that these products cause sufficient malabsorption of fat or calories to result in substantial weight loss. The FTC has challenged deceptive fat-blocker claims for some of the most popular diet products on the market. The evidence supports the position that consumers cannot lose substantial weight through the blockage of absorption of fat. It is not scientifically feasible for a nonprescription drug, dietary supplement, cream, wrap, device, or patch to cause substantial weight loss through the blockage of absorption of fat or calories.

Quick Weight Loss

CLAIM. The user of the advertised product can safely lose more than 3 pounds (1.4 kg) per week for periods exceeding four weeks. Table 9.3 shows claims that promise unbelievably rapid results.

EXAMPLE. "Lose three pounds per week, naturally and without side effects."

ASSESSMENT. Significant health risks are associated with medically unsupervised, rapid weight loss over extended periods. Basically, "the more restrictive the diet, the greater are the risks of adverse effects associated with weight loss." One documented risk is the increased incidence of gallstones. The claim that consumers using products such as these without medical oversight can safely lose more than three pounds per week for a period of more than four weeks is not feasible.

Weight-Loss Creams and Patches

CLAIM. The advertised product that is worn on the body or rubbed into the skin causes substantial weight loss.

EXAMPLES. "Lose two to four pounds daily with the Diet Patch," and "Thigh Cream drops pounds and inches from your thighs."

ASSESSMENT. Diet patches and creams that are worn or applied to the skin have not been proven to be safe or effective. Furthermore, their alleged mechanisms of action are not scientifically credible.

Guaranteed Success

CLAIM. The advertised product causes substantial weight loss for all users.

EXAMPLE. "Lose excess body fat. No willpower required. Works for everyone no matter how many times you've tried and failed before."

ASSESSMENT. This claim assumes that overweight and obesity arise from a single cause or are amenable to a single solution. Because the causes of overweight and obesity are thought to be genetic factors and environmental conditions, and contributing factors such as diet, metabolic rate, level of physical activity, and adherence to weight-loss treatment vary, it is unlikely that one product will be effective for all users. Even FDA-approved prescription drugs for weight loss have a high level of nonresponders, and surgical treatment for obesity is not successful 100% of the time. The claim that a nonprescription drug, dietary supplement, cream, wrap, device, or patch will cause substantial weight loss for all users is not scientifically feasible.

Targeted Weight-Loss Products

CLAIM. Users of the advertised product can lose weight from only those parts of the body where they wish to lose weight.

EXAMPLE. "And it has taken off quite some inches from my butt (5 inches) and thighs (4 inches), my hips now measure 35 inches. I still wear the same bra size though. The fat has disappeared from exactly the right places."

ASSESSMENT. Small published studies of aminophylline cream indicate that its use may cause the redistribution of fat from the thighs to other fat stores; it has not, however, been shown to cause fat loss. Even if some products were capable of causing more weight loss from certain areas of the body, no part would be spared completely—fat is lost from all fat stores throughout the body.

Campaign Targets Phony Weight-Loss Claims

Another FTC education initiative aims to assist the media to voluntarily screen weight-loss product ads containing claims that are "too good to be true." The media were targeted for intensive education not only because broad-based public education has proven largely inadequate to protect consumers from persuasive messages trumpeting easy weight loss but also to acknowledge the media's powerful ability to reduce weight-loss fraud by sharply limiting the dissemination of obviously false weight-loss advertising. In December 2003 the FTC launched its Red Flag campaign to assist the media to reduce deceptive weight-loss advertising and promote positive, reliable advertising messages about weight loss. The FTC (http://www.ftc.gov/news-events/press-releases/2003/12/ftc-releases-guidance-media-false-weight-loss-claims) defines Red Flag claims as those that promise to:

- Cause weight loss of two pounds or more a week for a month or more without dieting or exercise
- Cause substantial weight loss no matter what or how much the consumer eats
- Cause permanent weight loss (even when the consumer stops using product)
- Block the absorption of fat or calories to enable consumers to lose substantial weight
- Safely enable consumers to lose more than three pounds per week for more than four weeks
- Cause substantial weight loss for all users
- Cause substantial weight loss by wearing it on the body or rubbing it into the skin

The FTC also launched a website (http://www.consumer.ftc.gov/articles/0061-weighing-claims-diet-ads#the truth) to help consumers identify false weight-loss claims.

The FTC continues to file actions to stop false and unsupported weight-loss claims. For example, the FTC reports in a media release, "FTC Charges Marketers with Misleading Claims That Their Supplement Causes Weight Loss, Fat Loss, and Increased Metabolism in Women over Forty" (May 12, 2015, https://www.ftc.gov/news-events/press-releases/2015/05/ftc-charges-marketers-misleading-claims-their-supplement-causes) that it filed a federal court complaint to prohibit Lunada Biomedical, Inc. and its principals from advertising that their dietary supplement Amberen causes substantial and clinically proven weight loss for women age 40 and older. Amberen was advertised on radio, television, websites, and via email and claimed that Amberen is "the ONLY product on the market today clinically proven to cause sustained weight loss for women over 40." The FTC asserts that a clinical trial did not find a statistically significant difference in weight loss between the women who took the product and a control group that did not take the product. The FTC complaint also notes that the company advertised misleading success and consumer satisfaction rates and falsely claimed that consumers could try Amberen risk-free for 30 days.

FTC actions not only stop purveyors of weight-loss products from making unsubstantiated claims but also seek compensation for consumers. For example, in the media release "FTC Returns Money to Consumers Who Bought Allegedly Bogus Weight-Loss Products" (October 1, 2015, https://www.ftc.gov/news-events/press-releases/2015/10/ftc-returns-money-consumers-who-bought-allegedly-bogus-weight), the FTC reports that 23,406 checks totaling more than $3.7 million were mailed to consumers who bought LeanSpa, a supplement whose marketers made deceptive weight-loss claims. The FTC charged the company with using fake websites that promised free trials to consumers who paid shipping and handling fees. Instead, consumers paid nearly $80 for the trial and paid for recurring shipments that were difficult to cancel.

Although the FTC has taken aim at deceptive weight-loss advertising, some industry observers feel this effort should be intensified. In "Waving the Red Flag: FTC Regulation of Deceptive Weight-Loss Advertising 1951–2009" (*Health Communication*, vol. 31, no. 1, 2016), Julie C. Ellis asserts that while the number of complaints and financial penalties applied, "the FTC lacks systematic and specific policies to adequately deter advertisers and address what continues to be a growing problem."

DO VERY-LOW-CALORIE DIETS INCREASE LONGEVITY?

Although many Americans are overweight, some people are experimenting with very-low-calorie diets in the hope that by remaining extremely thin they will stave off disease and live longer. Advocates of extreme caloric restriction (CR) contend that sharply reducing caloric intake creates biochemical changes that slow the aging process, which theoretically should increase life expectancy.

Most people would find it impossible to adhere to semi-starvation diets, but there is scientific evidence—such as Luigi Fontana and Samuel Klein's "Aging, Adiposity, and Calorie Restriction" (*Journal of the American Medical Association*, vol. 297, no. 9, March 7, 2007) and Arthur V. Everitt and David G. Le Couteur's "Life Extension by Calorie Restriction in Humans" (*Annals of the New York Academy of Sciences*, vol. 1114, October 2007)—that subsistence diets increase the life span of fruit flies, worms, spiders, guppies, mice, and hamsters by between 10% and 40%. In theory, semi-starvation prolongs life by reducing metabolism (how quickly glucose is used for energy) in an evolutionary adaptation to conserve calories during periods of famine. Dieters are

familiar with this process—they know from experience that as they eat less, their metabolic rate drops, which makes losing weight increasingly more difficult. CR adherents experience comparable drops in metabolic rate—one study found that their body temperature dropped by a full degree. Proponents of CR assert that although metabolism is vital for life, it is also destructive because it produces unstable molecules known as free radicals that can damage cells through a process called oxidation.

CR adherents report immediate health benefits including increased mental acuity, reduced need for sleep, sharply reduced cholesterol and fasting blood sugar levels, weight loss, and reduced blood pressure. The regimen is clearly not easy, and even its staunchest advocates, such as members of the Caloric Restriction Society, concede that many people who practice CR experience constant hunger, obsessions with food, irritability and depression, and lowered libido (sex drive). CR can also cause people to feel cold, and even with adequate vitamin and mineral supplementation it can cause some people to suffer from osteoporosis (decreased bone mass) and hair loss. Jon Gertner reports in "The Calorie-Restriction Experiment" (NYTimes.com, October 7, 2009) that the majority of subjects in a study by the National Institutes of Health achieved their weight-loss goals and were maintaining their weight loss by sticking to their diet. He notes, however, that CR is a challenging undertaking and one that most Americans would forgo. Gertner opines that "living a life of less in a culture of more—is extremely difficult to achieve and even more difficult to maintain. Americans' seemingly inexorable slide toward obesity tends to indicate as much: for the majority of us, the desire to eat can easily overwhelm personal willpower and (so far) any messages from public-health campaigns."

Everitt and Le Couteur confirm that although short-term CR does improve specific markers that are associated with longevity, such as deep body temperature and plasma insulin levels, CR is unlikely to offer markedly increased longevity. The researchers cite as evidence the Okinawans, the longest-lived people on the earth, who consume 40% fewer calories than the average American and live just four years longer. Everitt and Le Couteur surmise that "the effects of CR on human life extension are probably much smaller than those achieved by medical and public health interventions, which have extended life by about 30 years in developed countries in the 20th century, by greatly reducing deaths from infections, accidents, and cardiovascular disease."

Although model organism and animal studies demonstrate positive responses to CR, it is not yet known whether CR will extend the human life span. Daniel L. Smith Jr., Tim R. Nagy, and David B. Allison of the University of Alabama, Birmingham, observe in "Calorie

Restriction: What Recent Results Suggest for the Future of Ageing Research" (*European Journal of Clinical Investigation*, vol. 40, no. 5, May 2010) that preliminary data from a seven-year study confirm many of the metabolic and physiologic responses that have been observed in animals. These responses include reductions in body weight, subcutaneous fat, visceral fat, lean muscle mass, insulin, energy expenditure, and core body temperature and improved lipid profiles. Smith, Nagy, and Allison opine that independent of whether CR confers longevity benefits, it is likely to play a role in disease prevention and healthy aging.

In "Ageing: Mixed Results for Dieting Monkeys" (*Nature*, vol. 489, no. 7415, September 2012), Steven N. Austad of the University of Texas Health Science Center at San Antonio's Barshop Institute for Longevity and Aging Studies reports the results of calorie restriction in rhesus monkeys. Although the 57 calorie-restricted monkeys were healthier in terms of cholesterol and triglyceride levels (indicators of reduced risk for cardiovascular disease) and muscle loss and suffered lower rates of diseases, they did not live longer than the 64 monkeys in the control group that were not calorie restricted.

Wanda Rizza, Nicola Veronese, and Luigi Fontana observe in "What Are the Roles of Calorie Restriction and Diet Quality in Promoting Healthy Longevity?" (*Ageing Research Reviews*, vol. 13, January 2014) that while long-term CR acts to reduce the risk of developing type 2 diabetes, hypertension, cardiovascular disease, and cancer, it is possible that some of this risk reduction may be attributable to the composition and quality of the diets consumed by CR adherents rather than calorie restriction alone. The researchers note that long-term CR is associated with lower levels of serum triiodothyronine (a hormone made by the thyroid gland) and core body temperature, independent of adiposity, and these changes also may contribute to longevity. Rizza, Veronese, and Fontana call for more studies to "understand the interactions among single nutrient modifications, CR and regular exercise and longevity.

CHAPTER 10
PREVENTING OVERWEIGHT AND OBESITY

Many obesity researchers and health professionals believe the most effective way to win the war on obesity is to intensify efforts to prevent overweight and obesity among children, adolescents, and adults. They assert that over time prevention is far more cost effective than the expenditures that are associated with weight-loss efforts and medical treatment of obesity-related diseases. They also observe that prevention is a preferable strategy because there is no universally effective long-term treatment that consistently produces and maintains weight loss.

The landmark report *Surgeon General's Call to Action to Prevent and Decrease Overweight and Obesity, 2001* (2001, http://www.cdc.gov/nccdphp/dnpa/pdf/CalltoAction.pdf) calls for the design and implementation of interventions to prevent and decrease overweight and obesity, both individually and collectively. It asserts that effective actions must occur at many levels and acknowledges that—although individual behavioral change is at the core of all strategies to reduce overweight and obesity—to be optimally effective, efforts must not be limited to individual behavioral change.

The report recommends actions to modify group influences by initiating prevention programs that target families, communities, employers and workers, the health care delivery system, and the media, as well as changes in public policy. Furthermore, the report calls for concerted efforts and predicts that actions to prevent and reduce overweight and obesity will fail unless changes are made at every level of U.S. society. Characterizing these problems as societal rather than as individual, the report observes that individual behavioral change is possible only in "a supportive environment with accessible and affordable healthy food choices and opportunities for regular physical activity." The report also warns that actions aimed exclusively at individual behavioral change that do not consider social, cultural, economic,

and environmental influences will be counterproductive, serving only to reinforce negative stereotypes, bias, and stigmatization of people who are overweight or obese.

Many public health professionals believe environmental and policy interventions are the most promising strategies for generating and maintaining healthy nutrition and physical activity behaviors in Americans. Environmental interventions are those actions that modify availability of, access to, pricing of, or education about foods at the places where they are purchased. Policy interventions legislate, regulate, or, through formal or informal rules, serve to guide individual and collective behavior. Examples of environmental and policy initiatives that have met with success include:

- Increasing the availability of fruits and vegetables at school and workplace cafeterias and adding fresh fruit to refrigerated vending machines

- Replacing soft drinks in school vending machines with fruit juices and water

- Instituting daily physical education requirements for students

- Providing point-of-purchase nutrition information at restaurants and grocery stores to encourage healthful food choices

- Allowing workers adequate break time and a location where nursing mothers can express milk so their babies can continue to accrue the health benefits of breast-feeding even after their mothers return to work

At the federal level, there are at least 14 prevention initiatives that address nutrition and weight status, including:

- Aim for a Healthy Weight, a National Institutes of Health (NIH) resource on healthy eating and physical activity

- Bright Futures for Women's Health and Wellness, an initiative to develop, implement, and evaluate consumer, provider, and community tools for women

- Dietary Guidelines for Americans, a set of recommendations for food choices that promote good health, a healthy weight, and disease prevention

- Healthy Communities, a Centers for Disease Control and Prevention (CDC) program that works with schools, employers, health care sites, and other community settings to prevent chronic diseases

- Let's Move!, an education program that informs parents, supports healthful food choices, and helps children become more physically active

- Maternal, Infant, and Early Childhood Home Visiting, a program aimed at improving the health of at-risk children

- Million Hearts, an initiative focused on heart disease prevention and reducing sodium in the food supply

- National Initiative to Improve Adolescent Health (NIIAH), an effort to improve the health, safety, and well-being of adolescents and young adults ages 10 to 24

- National Prevention Strategy, a set of guidelines outlining the most effective and achievable ways to improve national health and well-being

- National Stakeholder Strategy for Achieving Health Equity, a set of goals aimed at helping racial and ethnic minorities reach their full health potential

- Public Health System, Finance, and Quality Program, an organizational center to connect federal agencies and partners on public health system issues

- Surgeon General's Vision for a Healthy and Fit Nation, a set of actions to combat overweight and obesity and resultant disease

- We Can!, a national campaign to support parents, caregivers, and communities to help children ages eight to 13 remain at a healthy weight

- Well-Integrated Screening and Evaluation for Women across the Nation (WISEWOMAN), a program providing low-income, underinsured, or uninsured women ages 40 to 64 with screening, lifestyle programs, and referral services to prevent cardiovascular disease.

PREVENTION EFFORTS TARGET FAMILIES, COMMUNITIES, WORKSITES, AND SCHOOLS

Public health education, communication, and other programs aimed at families and communities are identified as the cornerstone of prevention efforts. The *National Prevention, Health Promotion and Public Health Council* describes various national prevention programs. For example, the Corporation for National and Community Service promotes healthy communities via programs that involve youth in physical activity and teach them the importance of nutrition. The U.S. Department of Health and Human Services (HHS) Community Transformation Grant program helps create safe recreational spaces to provide children with increased opportunities for physical activity and improve access to healthful food and beverages in school vending machines.

In the community, schools offer ideal settings and multiple opportunities for preventing overweight and obesity by educating children about, and engaging them in, healthful eating and physical activity. To reinforce their messages concerning the importance of school physical activity and nutrition programs, schools can ensure that breakfast and lunch programs meet nutrition standards and provide food options that are low in fat, calories, and added sugars. Other ways to improve student health and nutrition include offering healthful snacks in vending machines and school stores and providing all students with quality daily physical education to cultivate the knowledge, attitudes, skills, behaviors, and confidence needed to be physically active for life.

One way to consider how Americans relate to food and physical activity and how to improve diet and activity levels is to use a social-ecological model that looks at the population demographics, environments, organizations, values, and culture that influence nutrition and activity decisions. Public health officials use this model to show how all elements of society combine to shape an individual's food and physical activity choices, which in turn influence calorie balance and risk for overweight and obesity. Figure 10.1 displays the myriad influences on an individual's food and physical activity decisions.

Community Strategies to Prevent Obesity

In *Strategies to Prevent Obesity and Other Chronic Diseases: The CDC Guide to Strategies to Increase the Consumption of Fruits and Vegetables* (2011, http://www.cdc.gov/obesity/downloads/FandV_2011_WEB_TAG508.pdf), the CDC identifies the following 10 environmental- and policy-level strategies that communities and local governments can use to plan and monitor changes to help prevent obesity:

1. Promote food policy councils as a way to improve the food environment at state and local levels

2. Improve access to retail stores that sell high-quality fruits and vegetables or increase the availability of high-quality fruits and vegetables at retail stores in underserved communities

3. Start or expand farm-to-institution programs in schools, hospitals, workplaces, and other institutions

4. Start or expand farmers' markets in all settings

FIGURE 10.1

Factors shaping nutrition and physical activity decisions

SOURCE: "Figure 6-1. A Social Ecological Framework for Nutrition and Physical Activity Decisions," in *Dietary Guidelines for Americans, 2010*, 7th ed., U.S. Department of Health and Human Services and U.S. Department of Agriculture, December 2010, http://origin.www.cnpp.usda.gov/Publications/DietaryGuidelines/2010/PolicyDoc/Chapter6.pdf (accessed November 3, 2015)

5. Start or expand community-supported agriculture programs in all settings

6. Ensure access to fruits and vegetables in workplace cafeterias and other food service venues

7. Ensure access to fruits and vegetables at workplace meetings and events

8. Support and promote community and home gardens

9. Establish policies to incorporate fruit and vegetable activities into schools as a way to increase consumption

10. Include fruits and vegetables in emergency food programs

Similarly, in *Strategies to Prevent Obesity and Other Chronic Diseases: The CDC Guide to Strategies to Increase Physical Activity in the Community* (2011, http://www.cdc.gov/obesity/downloads/PA_2011_WEB.pdf), the CDC presents 10 strategies aimed at increasing physical activity:

1. Community-wide campaigns—large-scale multimedia campaigns in concert with support and self-help groups, physical activity counseling, and risk-factor screening and education at worksites, schools, and community health fairs

2. Point-of-decision prompts to encourage use of stairs—signs posted beside elevators and escalators to encourage people to use nearby stairs instead

3. Individually adapted health behavior change programs—custom-tailored strategies that respond to an individual's interests and preferences

4. Enhanced school-based physical education—engaging students in moderate to vigorous physical activity

5. Social support interventions in community settings—building, strengthening, and maintaining social networks that support physical activity behavior change

6. Creation of or enhanced access to places for physical activity combined with informational outreach activities—creating or improving access to exercise facilities and walking trails, providing programs that educate people about physical exercise, and offering screenings and referrals to other types of services

7. Street-scale urban design and land-use policies—activities include improving street lighting and increasing ease and safety of street crossings

8. Community-scale urban design and land-use policies—actions include improving the continuity and connectivity of streets, sidewalks, and bicycle lanes

9. Active transport to school—interventions designed to encourage and support youth walking, bicycling, or skating to school

10. Transportation and travel policies and practices—encouraging walking, bicycling, and public transportation use, increasing the safety of walking and bicycling, reducing car use, and improving air quality

Federally Funded National Nutrition Education

Together, the U.S. Department of Agriculture (USDA) and the HHS update *Nutrition and Your Health: Dietary Guidelines for Americans* every five years. First published in 1980, the guidelines serve as the basis for federal food and nutrition education programs.

The eighth version of the dietary guidelines, *Dietary Guidelines for Americans, 2015*, takes aim at obesity, diabetes, and cardiovascular health. In "What the New Dietary Guidelines Mean for You" (Health.usnews.com, March 4, 2015), Lisa Esposito reports that the updated guidelines urge Americans to limit added sugars to no more than 10% of their daily calories and to replace saturated fats with unsaturated fats. Figure 10.2 shows commonly used solid fats and oils and their composition in terms of saturated fat, monounsaturated fat, and polyunsaturated fat.

U.S. Secretary of Agriculture Tom Vilsack (1950–) and Secretary of Health and Human Services Sylvia Burwell (1965–) explain in "2015 Dietary Guidelines: Giving You the Tools You Need to Make Healthy Choices" (October 6, 2015, http://blogs.usda.gov/2015/10/06/2015-dietary-guidelines-giving-you-the-tools-you-need-to-make-healthy-choices/) that the 2015 guidelines are similar to those issued in years past, advising Americans to increase the consumption of:

- Nutrient-dense foods (e.g., fruits, lean meats and poultry, and eggs prepared without added solid fats, sugars, starches, and sodium) that provide the full range of essential nutrients and fiber, without excessive calories (see Figure 10.3, which compares the calorie content in some commonly consumed nutrient-dense foods with foods that are not nutrient dense)

- Vegetables (especially dark green, red, and orange vegetables), beans, peas, and fruits

FIGURE 10.2

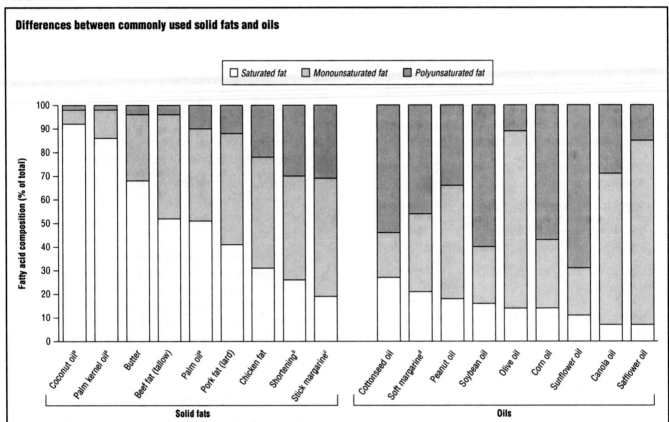

Differences between commonly used solid fats and oils

[a]Coconut oil, palm kernel oil, and palm oil are called oils because they come from plants. However, they are semi-solid at room temperature due to their high content of short-chain saturated fatty acids. They are considered solid fats for nutritional purposes.
[b]Partially hydrogenated vegetable oil shortening, which contains transfats.
[c]Most stick margarines contain partially hydrogenated vegetable oil, a source of transfats.
[d]The primary ingredient in soft margarine with no transfats is liquid vegetable oil.

SOURCE: "Figure 3-3. Fatty Acid Profiles of Common Fats and Oils," in *Dietary Guidelines for Americans, 2010*, 7th ed., U.S. Department of Health and Human Services and U.S. Department of Agriculture, December 2010, http://health.gov/dietaryguidelines/dga2010/dietaryguidelines2010.pdf (accessed November 3, 2015)

FIGURE 10.3

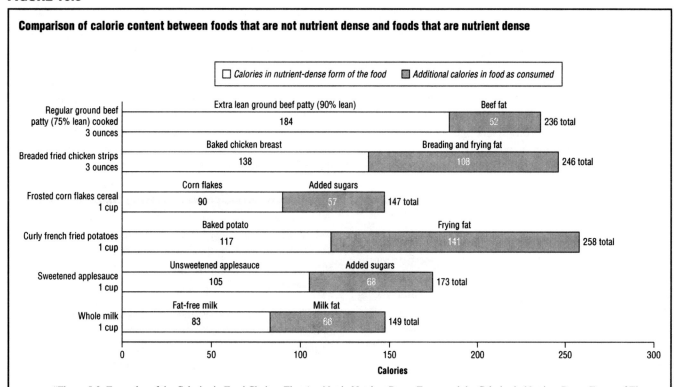

Comparison of calorie content between foods that are not nutrient dense and foods that are nutrient dense

☐ Calories in nutrient-dense form of the food   ▨ Additional calories in food as consumed

Food		
Regular ground beef patty (75% lean) cooked 3 ounces	Extra lean ground beef patty (90% lean) — 184	Beef fat — 52 — 236 total
Breaded fried chicken strips 3 ounces	Baked chicken breast — 138	Breading and frying fat — 108 — 246 total
Frosted corn flakes cereal 1 cup	Corn flakes — 90	Added sugars — 57 — 147 total
Curly french fried potatoes 1 cup	Baked potato — 117	Frying fat — 141 — 258 total
Sweetened applesauce 1 cup	Unsweetened applesauce — 105	Added sugars — 68 — 173 total
Whole milk 1 cup	Fat-free milk — 83	Milk fat — 66 — 149 total

Calories (0, 50, 100, 150, 200, 250, 300)

SOURCE: "Figure 5-2. Examples of the Calories in Food Choices That Are Not in Nutrient Dense Forms and the Calories in Nutrient Dense Forms of These Foods," in *Dietary Guidelines for Americans, 2010*, 7th ed., U.S. Department of Health and Human Services and U.S. Department of Agriculture, December 2010, http://health.gov/dietaryguidelines/dga2010/dietaryguidelines2010.pdf (accessed November 3, 2015)

- Whole grains and fat-free or low-fat dairy or fortified soy beverages

- Fish and other seafood

- A variety of foods high in protein, including eggs, beans, peas, soy products, and unsalted nuts and seeds

- Foods that are rich in potassium, dietary fiber, calcium, and vitamin D, including vegetables, fruits, whole grains, and dairy

The guidelines advise "appropriate calorie balance during each stage of life—childhood, adolescence, adulthood, pregnancy and breastfeeding, and older age." Women who may become pregnant are advised to choose foods that are rich in iron and folate and to take 400 micrograms of folic acid per day. Women who are pregnant are advised to take an iron supplement and those who are pregnant or breast-feeding are cautioned to limit their consumption of white tuna to just 6 ounces per week and to avoid eating tilefish, shark, swordfish, and mackerel, because these fish contain high mercury content. Adults aged 50 years and older are encouraged to choose foods that are fortified with vitamin B_{12}, such as fortified cereals, or to take dietary supplements to ensure adequate B_{12} intake.

Vilsack and Burwell explain that sustainability (the environmental impact of a food source) is an important issue and the USDA invests heavily in sustainable food production, sustainable and renewable energy, sustainable water systems, preserving and protecting our natural resources and lands, and research into sustainable practices. During the formulation of the 2015 guidelines there was discussion about including sustainability considerations and goals, but a decision was made to limit the scope of the guidelines to "nutritional and dietary information … based on the preponderance of scientific and medical knowledge."

MyPlate Is Also for Children

In 2011 MyPlate replaced MyPyramid for Kids, which, like the food pyramid for adults, provided guidance for children's diets. (See Figure 5.2 in Chapter 5.) The website ChooseMyPlate.gov replaces much of the information that was formerly available on MyPyramid.gov and, to engage children, includes a coloring sheet for children. It also has an interactive feature to help with meal planning. MyPlate is part of a larger communications initiative based on the 2010 dietary guidelines to help consumers of all ages make better food choices.

The dietary guidelines observe that healthy diets and adequate physical activity are vitally important for children in view of the fact that risk factors for adult chronic diseases are increasingly found in younger ages. The guidelines assert that "eating patterns established in childhood often track into later life, making early intervention on adopting healthy nutrition and physical activity behaviors a priority." The guidelines advise that young children consume between 1,000 and 2,000 calories per day and older children and adolescents between 1,400 and 3,200 calories per day. Table 10.1 shows the estimated calories needed for children, adolescents, and adults by sex and physical activity level. The proportion of recommended macronutrients (carbohydrate, fat, and protein) changes with advancing age. For example, children aged one to three years require less protein and more fat in their diet than do older children. (See Table 5.1 in Chapter 5.)

Children aged six years and older are encouraged to play hard and be more physically active to meet the government's recommended 60 minutes of exercise per day. Although the guidelines do not offer specific recommendations about the duration of physical activity for children aged two to five years, they advise that young children should play actively several times each day. Because children and teens are often active in short bursts of time rather than for sustained periods, these short bursts accumulate to meet physical activity requirements.

Praise and Criticism for MyPlate

Like the previous MyPyramid guidelines, MyPlate has garnered praise and criticism. In "Why It's Good That the Food Pyramid Became a Plate" (Atlantic.com,

June 3, 2011), Marion Nestle praised the new icon, explaining that it is easy enough for a child to use. Nestle approves of the fact that vegetables are the largest sector on the plate, that vegetables and fruits together consume half the plate, and that dairy foods are off to the side so they may be considered discretionary. Nestle also likes the fact that unless one chooses a very large plate, there's no need to count servings or measure portion sizes. She has just one criticism of MyPlate: its categorization of protein as a food group. Nestle explains that "protein is a nutrient, not a food," and observes that "protein is not exactly lacking in American diets. The average American consumes twice the protein needed." Nestle is concerned that Americans may equate protein exclusively with meat rather than with a larger group of foods including beans, nuts, poultry, fish, grains, and dairy (which have separate sectors on the plate) that are also sources of protein in American diets.

The Physicians Committee for Responsible Medicine (PCRM) concurs with Nestle in "Breaking News! USDA Replaces Food Pyramid with MyPlate" (June 2011) about the protein portion of the plate, observing that beans, whole grains, and vegetables contain protein but objects to the inclusion of dairy, which is often a source of fat and cholesterol, and opines that there are more healthful sources of dietary calcium. Furthermore, PCRM nutritionist Kathryn Strong asserts that "the USDA's new

TABLE 10.1

Estimated calorie needs by age, sex, and physical activity

Estimated amounts of calories needed to maintain calorie balance for various gender and age groups at three different levels of physical activity. The estimates are rounded to the nearest 200 calories. An individual's calorie needs may be higher or lower than these average estimates.

| Gender | Age (years) | Physical activity level[a] | | |
		Sedentary	Moderately active	Active
Child (female and male)	2–3	1,000–1,200[b]	1,000–1,400[b]	1,000–1,400[b]
Female[c]	4–8	1,200–1,400	1,400–1,600	1,400–1,800
	9–13	1,400–1,600	1,600–2,000	1,800–2,200
	14–18	1,800	2,000	2,400
	19–30	1,800–2,000	2,000–2,200	2,400
	31–50	1,800	2,000	2,200
	51+	1,600	1,800	2,000–2,200
Male	4–8	1,200–1,400	1,400–1,600	1,600–2,000
	9–13	1,600–2,000	1,800–2,200	2,000–2,600
	14–18	2,000–2,400	2,400–2,800	2,800–3,200
	19–30	2,400–2,600	2,600–2,800	3,000
	31–50	2,200–2,400	2,400–2,600	2,800–3,000
	51+	2,000–2,200	2,200–2,400	2,400–2,800

Notes: Based on Estimated Energy Requirements (EER) equations, using reference heights (average) and reference weights (healthy) for each age/gender group. For children and adolescents, reference height and weight vary. For adults, the reference man is 5 feet 10 inches tall and weighs 154 pounds. The reference woman is 5 feet 4 inches tall and weighs 126 pounds. EER equations are from the Institute of Medicine's *Dietary Reference Intakes for Energy, Carbohydrate, Fiber, Fat, Fatty Acids, Cholesterol, Protein, and Amino Acids.* Washington (DC): The National Academies Press; 2002.
[a]Sedentary means a lifestyle that includes only the light physical activity associated with typical day-to-day life. Moderately active means a lifestyle that includes physical activity equivalent to walking about 1.5 to 3 miles per day at 3 to 4 miles per hour, in addition to the light physical activity associated with typical day-to-day life. Active means a lifestyle that includes physical activity equivalent to walking more than 3 miles per day at 3 to 4 miles per hour, in addition to the light physical activity associated with typical day-to-day life.
[b]The calorie ranges shown are to accommodate needs of different ages within the group. For children and adolescents, more calories are needed at older ages. For adults, fewer calories are needed at older ages.
[c]Estimates for females do not include women who are pregnant or breastfeeding.

SOURCE: "Table 2-3. Estimated Calorie Needs per Day by Age, Gender, and Physical Activity Level," in *Dietary Guidelines for Americans, 2010,* 7th ed., U.S. Department of Health and Human Services and U.S. Department of Agriculture, December 2010, http://health.gov/dietaryguidelines/dga2010/dietaryguidelines2010.pdf (accessed November 3, 2015) plate icon couldn't be more at odds with federal food subsidies. The plate icon advises Americans to limit high-fat products like meat and cheese, but the federal government is subsidizing these very products with billions of tax dollars and giving almost no support to fruits and vegetables." Nearly two-thirds (63%) of federal agricultural subsidies support meat and dairy production and less than 1% of subsidies support the cultivation of fruits and vegetables.

Some of these criticisms were addressed in updated MyPlate educational materials. For example, an August 2013 publication, "Eat the MyPlate Way," specified whole grains and added physical activity to the dietary recommendations. (See Figure 10.4.) In addition, Americans' awareness of the MyPlate graphic has increased over time. The International Food Information Council (IFIC) *Food and Health Survey 2015* (http://www.food insight.org/sites/default/files/2015-Food-and-Health-Survey-Full-Report.pdf) finds that Americans' recognition of the MyPlate graphic increased from 2014 to 2015, with 42% of Americans indicating that they "know something about the graphic."

Texting MyPlate Guidelines Proves Effective

In "Mobile MyPlate: A Pilot Study Using Text Messaging to Provide Nutrition Education and Promote Better Dietary Choices in College Students " (*Journal of American College Health*, vol. 62, no, 5, March 2014), Onikia N. Brown, Lauren E. O'Connor, and Dennis Savaiano sought to determine the effectiveness of nutrition education via repeated text messages about college students' fruit and vegetable consumption. The researchers sent twice weekly text messages containing the MyPlate graphic and USDA guidelines to 150 college students for seven weeks. A control group received the same information in a mailed brochure. The students' knowledge and behavior were assessed before and after the nutrition education initiative. The students who received the text messages had greater recognition of the MyPlate food groups and better knowledge of the guidelines than did the control group. Students who received the text messages consumed more fruits than those in the control group and also may have consumed more vegetables. The researchers conclude, "Texting repeated messages appears to be an acceptable and effective way to increase nutrition knowledge and promote positive diet-related behaviors in college students."

Fruits & Veggies: More Matters

Founded in 1991, the 5 a Day for Better Health Program was jointly sponsored by the National Cancer Institute and the Produce for Better Health Foundation (PBH), a nonprofit consumer-education foundation representing the fruit and vegetable industry. To reflect the changes and recommendations made in the dietary guidelines that were released in 2010, the PBH revamped the program and gave it a new name: Fruits & Veggies: More Matters.

The Fruits & Veggies: More Matters initiative (2015, http://www.fruitsandveggiesmorematters.org) aims to increase fruit and vegetable consumption. Its objective is to help "Americans increase fruit & vegetable consumption for better health." Studies indicate that the majority of U.S. adults and adolescents are not eating the recommended two or more servings of fruit and three or more servings of vegetables per day. For example, in "Fruit and Vegetable Consumption of U.S. Youth, 2009–2010" (*NCHS Data Brief*, no. 156, July 2014), Samara Joy Nielsen et al. report that about one-quarter of youth do not consume any fruit on a given day, let alone the recommended minimum of one cup of fruit and one cup of vegetables.

Along with reducing the risk for heart disease, high blood pressure, stroke, many cancers, and diabetes, diets rich in fruits and vegetables can help prevent overweight and obesity. Fruits and vegetables are naturally low in calories and fat, and their high water and fiber content produce feelings of satiety (the feeling of fullness or satisfaction after eating). Combined with an active lifestyle and a low-fat diet, eating greater amounts of fruits and vegetables and fewer high-calorie foods at meals can help control weight.

The Fruits & Veggies: More Matters initiative offers information about the benefits of eating fruits and vegetables, recipes, interactive tools, and information about how to use fruits and vegetables to help consumers manage their weight. For example, Table 10.2 shows fruit and vegetable choices that total 100 calories or fewer. In "100-Calorie Comparison Chart" (2014, http://www.fruit sandveggiesmorematters.org/100-calorie-comparison), the PBH illustrates how substituting fruits or vegetables for high-calorie snacks such as muffins, corn chips, or cookies enables dieters to eat more. For example, two cups of strawberries or cantaloupe contain the same 100 calories as two 2-inch (5-cm) chocolate chip cookies or three-eighths of a doughnut.

State and Community Funding for Prevention Efforts

The CDC Division of Nutrition, Physical Activity, and Obesity aims to help states prevent obesity and other chronic diseases by focusing on poor nutrition and inadequate physical activity. The division assists states in developing and implementing nutrition and physical activity interventions, and sponsoring initiatives to help populations balance caloric intake and expenditure, increase physical activity, improve nutrition by increasing consumption of fruits and vegetables, reduce television time, and increase breast-feeding.

In "CDC's State Public Health Actions to Prevent and Control Diabetes, Heart Disease, Obesity and Associated Risk Factors and Promote School Health (State

FIGURE 10.4

How to use MyPlate, 2013

Enjoy your food but eat less.

Avoid oversized portions.

Make half your plate fruits and vegetables.

Make at least half your grains whole.

Compare sodium, sugars, and saturated fats in foods and choose the foods with lower numbers.

Drink water instead of sugary drinks.

Switch to fat-free or low-fat (1%) milk.

Be active your way.

How to fill my plate

Apples • Bananas • Grapefruit • Lemons • Oranges • Strawberries
Cantaloupe • 100% apple juice • 100% grape juice

Dark green leafy lettuce • Broccoli • Potatoes • Corn
Butternut squash • Red pepper • Garbanzo beans • Zucchini

Brown rice • Rolled oats • Popcorn • Whole-wheat flour
Whole-wheat spaghetti • Bulgur • Whole rye • Quinoa

Lean cuts of beef, pork, chicken • Eggs • Black beans • Lentils
Soy beans • Almonds • Walnuts • Haddock • Salmon • Shrimp • Tuna

Fat-free or Low-fat (1%) Milk, Yogurt, Cheese
Calcium-fortified soy milk

Walking • Jogging • Biking • Hiking • Tennis • Basketball
Soccer • Swimming

Get started!

1. Use ChooseMyPlate.gov for health tips and resources.

2. Select your daily food plan on ChooseMyPlate.gov. Use it as a guide to building a healthy plate.

3. Determine how many calories you should consume per day using SuperTracker.usda.gov

SOURCE: "Eat the MyPlate Way," U.S. Department of Agriculture, Center for Nutrition Policy and Promotion, August 2013, http://www.choosemyplate .gov/sites/default/files/printablematerials/2013-EatTheMyPlateWay.pdf (accessed November 4, 2015)

Public Health Actions)" (September 22, 2015, http://www .cdc.gov/nccdphp/dnpao/state-local-programs/funding.html), the CDC lists examples of initiatives intended to prevent or reduce obesity, including programs to reduce obesity in counties with more than 40% prevalence of adult obesity. In 2015 State Public Health Actions grants awarded $6.2 million to eight programs that perform outreach at the community level in Alabama, Arkansas, Kentucky, Louisiana, South Dakota, Tennessee, Texas, and West Virginia.

TABLE 10.2

Servings of fruit and vegetables with 100 calories or less

- a medium-size apple (72 calories)
- a medium-size banana (105 calories)
- 1 cup steamed green beans (44 calories)
- 1 cup blueberries (83 calories)
- 1 cup grapes (100 calories)
- 1 cup carrots (45 calories), broccoli (30 calories), or bell peppers (30 calories) with 2 tbsp. hummus (46 calories)

SOURCE: "About 100 Calories or Less," in *How to Use Fruits and Vegetables to Help Manage Your Weight*, Centers for Disease Control and Prevention, National Center for Chronic Disease Prevention and Health Promotion, July 13, 2012, http://www.cdc.gov/nccdphp/dnpa/nutrition/pdf/CDC_5-A-Day .pdf (accessed November 4, 2015)

There is evidence that state and community antiobesity initiatives are effective. In "Implementation and Evaluation of the HEROES Initiative: A Tri-state Coordinated School Health Program to Reduce Childhood Obesity" (*Health Promotion Practice*, vol. 15, no. 3, May 2014), Mindy H. King et al. report the results of a coordinated school health approach involving 17 schools in southern Indiana, northwestern Kentucky, and southeastern Illinois. King et al. find that the initiative was "successful in reducing the percentage of overweight children in participating schools and healthfully modifying their dietary, physical activity, and sedentary behaviors."

IS NUTRITION EDUCATION WORKING TO IMPROVE AMERICANS' DIETS?

The Healthy Eating Index (HEI) is a measure developed in 1990 by the USDA to assess the overall health value of Americans' diets. It captures the type and quantity of foods people eat and the degree to which diets comply with specific recommendations in the USDA dietary guidelines. The HEI assigns points for eating consistently within USDA guidelines. It assesses 10 dietary components—grains, vegetables, fruits, milk, meat, total fat, total saturated fat, cholesterol, sodium, and a varied diet—on a scale of 0 to 10. Individuals who eat grains, vegetables, fruits, milk, meat (including chicken and fish), as well as a variety of foods at or above the USDA-recommended levels, receive a maximum score of 10. A score of 0 is assigned when the recommended amount of those components is not eaten. For fat, saturated fat, cholesterol, and sodium, a score of 10 is awarded for eating the recommended amount or less. The highest possible score is 100; a score of 80 or above is considered a healthy diet, scores between 51 and 80 show a need for dietary improvement, and scores below 50 indicate a poor diet.

Researchers use the HEI to evaluate Americans' diets. For example, Emilyn C. Banfield et al. used the HEI to assess children's diet quality and reported their findings in "Poor Adherence to U.S. Dietary Guidelines for Children and Adolescents in the National Health and

Nutrition Examination Survey Population" (*Journal of the Academy of Nutrition and Dietetics*, September 19, 2015). The researchers find that children aged four to eight years had the highest overall diet quality due to significantly greater scores for total fruit, whole fruit, dairy, and whole grains, but these younger children also had the highest scores for sodium, refined grains, and empty calories. Overall, HEI scores ranged from 43.59 to 52.11 out of 100, much lower than the minimum score of 80 that is considered indicative of a healthy diet.

Americans' Snack Food Choices

The NPD Group observes in "Consumers Like Their Snacks with a 'Healthy' Twist" (June 9, 2015, https://www .npd.com/wps/portal/npd/us/news/press-releases/2015/con sumers-like-their-snacks-with-a-healthy-twist/) that consumers, especially youth and people ages 23 to 48, are seeking more healthful snacks. Consumers are looking for snacks that are natural and contain protein and no sugar or only a small amount. The NPD Group reports that consumption of more healthful snack foods such as fresh fruit, breakfast/sports bars, and yogurt has increased 14% since 2006 and that more healthful snacks are the fastest-growing segment of the snack market.

The NPD Group also finds that consumer preference for sweet and savory snacks is determined by the time of day, but more healthful snack choices are determined by location. In "Time of Day Dictates Sweet and Savory Snack Consumption, but Place Is Predictor for Eating Better-for-You Snacks" (October 27, 2015, https://www .npd.com/wps/portal/npd/us/news/press-releases/2015/time-of-day-dictates-sweet-and-savory-snack-consumption/), NPD observes that more than 40% of snacks brought from home and consumed at school, work, in the car, or at other locations are in the "better-for-you" category.

Snacking May Help to Promote Weight Management

In the press release "The Right Snack May Aid Satiety, Weight Loss" (July 16, 2013, http://www.ift.org/ newsroom/news-releases/2013/july/16/the-right-snack-may-aid-satiety.aspx), the Institute of Food Technologists observes that healthful snacks that promote satiety may reduce the quantity of food consumed at subsequent meals. In a presentation at the 2013 Institute of Food Technologists Annual Meeting & Food Expo, Roberta Re of Leatherhead Food Research in Surrey, England, explained that the food industry is trying to offer consumers snacks that improve satiety to help them reduce their total daily food intake. Re reports that midmorning snacks of cereal or nuts reduced food consumption at lunch and dinner, effectively decreasing the total daily food intake.

For example, Sarah Hull et al. report in "A Midmorning Snack of Almonds Generates Satiety and Appropriate Adjustment of Subsequent Food Intake in Healthy

Women" (*European Journal of Nutrition*, vol. 54, no. 5, August 2015) that a midmorning snack of almonds decreased consumption at lunch and dinner such that total calories consumed were not increased by the snack.

Portion-controlled snacks, such as Nabisco 100-Calorie Packs, aim to help dieters control their caloric intake while still enjoying their favorite snacks, which are often sweet, salty, or low-nutrient-value foods. Brian Wansink, Collin R. Payne, and Mitsuru Shimizu conducted research to determine whether the 100-calorie packages reduced the caloric intake of normal-weight and obese people and whether they enabled people to accurately track their caloric intake. The results of the study were published in "The 100-Calorie Semi-solution: Sub-packaging Most Reduces Intake among the Heaviest" (*Obesity*, vol. 19, no. 5, May 2011). The researchers asked 42 college students to eat snack crackers while watching television. Half of the study subjects were given a large 400-calorie package of crackers and the other half were given four 100-calorie packages. After the show, the subjects were asked to estimate how many crackers they had consumed, and then their actual consumption was calculated. Subjects ate an average 25% less when given four 100-calorie packages of crackers than when given one 400-calorie package, and overweight subjects' intake decreased 54%. Nonetheless, all of the subjects underestimated their consumption by 60% or more, which suggests that portion-controlled packaging does not improve the accuracy of estimated intake.

Interventions to Promote Healthy Weight

In "Obesity Prevention and Control: Interventions in Community Settings" (August 14, 2015, http://www.the communityguide.org/obesity/communitysettings.html), the CDC's Community Preventive Services Task Force reviews the effectiveness of interventions that prevent obesity and promote healthy eating and physical activity. The task force considers the effectiveness of population-based interventions that promote healthy growth and development of children and adolescents and that support healthy weights among adults. It also focuses on school-based strategies, worksite programs, health care system interventions, and community initiatives.

The task force recommends interventions that reduce the time children and teens spend watching television, playing video or computer games, and surfing the Internet. It endorses worksite programs that combine nutrition and physical activity as effective strategies to reduce and control overweight and obesity. It also indicates that more research is needed to determine the extent to which school-based programs help control overweight and obesity. Table 10.3 is an overview of the interventions and task force ratings.

Proven Community-Based Prevention Programs

In October 2013 the Trust for America's Health and the New York Academy of Medicine published *A Compendium of Proven Community-Based Prevention Programs* (http://healthyamericans.org/assets/files/Compendium _Report_1016_1131.pdf), which details 79 community-based prevention programs that have demonstrated the ability to improve health and save lives. Examples of programs that have increased physical activity include the installation of a six-block walking path and school playground in a low-income African American neighborhood in New Orleans, Louisiana, and a comprehensive nutrition and health education program in Somerville, Massachusetts, that helps prevent overweight in elementary school students.

PREVENTION PROGRAMS AT THE WORKSITE

Along with school-based nutrition programs and education initiatives aimed at the public at large, several notable obesity-prevention efforts involve developing and implementing strategies to integrate physical activity and healthful food choices into routine worksite activities. Examples of such activities include incorporating planned activity breaks with music into long meetings, offering healthful food choices during meetings and breaks and in employee cafeterias, and hosting walking meetings.

Because more than 100 million Americans (over one out of every three people in the United States) spend a large number of their waking hours at work, the worksite presents another opportunity for prevention programs. In "Obesity Prevention and Control: Interventions in Community Settings," the Community Preventive Services Task Force advises moving beyond traditional workplace health education programs. It recommends more intensive and comprehensive efforts, such as modifying physical and social environments, instituting policies consistent with the objective of preventing overweight and obesity, and extending worksite prevention efforts not only to employees but also to the families of employees and their communities.

Examples of worksite obesity-prevention and weight-control strategies include:

- Educating workers using lectures, written materials provided in print or online, and educational software

- Ensuring that healthful food options are available in cafeterias and vending machines

- Establishing worksite exercise facilities or creating incentives for employees to join local fitness centers

- Developing incentives, rewards, and reinforcements for workers to achieve and maintain a healthy body weight

TABLE 10.3

Obesity prevention interventions and task force ratings

	Ratings
Interventions to reduce screen time (e.g., time in front of a TV, computer monitor)	
Behavioral interventions to reduce screen time	Recommended
These interventions may include:	
• Skills building, tips, goal setting, and reinforcement techniques	
• Parent or family support through provision of information on environmental strategies to reduce access to television, video games, and computers	
• A "TV turnoff challenge" in which participants are encouraged not to watch TV for a specified number of days	
Mass media interventions to reduce screen time	Insufficient evidence
In these campaigns, one or more components is designed to:	
• Increase knowledge about screen time	
• Influence attitudes	
• Change behavior by transmitting messages through newspapers, radio, television, and billboards	
Technology-supported interventions (e.g., computer or web applications)	
Technology-supported components may include use of the following:	
• Computers (e.g., internet, CD-ROM, e-mail, kiosk, computer program)	
• Video conferencing	
• Personal digital assistants	
• Pagers	
• Pedometers with computer interaction	
• Computerized telephone system interventions that target physical activity, nutrition, or weight.	
Non-technological components may include use of the following:	
• In-person counseling	
• Manual tracking	
• Printed lessons	
• Written feedback	
Multicomponent coaching or counseling interventions:	
• To reduce weight	Recommended
• To maintain weight loss	Recommended
Interventions in specific settings	
Worksite programs	Recommended
• Informational and educational strategies aim to increase knowledge about a healthy diet and physical activity. Examples include:	
Lectures	
Written materials (provided in print or online)	
Educational software	
• Behavioral and social strategies target the thoughts (e.g. awareness, self-efficacy) and social factors that effect behavior changes. Examples include:	
Individual or group behavioral counseling	
Skill-building activities such as cue control	
Rewards or reinforcement	
Inclusion of co-workers or family members to build support systems	
• Policy and environmental approaches aim to make healthy choices easier and target the entire workforce by changing physical or organizational structures. Examples of this include:	
Improving access to healthy foods (e.g. changing cafeteria options, vending machine content)	
Providing more opportunities to be physically active (e.g. providing on-site facilities for exercise)	
• Policy strategies may also change rules and procedures for employees such as health insurance benefits or costs or money for health club membership.	
• Worksite weight control strategies may occur separately or as part of a comprehensive worksite wellness program that addresses several health issues (e.g., smoking cessation, stress management, cholesterol reduction).	
School-based programs	Insufficient evidence
These interventions are conducted in the classroom and may seek to increase physical activity and/or improve nutrition, both in school and at home. Classroom and physical education teachers may receive special training to carry out the programs.	

SOURCE: Adapted from "Summary of Task Force Recommendations," in *Obesity Prevention and Control: Interventions in Community Settings*, Guide to Community Preventive Services, September 27, 2013, http://www.thecommunityguide.org/obesity/communitysettings.html (accessed November 5, 2015)

• Encouraging employers to require weight management and physical activity counseling as covered benefits in health insurance contracts

• Providing individual or group behavioral counseling

Dorte Eriksen et al. observe in "Sedentary Work—Associations between Five-Year Changes in Occupational Sitting Time and BMI" (*Preventive Medicine*, vol. 73, April 2015) that there is evidence of a link between a sedentary lifestyle and BMI. Many office workers, move an average of two hours less per day and as a result expend less energy than their more active peers, increasing their risk for obesity, chronic metabolic disease, and cardiovascular death. Eriksen et al. looked at changes in occupational sitting time and confirmed a positive relationship between changes in sitting time and BMI in women but not men. Eriksen et al. speculate that the reduced energy expenditure associated with sitting likely affects men, but BMI may not be the correct measure for men since they have greater muscle mass than women and BMI does not distinguish between fat and muscle. The researchers suggest that future studies consider fat percentage of body composition instead of BMI.

Offices and Worksites Can Improve Health and Fitness

Mary MacVean notes in "'Get Up!' or Lose Hours of Your Life Every Day, Scientist Says" (LATimes.com,

July 31, 2014) that James Levine, who studies nonexercise activity thermogenesis (NEAT; the calories people burn during everyday activities such as standing, walking, or even fidgeting; low NEAT is linked to weight gain), believes that sitting imperils health. Levine asserts that people lose two hours of life for every hour they sit, and even a daily workout at the gym does not counteract the harmful effects of sitting all day long. He says it is crucial to break up the hours of sitting and suggests walking at lunchtime and moving more at work.

Levine explains in *Get Up!: Why Your Chair Is Killing You and What You Can Do about It* (2014) that Americans' reliance on electronics and especially the Internet has deprived them of the opportunity to be physically active and burn calories. He asserts that changing office workers' routines to include more standing, turning, and bending throughout the course of the workday not only burns calories, boosts metabolism, reduces blood pressure, and increases mental clarity but also increases productivity.

In "Effects of a Worksite Physical Activity Intervention for Hospital Nurses Who Are Working Mothers" (*AAOHN Journal*, vol. 59, no. 9, September 2011), Sharon J. Tucker et al. report the results of a study that tested an innovative 10-week worksite physical activity intervention that was incorporated into the workflow of hospital-based nurses. The intervention involved redesigning and changing the physical environment and providing social reinforcements and strategies for engaging in physical activities while at work and away from work. The nurses were given an intervention toolkit that contained a water bottle, tote bag, research-grade pedometer, resistance band, relaxation ball, relaxation CD, exercise DVD, brochure offering nutrition and activity tips, nutritious snack, walking meeting tag, and wellness journal. After a 30- to 60-minute introductory session, the nurses were asked to increase their overall physical activity for 10 weeks by one hour each workday, 30 minutes of which were to be through walking. The study met its objective, increasing overall daily hours of physical activity by one hour per day over the study period. Tucker et al. conclude that "it is feasible to target the worksite of hospital-based registered nurses to improve body composition and physical activity."

DOES PARTICIPATION IN WORKSITE HEALTH PROMOTION PROGRAMS INCREASE PHYSICAL ACTIVITY?
Worksite health promotion programs have demonstrated the ability to help workers improve their health, increase productivity, and manage health care costs. Lisa J. Leininger et al. compared the physical activity of state university workers on campuses with formal health promotion programs to the physical activity levels of workers on campuses without such programs to determine if the programs served to increase physical activity levels. The research and its

results were described in "Differences in Physical Activity Participation between University Employees with and without a Worksite Health Promotion Program" (*Californian Journal of Health Promotion*, vol. 11, no. 1, March 2013). The researchers find that the presence of a health promotion program was only associated with more walking days per week and made no difference in the amount of vigorous physical activity workers engaged in. Leininger et al. conclude, "Overall findings of this study indicate that if health promotion programs are to carry out their mission of improved health behaviors and increased [physical activity] levels, best practices must be implemented and further research must be conducted."

INTENSIFYING THE PREVENTION AGENDA IN THE HEALTH CARE SYSTEM

Interactions with health care professionals are important opportunities to deliver powerful prevention messages. Physicians' and other health professionals' prescriptions and recurring advice to maintain a healthy weight to prevent disease or reduce symptoms of existing disease are often powerful inducements for behavioral change. Most Americans have at least annual contact with a health care professional, and if this contact includes information about the importance of weight management, then it may reinforce prevention messages received in other settings such as schools and worksites. Furthermore, health care professionals are instrumental in shaping public policy and can leverage their expertise and credibility to present accurate messages in the media and catalyze sweeping changes in the community at large.

Examples of strategies to expand on prevention efforts in the health care delivery system include:

- Training health care providers and health profession students to use effective techniques to prevent and treat overweight and obesity

- Cultivating partnerships between health care providers, schools, faith-based groups, and other community organizations to target social and environmental causes of overweight and obesity

- Classifying obesity as a disease to enable reimbursement for prevention efforts

- Partially or fully covering weight-management services including nutrition education and physical activity programs as health plan benefits

The Patient Protection and Affordable Care Act (ACA), the 2010 health reform legislation that expands health care coverage, emphasizes community prevention as an important strategy for improving the nation's health and curbing the costs associated with untreated chronic disease. The act requires health plans to fully cover obesity screening and counseling for adults and children, appropriates funds for demonstration projects to develop model programs for reducing childhood obesity, and, as described in Chapter 8, requires the disclosure of specified nutrient information for food sold in many chain restaurants and vending machines.

In "Calorie Changes in Chain Restaurant Menu Items" (*American Journal of Preventive Medicine*, vol. 48, no. 1, January 2015), Sara N. Bleich, Julia A. Wolfson, and Marian P. Jarlenski note that the ACA requirement that chain restaurants with 20 or more locations provide calorie information on their menus and menu boards has prompted large restaurant chains to offer menu items with fewer calories. The researchers find new main course items had 10% fewer calories in 2013 than they did in 2012. New beverage calorie counts decreased 8%, and calories in children's items were down 20%.

USING THE MEDIA TO COMMUNICATE THE PREVENTION MESSAGE

The media play a pivotal role in prevention efforts. The media can communicate and educate the public about healthy behaviors and health risks that are associated with overweight and obesity, introduce and reinforce prevention messages from health care professionals, and assist to alter attitudes and perceptions by celebrating healthy eating and physical activity.

The IFIC has tracked media coverage of diet, nutrition, and food safety since 1995. In its first report, *Food for Thought* (1995), the IFIC noted that the leading nutrition and food issues receiving newspaper, television, and other media coverage during the previous 12 months were reducing fat intake; the impact of diet on disease risks; and discussions of foodborne illnesses, vitamin and mineral intake, disease causation, caloric intake, antioxidants, cholesterol intake, sugar intake, and fiber intake. As obesity became a more prominent issue during the late 1990s, the IFIC reports in "Executive Summary" (*Food for Thought VI* [December 2005, http://www.foodinsight.org/Content/3651/ExecSummaryFFTVI.pdf]) that the number of stories about diet, weight loss, nutrition, and obesity increased from 1,270 in 1995 to 2,412 in 2005. This increase reflected both a rising volume of coverage and an escalation in the number of media outlets reporting about diet, overweight, and obesity. In *Food for Thought VI*, the IFIC reports that obesity was the leading topic in food and nutrition media stories during 2004, followed by disease prevention, physical activity, weight management, disease causation, vitamin and mineral intake, fat intake, functional foods, mad cow disease, caloric intake, and biotechnology.

Ten years later, in *Food and Health Survey 2015*, the IFIC notes that although the majority of Americans trust their health care professionals for advice about diet and nutrition (70%), about one-quarter (24%) of Americans trust food experts on television for information about

food and nutrition, and the same proportion look to health, food, and nutrition bloggers (24%) or to U.S. government agencies (26%).

The media have responded with advertising and public service campaigns intended to heighten awareness of the risks that are associated with obesity and help Americans make healthier choices. For example, in "Patchy Progress on Obesity Prevention: Emerging Examples, Entrenched Barriers, and New Thinking" (*Lancet*, vol. 385, no. 9985, June 13, 2015), Christina A. Roberto et al. describe public service campaigns such as the "pouring on the pounds" public education campaign that informs New Yorkers about the risks of overconsumption of sugar-sweetened beverages and the "sugar pack" campaign in Los Angeles that shows consumers the number of sugar packets in sugar-sweetened beverages make use of transit and billboard advertising as well as social media. By early 2016, however, it was not yet known if these antiobesity advertising campaigns were effective.

Further, Rebecca M. Puhl, Joerg Luedicke, and Jamie Lee Peterson caution in "Public Reactions to Obesity-Related Health Campaigns: A Randomized Controlled Trial" (*American Journal of Preventive Medicine*, vol. 45, no. 1, July 2013) that public health campaigns that consumers perceive as stigmatizing obese people are considered less motivating for improving lifestyle behaviors and promoting healthy behavior change than those that have neutral or less stigmatizing messages.

TARGETING CHILDHOOD OBESITY

We are seeing promising signs that childhood obesity rates, though still far too high, are leveling off in certain populations. I'm proud to recognize the incredible work of our nation's schools, corporations, and community organizations who are working with the Alliance for a Healthier Generation to make our children's health a priority.

—Mark Creager, M.D., president of the American Heart Association and director of the Heart and Vascular Center, Dartmouth-Hitchcock Medical Center, Lebanon, New Hampshire, October 2, 2015

In 2005 the American Heart Association and the William J. Clinton Foundation launched a new initiative, the Alliance for a Healthier Generation (2015, https://www.healthiergeneration.org/about_us/), to combat childhood obesity. The mission of the alliance is to "reduce the prevalence of childhood obesity and to empower kids to develop lifelong, healthy habits." Working with companies that influence children's lives—food, beverage, fitness, gaming, and technology—the alliance seeks to improve children's health and nutrition at home, in school, in physicians' offices, and in the community at large.

The alliance's Healthy Schools Program works with more than 29,000 schools and supports administrators, teachers, parents, and students to institute policies and programs that enable students to eat better and move more. It also involves insurers, employers, and health care providers to encourage reimbursement to physicians and registered dietitians for obesity prevention–related services. The alliance has helped forge voluntary agreements with the beverage, snack food, and dairy industries to significantly reduce the amount of high-calorie foods that are available to students in schools.

According to the October 21, 2015, press release "The Urban School Food Alliance and the Alliance for a Healthier Generation Leverage $3 Billion in Purchasing Power for Market-Driven Change in School Meals" (https://www .healthiergeneration.org/news__events/2015/10/21/1383/ the_urban_school_food_alliance_and_the_alliance_for_a _healthier_generation_leverage_3_billion_in_purchasing _power_for_market-driven_change_in_school_meals/), the Urban School Food Alliance, a nonprofit coalition of the largest school districts in the United States, and the Alliance for a Healthier Generation have joined forces and with a combined budget of more than $3 billion plan to provide 30 million students with meals that are "nutritionally wholesome, ecologically sound, economically viable and socially responsible."

CHAPTER 11
PUBLIC OPINION AND ACTION ABOUT DIET, WEIGHT, NUTRITION, AND PHYSICAL ACTIVITY

Knowledge may or may not translate into power. Obliviousness far more reliably translates into powerlessness. Parents cannot ignore the threat of obesity to our children and still hope to fix it. We can, however, fix it, without fixating on it. The BMI is just a measure of potential health risk, like a dashboard indicator light. When it flashes, it is not an indication of failure or neglect, but an invitation for corrective action before things go from bad to worse.

—David L. Katz, " Oblivobesity: Looking over the Overweight That Parents Keep Overlooking" (*Childhood Obesity*, vol. 11, no. 3, June 2015)

Obesity in America is increasing. According to Jenna Levy of the Gallup Organization, in *U.S. Obesity Rate Inches Up to 27.7% in 2014* (January 26, 2015, http://www.gallup.com/poll/181271/obesity-rate-inches-2014.aspx), in 2015 the adult obesity rate was 27.7%, up from 27.1% in 2013. (See Figure 11.1.) Worse still, 4% are people with a BMI of 40 or greater, termed class III obesity, and this percentage is the highest Gallup has found in seven years of surveying Americans' weight. (See Figure 11.2.)

In the United States obesity rates rose between 2008 and 2014 in every age and socioeconomic group, in every geographic region, and among people of all races and ethnicities, except Hispanics. The greatest increases were among adults aged 65 years and older and those aged 45 to 64 years. (See Table 11.1.)

Obesity takes a toll on Americans' well-being. In 2014 individuals with class III obesity had the lowest self-perceived well-being scores on a scale of 0 to 100 in five areas that contribute to well-being: purpose, social relationships, finances, community engagement, and physical health. Interestingly, people who were underweight had lower well-being scores than those who were overweight. Not surprisingly, people of normal weight reported the highest levels of well-being. (See Table 11.2.)

AMERICANS ARE WORRIED ABOUT THEIR WEIGHT

In *Nearly Half in U.S. Remain Worried about Their Weight* (July 25, 2014, http://www.gallup.com/poll/174089/nearly-half-remain-worried-weight.aspx), Joy Wilke of the Gallup Organization observes that 45% of Americans worry about their weight "all or some of the time." About two-thirds (67%) of people who describe themselves as overweight worry about their weight compared with 32% of those who consider their weight "about right." (See Figure 11.3.)

The percentage of Americans worried about their weight is considerably higher than the 34% who were worried about their weight in 1990. In a 2014 Gallup survey women (55%) were much more likely to worry about their weight than were men (35%). At that time one-fifth (21%) of women worried "all of the time" and a third (34%) of women worried "some of the time" about their weight, compared with 9% of men who worried about their weight all of the time and 26% of men who worried some of the time. In 2014 concern about weight was highest among those aged 30 to 64 years. (See Table 11.3.)

Although 45% of Americans reported being worried about their weight in 2014, just 29% were seriously trying to lose weight. (See Figure 11.4.) Women (35%) and nonwhite Americans (41%) were more likely to be making serious attempts to lose weight than were men (22%) and whites (24%). (See Table 11.4.) About half (49%) of those trying to lose weight said it is to improve their health, 29% want to lose weight to address a medical problem such as diabetes or hypertension, and 23% want to look better. (See Table 11.5.)

CONSUMER ATTITUDES AND BEHAVIORS TOWARD DIET AND HEALTH

The International Food Information Council reports in the 10th annual *Food and Health Survey 2015* (2015,

FIGURE 11.1

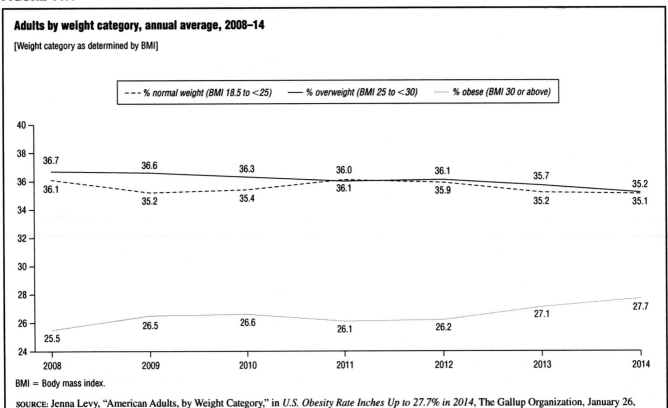

Adults by weight category, annual average, 2008–14

[Weight category as determined by BMI]

--- % normal weight (BMI 18.5 to <25) ——— % overweight (BMI 25 to <30) ········· % obese (BMI 30 or above)

BMI = Body mass index.

FIGURE 11.2

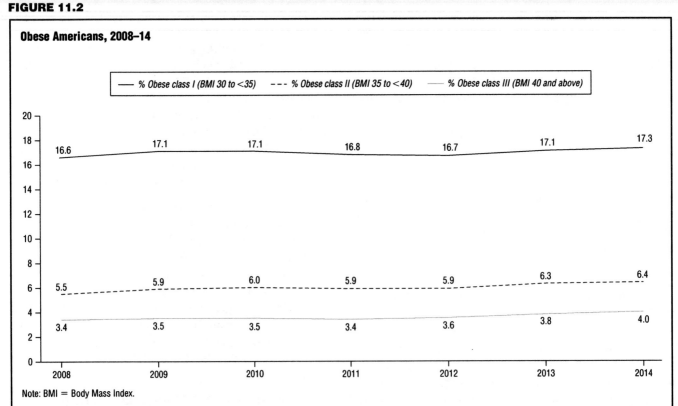

Obese Americans, 2008–14

——— % Obese class I (BMI 30 to <35) --- % Obese class II (BMI 35 to <40) ········· % Obese class III (BMI 40 and above)

Note: BMI = Body Mass Index.

TABLE 11.1

Obesity by demographic characteristics, 2008 and 2014

[Among adults aged 18 and older]

	2008	2014	Difference
	%	%	(pct. pts.)
National adults	25.5	27.7	2.2
Aged 65+	23.4	27.4	4.0
Aged 45 to 64	29.5	33.0	3.5
Midwest	26.8	29.7	2.9
Women	23.9	26.7	2.8
Whites	24.3	26.7	2.4
Aged 30 to 44	27.0	29.3	2.3
South	26.9	29.2	2.3
Annual income less than $36,000	30.0	32.3	2.3
Annual income $90,000+	21.1	23.1	2.0
East	24.7	26.6	1.9
Annual income $36,000 to $89,999	25.8	27.7	1.9
West	22.8	24.6	1.8
Men	27.0	28.7	1.7
Blacks	35.0	35.5	0.5
Aged 18 to 29	17.4	17.7	0.3
Hispanics	28.8	28.3	−0.5

SOURCE: Jenna Levy, "Percentage Obese in U.S. among Various Demographic Groups," in *U.S. Obesity Rate Inches Up to 27.7% in 2014*, The Gallup Organization, January 26, 2015, http://www.gallup.com/poll/181271/obesity-rate-inches-2014.aspx?g_source=weight&g_medium=search&g_campaign=tiles (accessed November 6, 2015). Copyright © 2015 Gallup, Inc. All rights reserved. The content is used with permission; however, Gallup retains all rights of republication.

TABLE 11.2

Well-being by weight category, 2014

[Well-Being Index scores on a scale of 0–100]

	WBI mean score
Underweight	62.2
Normal weight	64.5
Overweight	63.0
Obese class I	57.5
Obese class II	54.7
Obese class III	50.9

SOURCE: Jenna Lèvy, "Average Well-Being Index Scores, by Weight Category, 2014," in *U.S. Obesity Rate Inches Up to 27.7% in 2014*, The Gallup Organization, January 26, 2015, http://www.gallup.com/poll/181271/obesity-rate-inches-2014.aspx?g_source=weight&g_medium=search&g_campaign=tiles (accessed November 6, 2015). Copyright © 2015 Gallup, Inc. All rights reserved. The content is used with permission; however, Gallup retains all rights of republication.

http://www.foodinsight.org/sites/default/files/2015-Food-and-Health-Survey-Full-Report.pdf) that in 2015 nearly half of Americans gave a lot of thought to the healthfulness of the foods and beverages they consume and about the same proportion think about their level of physical activity. Other key survey findings include:

- Taste, price, and healthfulness continue to drive food choices, but Americans feel less strongly about these—healthfulness in particular—than they did in 2014.

- One in five Americans spends less than 15 minutes cooking or preparing dinner on the average weekday.

- Those who already spend more time cooking/preparing dinner also are more likely to spend any extra time they have on food- or diet-related activities.

- Given the choice of losing money or gaining weight, women would rather lose money while men are evenly split between the two options.

- Four out of five Americans are trying to lose weight or maintain their current weight.

- About half of Americans use nutrition information at least occasionally to decide what to choose when eating out and six in 10 want to be able to customize their food at restaurants.

Interestingly, more than half of Americans who rate their health as "excellent" or "very good" are overweight or obese. The top reasons offered for weight management were improvement in physical appearance (56%); increased energy, physical mobility, less tired (55%); improvement in health/overall well-being (53%); increased self-esteem (36%); compliments from friends and family (30%), and stress relief (25%).

When asked in the *Food and Health Survey 2015* which actions would contribute or have contributed to their success in losing weight or maintaining their weight, about half of the survey respondents cited "changing the types of food eaten" (51%) and "making sure I get enough physical activity" (50%), 41% said "eating smaller meals or snacks," 30% said "controlling higher calorie food and beverages," and 24% cited "changing how often I eat throughout the day."

When respondents were asked which methods they would use to manage their weight, the top responses were to eat smaller portions (75%), snack less frequently (68%), track physical activity (67%), eat smaller, more frequent meals and snacks (65%), substitute lower-calorie foods for full-calorie foods (59%), track calories consumed (55%), and eat meals less frequently (46%). About one-third of Americans (32%) say they use support from family and friends to improve the healthfulness of their diet, and more than one in five use a weight-loss plan, an app, or another tracking tool.

The *Food and Health Survey 2015* reveals that the changes Americans made to improve their diets include eating more fruits and vegetables (82%), reducing calorie consumption by drinking water or low- and no-calorie beverages (76%), eating more whole grains (70%), limiting foods with added sugars (69%), consuming smaller portions (68%), and cutting back on foods high in salt (65%).

Americans say that they eat more healthfully at home than at restaurants. Only about half of respondents use nutrition information when deciding what to choose when eating out and about one-quarter either have noticed

FIGURE 11.3

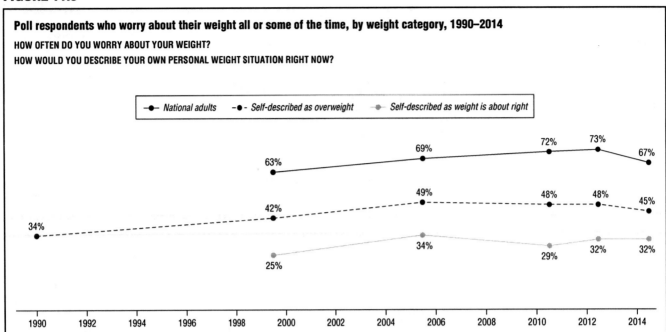

Poll respondents who worry about their weight all or some of the time, by weight category, 1990–2014

HOW OFTEN DO YOU WORRY ABOUT YOUR WEIGHT?

HOW WOULD YOU DESCRIBE YOUR OWN PERSONAL WEIGHT SITUATION RIGHT NOW?

SOURCE: Joy Wilke, "Percentage of Americans Who Worry about Their Weight All or Some of the Time," in *Nearly Half in U.S. Remain Worried about Their Weight*, The Gallup Organization, July 25, 2014, http://www.gallup.com/poll/174089/nearly-half-remain-worried-weight.aspx?g_source=worry%20about%20weight&g_medium=search&g_campaign=tilesx (accessed November 6, 2015). Copyright © 2015 Gallup, Inc. All rights reserved. The content is used with permission; however, Gallup retains all rights of republication.

TABLE 11.3

Poll respondents who worry about their weight, by age and sex, 2014

HOW OFTEN DO YOU WORRY ABOUT YOUR WEIGHT?

	All of the time	Some of the time	Not too often	Never
Gender				
Men	9%	26%	33%	32%
Women	21%	34%	29%	16%
Age				
18–29 years	21%	18%	33%	28%
30–49 years	14%	34%	29%	24%
50–64 years	14%	39%	32%	14%
65+ years	12%	25%	32%	30%

SOURCE: Joy Wilke, "How Often Do You Worry about Your Weight?" in *Nearly Half in U.S. Remain Worried about Their Weight*, The Gallup Organization, July 25, 2014, http://www.gallup.com/poll/174089/nearly-half-remain-worried-weight.aspx?g_source=worry%20about%20weight&g_medium=search&g_campaign=tilesx (accessed November 6, 2015). Copyright © 2015 Gallup, Inc. All rights reserved. The content is used with permission; however, Gallup retains all rights of republication.

nutrition information but have not paid attention to it (35%) or have not noticed or seen nutrition information in restaurants (23%).

As reported in the *Food and Health Survey 2015*, Americans are thinking about physical activity; 53% think about it a lot, and 41% think about it a little. About one-quarter of Americans (25%) try a great deal to control their physical activity, down from 31% in 2013. Those with higher incomes, in better health, and with lower BMI are making more of an effort to control their physical activity, diet, and weight.

Americans in the *Food and Health Survey 2015* cited lack of willpower (37%), lack of time (31%), not seeing results quickly (28%), stress, demanding work or travel schedule (27%), lack of energy (26%), and the cost of healthful foods, weight-loss programs or gym memberships (26%) as major reasons that they do not assume more control over their weight. Younger adults, aged 18 to 34 years, are more likely to name time (45%), stress, demanding work and travel (35%), and cost (33%) as barriers to weight loss and weight management.

Are Americans Getting Enough Exercise to Help Them Manage Their Weight?

In *So Far in 2015, More Americans Exercising Frequently* (July 29, 2015, http://www.gallup.com/poll/184403/far-2015-americans-exercising-frequently.aspx), Rebecca Riffkin of the Gallup Organization reports that more than half (55.5%) of Americans were exercising at least 30 minutes on three or more days per week in mid-2015. According to Mendes, the rate is the highest it has been since Gallup starting tracking it in 2008. (See Figure 11.5.) Younger adults aged 18 to 29 years and upper-income Americans were more likely to exercise frequently. Hispanics were slightly more likely than were whites and African Americans to report exercising frequently. (See Table 11.6.)

FIGURE 11.4

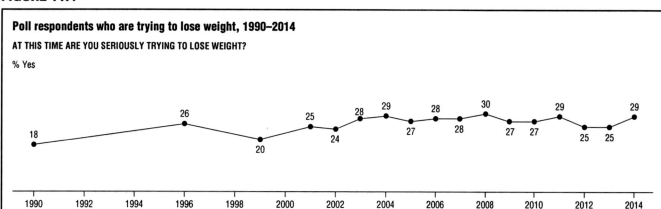

Poll respondents who are trying to lose weight, 1990–2014

AT THIS TIME ARE YOU SERIOUSLY TRYING TO LOSE WEIGHT?

% Yes

SOURCE: Joy Wilke, "At This Time Are You Seriously Trying to Lose Weight?" in *Nearly Half in U.S. Remain Worried about Their Weight*, The Gallup Organization, July 25, 2014, http://www.gallup.com/poll/174089/nearly-half-remain-worried-weight.aspx?g_source=worry%20about%20weight&g_medium=search&g_campaign=tilesx (accessed November 6, 2015). Copyright © 2015 Gallup, Inc. All rights reserved. The content is used with permission; however, Gallup retains all rights of republication.

TABLE 11.4

Poll respondents who are trying to lose weight, by selected characteristics, 2014

AT THIS TIME ARE YOU SERIOUSLY TRYING TO LOSE WEIGHT?

	% Yes, trying to lose weight	% No, not trying
Current weight		
Overweight	54	45
About right	12	88
Underweight	5	95
Gender		
Men	22	78
Women	35	65
Race		
White	24	76
Nonwhite	41	59

SOURCE: Joy Wilke, "Trying to Lose Weight, among Select Groups," in *Nearly Half in U.S. Remain Worried about Their Weight*, The Gallup Organization, July 25, 2014, http://www.gallup.com/poll/174089/nearly-half-remain-worried-weight.aspx?g_source=worry%20about%20weight&g_medium=search&g_campaign=tilesx (accessed November 6, 2015). Copyright © 2015 Gallup, Inc. All rights reserved. The content is used with permission; however, Gallup retains all rights of republication.

TABLE 11.5

Poll respondents who are trying to lose weight, by reasons for weight loss, 2014

WHAT ARE ONE OR TWO OF THE MOST IMPORTANT REASONS WHY YOU ARE TRYING TO LOSE WEIGHT? (ASKED OF THOSE TRYING TO LOSE WEIGHT)

	%
To be healthier	49
For medical/health reasons (diabetes, high blood pressure, etc.)	29
To look better/improve physical appearance	23
To feel better	11
For family/loved ones	6
To be more fit/improve athleticism	5
To improve energy level	4
To prolong [my] life	4
Other	2

SOURCE: Joy Wilke, "Reasons Americans Are Trying to Lose Weight," in *Nearly Half in U.S. Remain Worried about Their Weight*, The Gallup Organization, July 25, 2014, http://www.gallup.com/poll/174089/nearly-half-remain-worried-weight.aspx?g_source=worry%20about%20weight&g_medium=search&g_campaign=tilesx (accessed November 6, 2015). Copyright © 2015 Gallup, Inc. All rights reserved. The content is used with permission; however, Gallup retains all rights of republication.

Americans Consider Obesity a Disease

The way people think about the causes of obesity can influence their views about it being a disease. According to a January 2014 national survey conducted by the Rudd Center for Food Policy and Obesity at the University of Connecticut, six months after the American Medical Association designated obesity as a disease, most Americans supported the disease classification and well over half (58%) thought that there was a medical basis for designating obesity as a disease. In "A National Survey of Public Views about the Classification of Obesity as a Disease" (*Obesity*, vol. 23, no. 6, June 23, 2015), Rebecca M. Puhl and Sai Liu report that most survey respondents agreed that classifying obesity as a disease will prompt more physicians to spend time discussing weight with their patients (61%), help people gain access to obesity treatment (59%), encourage allocation of additional resources to obesity research (58%), and improve reimbursement for weight-loss counseling (55%).

Survey respondents were divided about whether classifying obesity as a disease would serve to increase or reduce obesity-related stigma. More than one-third (37%) thought the disease classification would act to reduce stigma, but 31% thought that stigma might increase.

Few Know All the Risks Associated with Obesity

The results of an Associated Press–NORC Center for Public Affairs Research survey conducted in November

FIGURE 11.5

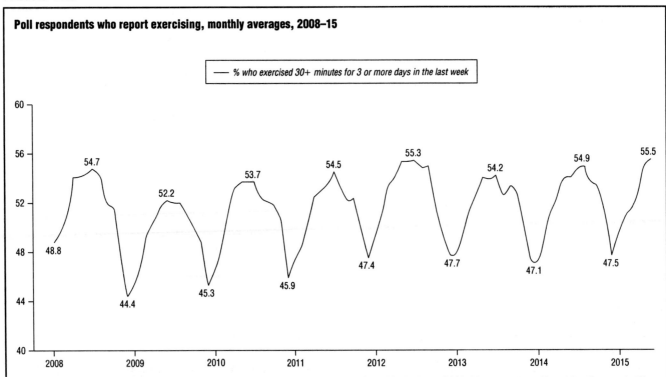

Poll respondents who report exercising, monthly averages, 2008–15

— % who exercised 30+ minutes for 3 or more days in the last week

SOURCE: Rebecca Riffkin, "Record Number of Americans Report Exercising in June 2015," in *So Far in 2015, More Americans Exercising Frequently*, The Gallup Organization, July 29, 2015, http://www.gallup.com/poll/184403/far-2015-americans-exercising-frequently.aspx?g_source=exercise&g_medium=search&g_campaign=tiles (accessed November 6, 2015). Copyright © 2015 Gallup, Inc. All rights reserved. The content is used with permission; however, Gallup retains all rights of republication.

and December 2012 reported in "Obesity in the United States: Public Perceptions" (January 2013, http://www.apnorc.org/PDFs/Obesity/AP-NORC-Obesity-Research-Highlights.pdf) by Trevor Tompson et al. found that although seven in 10 Americans accurately identify heart disease and diabetes as among the most serious consequences of obesity, other health consequences are not as well known. For example, just 15% knew that obesity increases risk for arthritis, 7% of survey respondents named increased cancer risk, only 5% mentioned respiratory disease, and other problems such as infertility were not even mentioned. The survey also found that only about half (52%) of Americans have talked about the health risks and consequences of obesity with their physicians.

Most Oppose Policies That Limit Food Choices

The Associated Press–NORC Center for Public Affairs Research survey also found that although Americans implicate inexpensive junk food as at least in part responsible for the nation's obesity epidemic, six in 10 oppose so called "sin taxes" that would make soda and junk food less affordable.

Many industry observers recommend imposing taxes on unhealthful foods, but others assert that such sin taxes discriminate against the poor and would not effectively change consumers' behavior. For example, in "Regressive Effects Causes and Consequences of

Selective Consumption Taxation" (March 2015, http://mercatus.org/sites/default/files/Hoffer-Selective-Consumption-Taxation.pdf), Adam Hoffer et al. explain that for individuals living in "food deserts" (communities without ready access to fresh, healthful, and affordable food), sin taxes will simply penalize people who have the fewest options and the most difficulty making ends meet. Hoffer et al. contend that consumers need more education about healthy diets and policies that enable grocery stores to open in low-income neighborhoods rather than economic sanctions.

Should Public Policy Stigmatize and Penalize People Who Are Obese?

In 2013 Albert Buitenhuis, a South African chef living in New Zealand—the third-most obese developed country (after the United States and Mexico)—faced deportation because the government of New Zealand determined that he did not have an "acceptable standard of health." When Buitenhuis moved to Christchurch, New Zealand, six years earlier, he weighed 350 pounds but had lost 60 pounds by the time he was to be deported. He worked as a chef, his wife worked as a waitress, and they paid taxes, yet the government argued that the demands Buitenhuis's obesity might place on New Zealand's health care system, which provides free medical care to all permanent residents, could be excessive.

TABLE 11.6

Poll respondents who exercise at least 30 minutes three or more days per week, by sex, age, race/ethnicity, income and region, 2015

[% who exercised for 30+ minutes 3 or more days in the last week]

	% Frequently exercised
Gender	
Male	58.4
Female	52.7
Age	
18–29	64.5
30–44	55.4
45–64	52.9
65+	49.7
Race/ethnicity	
Hispanic	58.5
White	55.7
Black	50.3
Annual household income	
Less than $36,000	51.4
$36,000–$90,000	56.5
$90,000+	59.4
Region	
West	61.9
Midwest	54.7
East	53.8
South	52.6

SOURCE: Rebecca Riffkin, "Frequent Exercise among Various Demographic Groups in June 2015," in *So Far in 2015, More Americans Exercising Frequently*, The Gallup Organization, July 29, 2015, http://www.gallup.com/poll/184403/far-2015-americans-exercising-frequently.aspx?g_source=exercise&g_medium=search&g_campaign=tiles (accessed November 6, 2015). Copyright © 2015 Gallup, Inc. All rights reserved. The content is used with permission; however, Gallup retains all rights of republication.

Some observers opined that the country had a right to protect its economy from the ravages of the obesity epidemic. Others, however, decried New Zealand's actions as unfair, observing that the country does not seek to deport smokers, who also may be costly for the health care system. Arthur L. Caplan declares in "New Zealand's Solution for Rising Health Costs? Deport Fat People" (NBCNews.com, August 11, 2013) that "deporting Albert, especially while he is losing weight, looks for all the world like a sudden attack of unbridled prejudice." In "Kick Out Fat People to Lower Healthcare Costs?" (Medscape.com, October 22, 2013), Caplan states, "There are many ways to wage war on obesity. Deporting people is not one of them. I think we have to take a lesson here. It's important to say that there are all kinds of weaknesses and temptations that have led to our obesity epidemic. We took a long time to eat ourselves into the problem. It will take a long time to work our way out of the problem. But I don't think citizens should have to worry that they are not going to get benefits, that they are going to be penalized or, at the far extreme, thrown out of the country because they have a medical problem."

Buitenhuis appealed the deportation and in September 2013 was granted a 23-month reprieve. In "'Too Fat'

South African Wins Reprieve from New Zealand Deportation" (News24.com, September 9, 2013), the New Zealand associate immigration minister Nikki Kaye (1980–) explains that although Buitenhuis has been granted a work visa, "under this arrangement he is not entitled to publicly-funded health care, and he will have to meet any health costs himself."

Buitenhuis continued to work on his interim visa but in September 2015 once again faced deportation for being clinically obese. Unable to work in New Zealand without a visa, he returned voluntarily to South Africa in December 2015.

NEW YORK CITY FAILS TO LIMIT SALES OF SUGAR-SWEETENED BEVERAGES

Former New York City mayor Michael Bloomberg (1942–) has had a long-standing interest in public health measures and was among the first to ban the use of trans fats and to require calorie counts on chain restaurant menus. In 2013, as mayor, Bloomberg moved to ban the sale of sodas and other sugary beverages larger than 16 ounces (473 ml) in restaurants, movie theaters, stadium concession stands, and other venues in New York City. Convenience stores, vending machines, and some newsstands were unaffected by the ban. In "Health Panel Approves Restriction on Sale of Large Sugary Drinks" (NYTimes.com, September 13, 2012), Michael M. Grynbaum reports that despite protests from some city council members, the former city comptroller, and groups funded by the soft-drink industry, the New York City Board of Health approved the measure.

In "Bloomberg's Ban on Big Sodas Is Unconstitutional: Appeals Court" (Reuters.com, July 30, 2013), Joseph Ax reports that in July 2013 the New York Supreme Court's Appellate Division deemed the mayor's proposed ban unconstitutional, declaring that it "violated the state principle of separation of powers." The appeals court explained that the ruling did not reflect disapproval of the effort to restrict the sale of large sodas. Rather it asked that only "the government body with the authority to do so" enact the laws.

In November 2013 Bloomberg's successor, Mayor-Elect Bill de Blasio (1961–), vowed to appeal the court rejection of the soda ban. In "Bill de Blasio Must Fight New York City's Legal Battles Left by Mike Bloomberg" (NYDailyNews.com, November 18, 2013), Dareh Gregorian and Daniel Beekman reported that de Blasio agreed with Bloomberg about the ban on supersized sodas and would take on the appeal when he assumed office in 2014.

In June 2014 the state's highest court refused to reinstate the Bloomberg ban on the sale of sugary drinks that are 16 ounces (473 ml) or larger, effectively ending the former mayor's effort to curb consumption of beverages associated with obesity. In "New York's Ban on Big Sodas Is Rejected by Final Court" (NYTimes.com, June 26, 2014), Michael M. Grynbaum reports that the New York State Court of Appeals decision represented "a major victory for the American soft-drink industry, which had fought the plan."

Americans Are Concerned about Childhood Obesity

In "Overweight in Children" (August 17, 2015, http://www.heart.org/HEARTORG/GettingHealthy/Over weight-in-Children_UCM_304054_Article.jsp#.Vj6jDo TMp84), the American Heart Association reports that childhood obesity is number one on parents' lists of health concerns, outpacing smoking and drug abuse.

Health professionals are concerned as well. The American Academy of Pediatrics (AAP) guidelines, updated in June 2015, emphasize prevention. The new guidelines exhort pediatricians to assume a more active role in managing children's weight, identifying children at risk for obesity early, and taking steps to prevent weight gain before it becomes a problem. In "Doctors: Childhood Obesity Prevention Must Start Sooner" (CBSNews.com, June 29, 2015), Bianca Seidman reports that although pediatricians can track children's weight, only about half of pediatricians routinely do so.

Many Parents Think Some Sugary Drinks Are Healthful

In March 2013 a panel of experts issued Recommendations for Healthier Beverages (Healthy Eating Research, a National Program of the Robert Wood Johnson Foundation, http://www.rwjf.org/content/dam/farm/reports/issue_briefs/2013/rwjf404852) advising that children aged 13 years and younger drink only water, low-fat and nonfat milk, and 100% juice, and that adolescents aged 14 to 18 years drink only water, low-fat and nonfat milk, 100% juice, and other non-caffeinated, non-fortified beverages with no more than 40 calories per container.

Despite widespread media and health education campaigns promoting the recommendations and emphasizing the importance of limiting children's consumption of added sugars, particularly sugar-sweetened beverages, many parents believe that sugary beverages such as sports drinks, fruit-flavored drinks, and flavored water are healthy choices for children. In "Parents' Beliefs about the Healthfulness of Sugary Drink Options: Opportunities to Address Misperceptions" (*Public Health Nutrition*, March 11, 2015), Christina R. Munsell et al. report that 96% of parents surveyed had given sugary drinks to their children in the month preceding the survey. More than three-quarters (77%) gave children fruit drinks, and 62% gave their children soda. Many parents noted that nutritional claims on packages such as "real"

or "natural," contained vitamin C or antioxidants, or "low in calories" influenced their purchasing behavior.

Are Parents to Blame for Children's Obesity?

There is no question that parents play a pivotal role in terms of preventing childhood obesity by shaping their children's early eating and physical activity habits. However, should overweight children be taken away from their parents?

In "State Intervention in Life-Threatening Childhood Obesity" (*Journal of the American Medical Association*, vol. 306, no. 2, July 13, 2011), Lindsey Murtagh and David S. Ludwig support the use of state intervention in cases of life-threatening obesity. Murtagh and Ludwig point out that "improper feeding practices, causing undernourishment and failure to thrive, have long been addressed through the child abuse and neglect framework." Murtagh and Ludwig assert that physicians are or should be obligated to inform child protective services in "cases of children for whom chronic parental neglect has resulted in severe weight-related health complications." In contrast, Susan Z. Yanovski, Jack A. Yanovski, and Mary Horlick note in "Life-Threatening Childhood Obesity and Legal Intervention" (*Journal of the American Medical Association*, vol. 306, no. 16, October 26, 2011) that obesity is highly heritable and that genetic factors play a key role in risk for obesity.

The article "200 Pound Child Removed from Home Because of Weight" (UPI.com, November 28, 2011) reports that in November 2011 an eight-year-old boy who weighed more than 200 pounds (91 kg) was removed from his home in Ohio and placed in foster care. This action was the first recorded instance of a government agency intervening to remove a child from his or her home because of concern about the child's physical health. According to a spokesperson for the Cuyahoga County Department of Children and Family Services, the third grader was removed because his mother had not done enough to help him lose weight and had failed to comply with his physician's orders. As a result, "case workers considered his mother's failure to reduce his weight a form of medical neglect." A lawyer representing the boy's mother argued that the boy's weight did not pose an imminent danger to his health and that removing him from his family, school, and friends could result in emotional distress.

According to Tara Dodrill in "Ohio Boy Removed from Home Because of Obesity Concerns" (Yahoo News.com, November 28, 2011), the case created a firestorm of commentary in the blogosphere via e-mail, Twitter, and other social media. Many people spoke out in favor of protecting the boy's health and preventing increasingly dire consequences of obesity, whereas others decried removing the child from his home because they feared that the trauma would only compound his problems. Still others called for support services and counseling to help parents and children who are overweight or obese.

In March 2012, after having lived in a foster care home and later with an uncle, the boy had lost 50 pounds and was returned to his mother. The article "200-lbs. Ohio Boy Returned to Mother's Custody after Losing 50 Pounds" (Associated Press, May 11, 2012) notes that despite having moved several times and having changed schools, the boy appeared to be doing well and was continuing to exercise to control his weight.

The United Kingdom also has separated children who are obese from their homes. A February 28, 2014, article in the *Telegraph*, "Obese Children Removed from Families," reports that as many as 74 children were removed from their families from 2011 to 2014 because their excessive weight threatened their health.

Parents Misjudge Children's Weight

Several studies find that parents often misperceive their children's weight and underestimate their risk for obesity in adulthood. For example, Dustin Duncan et al. analyzed National Health and Nutrition Examination Survey data from two groups of children over two periods, 1988–1994 and 2007–2012, and reported their results in "Change in Misperception of Child's Body Weight among Parents of American Preschool Children" (*Childhood Obesity*, vol. 11, no. 4, August 2015). The researchers queried parents' regarding whether they thought their children aged two to five years were overweight, underweight, or just about the right weight. They determined whether the parents' assessments were accurate by comparing their responses with reported information about their child's weight and height.

Nearly all parents of overweight boys from the first study group thought their sons were "about the right weight" (97%), as did parents in the second study group

(95%). Parents of overweight girls also misjudged their daughters' weight, with 88% in the first study describing their daughters as "about the right weight" and 93% in the second study group.

Especially concerning is the fact that the children in the second study group were significantly more overweight than the children in the first study group, yet the parents' misperceptions of their children's weight was not very different. Of parents surveyed, lower-income and African American parents had the most difficulty accurately gauging their children's weight. This finding is significant because low-income and African American children have the highest rates of obesity. Parents' misperceptions are important because they may delay intervention to help children achieve and maintain a healthy weight.

The researchers speculate that one reason parents misperceive their children's weight is their tendency to compare the children to others to judge their weight. As Americans have become heavier, the perception of a healthy weight also has changed. The researchers also attribute the misperception to the fact that many parents simply do not know how much their children should weigh.

In the editorial "Oblivobesity: Looking over the Overweight That Parents Keep Overlooking" (*Childhood Obesity*, vol. 11, no. 3, June 2015), David Katz observes that parental obliviousness to obesity in children hampers efforts to combat the problem, "We do not always fix what we know to be broken, but we virtually never fix what we are overlooking." Katz explains, "Parents cannot ignore the threat of obesity to our children and still hope to fix it. We can, however, fix it, without fixating on it. The BMI is just a measure of potential health risk, like a dashboard indicator light. When it flashes, it is not an indication of failure or neglect, but an invitation for corrective action before things go from bad to worse."

IMPORTANT NAMES
AND ADDRESSES

Academy for Eating Disorders
111 Deer Lake Rd., Ste. 100
Deerfield, IL 60015
(847) 498-4274
FAX: (847) 480-9282
E-mail: info@aedweb.org
URL: http://www.aedweb.org/

Academy of Nutrition and Dietetics
120 S. Riverside Plaza, Ste. 2000
Chicago, IL 60606-6995
(312) 899-0040
1-800-877-1600
URL: http://www.eatright.org/

American Academy of Sleep Medicine
2510 N. Frontage Rd.
Darien, IL 60561
(630) 737-9700
FAX: (630) 737-9790
URL: http://www.aasmnet.org/

American Cancer Society
250 Williams St. NW
Atlanta, GA 30303
1-800-227-2345
URL: http://www.cancer.org/

American Diabetes Association
1701 N. Beauregard St.
Alexandria, VA 22311
1-800-342-2383
URL: http://www.diabetes.org/

American Heart Association
7272 Greenville Ave.
Dallas, TX 75231
1-800-242-8721
URL: http://www.americanheart.org/

**American Society for Metabolic and
Bariatric Surgery**
100 SW 75th St., Ste. 201
Gainesville, FL 32607
(352) 331-4900
FAX: (352) 331-4975
URL: http://www.asmbs.org/

Arthritis Foundation
1355 Peachtree St. NE, Sixth Floor
Atlanta, GA 30309
(404) 872-7100
1-800-283-7800
URL: http://www.arthritis.org/

Atkins Nutritionals, Inc.
1050 17th St., Ste. 1500
Denver, CO 80265
1-800-628-5467
URL: http://www.atkins.com/

**Center for Science in the
Public Interest**
1220 L St. NW, Ste. 300
Washington, DC 20005
(202) 332-9110
FAX: (202) 265-4954
E-mail: cspi@cspinet.org
URL: http://www.cspinet.org/

**Centers for Disease Control and
Prevention**
1600 Clifton Rd.
Atlanta, GA 30329-4027
1-800-232-4636
URL: http://www.cdc.gov/

**Council on Size and Weight
Discrimination**
PO Box 305
Mt. Marion, NY 12456
(845) 679-1209
FAX: (845) 679-1206
E-mail: info@cswd.org
URL: http://www.cswd.org/

Eating Disorders Coalition
PO Box 96503-98807
Washington, DC 20090
(202) 543-9570
URL: http://www.eatingdisorderscoalition.org/

Federal Trade Commission
600 Pennsylvania Ave. NW
Washington, DC 20580

(202) 326-2222
1-877-382-4357
URL: http://www.ftc.gov/

International Food Information Council
1100 Connecticut Ave. NW, Ste. 430
Washington, DC 20036
(202) 296-6540
E-mail: info@foodinsight.org
URL: http://www.foodinsight.org/

**National Association of Anorexia
Nervosa and Associated Disorders**
750 E. Diehl Rd., Ste. 127
Naperville, IL 60563
(630) 577-1330
E-mail: anadhelp@anad.org
URL: http://www.anad.org/

**National Association of
Cognitive-Behavioral Therapists**
102 Gilson Ave.
Weirton, WV 26062
1-800-253-0167
URL: http://www.nacbt.org/

**National Association to Advance Fat
Acceptance**
PO Box 4662
Foster City, CA 94404-0662
(916) 558-6880
URL: http://www.naafa.org/

National Center for Health Statistics
3311 Toledo Rd., Rm. 5419
Hyattsville, MD 20782-2064
1-800-232-4636
URL: http://www.cdc.gov/nchs/

**National Diabetes Information
Clearinghouse**
One Information Way
Bethesda, MD 20892-3560
(301) 654-3327
1-800-860-8747
E-mail: ndic@info.niddk.nih.gov
URL: http://diabetes.niddk.nih.gov/

National Digestive Diseases Information Clearinghouse
Two Information Way
Bethesda, MD 20892-3570
(301) 654-3810
1-800-891-5389
E-mail: nddic@info.niddk.nih.gov
URL: http://digestive.niddk.nih.gov/

National Eating Disorders Association
165 W. 46th St., Ste. 402
New York, NY 10036
(212) 575-6200
1-800-931-2237
FAX: (212) 575-1650
E-mail: info@NationalEatingDisorders.org
URL: http://www.nationaleatingdisorders.org/

National Heart, Lung, and Blood Institute
PO Box 30105
Bethesda, MD 20824-0105
(301) 592-8573
E-mail: nhlbiinfo@nhlbi.nih.gov
URL: http://www.nhlbi.nih.gov/

National Institute of Diabetes and Digestive and Kidney Diseases
Bldg. 31, Rm. 9A06
31 Center Dr., MSC 2560
Bethesda, MD 20892-2560
(301) 496-3583
URL: http://www.niddk.nih.gov/

National Mental Health Association
2000 N. Beauregard St., Sixth Floor
Alexandria, VA 22311

(703) 684-7722
1-800-969-6642
FAX: (703) 684-5968
URL: http://www.nmha.org/

National Women's Health Information Center
PO Box 430
Red Bank, NJ 07701
(732) 530-3425
1-877-986-9472
FAX: (732) 865-7225
E-mail: info@healthywomen.org
URL: http://www.healthywomen.org/

Obesity Medicine Association
101 University Blvd., Ste. 330
Denver, CO 80206
(303) 770-2526
FAX: (303) 779-4834
E-mail: info@obesitymedicine.org
URL: http://www.asbp.org/

Obesity Society
8757 Georgia Ave., Ste. 1320
Silver Spring, MD 20910
(301) 563-6526
FAX: (301) 563-6595
URL: http://www.obesity.org/

Office on Women's Health U.S. Department of Health and Human Services
200 Independence Ave. SW, Rm. 712E
Washington, DC 20201
(202) 690-7650

1-800-994-9662
FAX: (202) 205-2631
URL: http://www.womenshealth.gov/

Rudd Center for Food Policy and Obesity University of Connecticut
One Constitution Plaza, Ste. 600
Hartford, CT 06103
(860) 380-1000
FAX: (860) 509-0009
E-mail: rudd.center@uconn.edu
URL: http://www.uconnruddcenter.org/

TOPS Club Inc.
4575 S. Fifth St.
Milwaukee, WI 53207
(414) 482-4620
URL: http://www.tops.org/

Weight Watchers International Inc.
175 Crossways Park West
Woodbury, NY 11797
(516) 390-1400
1-800-651-6000
FAX: (516) 390-1334
URL: http://www.weightwatchers.com/

Weight-Control Information Network
One WIN Way
Bethesda, MD 20892-3665
1-877-946-4627
FAX: (301) 634-0716
E-mail: win@info.niddk.nih.gov
URL: http://win.niddk.nih.gov/index.htm

RESOURCES

The Centers for Disease Control and Prevention (CDC) tracks nationwide health trends, including overweight and obesity, and reports its findings in several periodicals, especially its *Health, United States* and *Morbidity and Mortality Weekly Reports*. The *National Vital Statistics Reports*, which is issued by the CDC's National Center for Health Statistics (NCHS), gives detailed information on U.S. births, birth weights, and death data and trends. The NCHS also compiles and analyzes demographic data—the heights and weights of a representative sample of the U.S. population—to develop standards for desirable weights. The National Health Interview Surveys, the National Health Examination Surveys, the National Health and Nutrition Examination Surveys, and the Behavioral Risk Factor Surveillance System offer ongoing information about the lifestyles, health behaviors, and health risks of Americans. Working with other agencies and professional organizations, the CDC produced *Healthy People 2020*, which serves as a blueprint for improving the health status of Americans.

The U.S. Department of Agriculture provides nutrition guidelines for Americans, and the Federal Trade Commission (FTC) has launched initiatives to educate consumers and the media about false and deceptive weight-loss advertising. The FTC is one of about 50 members of the Partnership for Healthy Weight Management, a coalition of scientific, academic, health care, government, commercial, and public-interest representatives that aims to increase public awareness of the obesity epidemic and to promote responsible marketing of weight-loss products and programs.

The relationship between birth weight and future health risks has been examined by many researchers, and the studies cited in this text were reported in *American Journal of Epidemiology*, *American Journal of Obstetrics and Gynecology*, *Breast Cancer Research*, *Circulation*, *Journal of Clinical Endocrinology and Metabolism*,

Medicine and Science in Sports and Exercise, *Obesity*, *Pediatrics*, *PLoS One*, and *Seminars in Reproductive Medicine*. Data from the CDC Pregnancy Nutrition Surveillance System show that very overweight women benefit from reduced weight gain during pregnancy to help reduce the risk for high-birth-weight infants.

The World Health Organization and the National Institutes of Health provide definitions, epidemiological data, and research findings about a comprehensive range of public health issues, including diet, nutrition, overweight, and obesity. The Central Intelligence Agency's *World Factbook* provides longevity estimates. The National Heart, Lung, and Blood Institute conducts research about obesity and overweight. Weight-control information and updated weight-for-height tables that incorporate height, weight, and body mass index are published by the National Institute of Diabetes and Digestive and Kidney Diseases (the part of the National Institutes of Health that is primarily responsible for obesity- and nutrition-related research). The National Institute of Mental Health offers information about eating disorders as well as the mental health issues that are related to obesity.

The origins, causes, and consequences of the obesity epidemic and eating disorders have been described in numerous professional and consumer publications, including *Academic Pediatrics*; *American Journal of Clinical Nutrition*; *American Journal of Nutrition*; *American Journal of Preventive Medicine*; *American Journal of Public Health*; *Annual Review of Clinical Psychology*; *Archives of General Psychiatry*; *Archives of Pediatrics and Adolescent Medicine*; *Biological Psychiatry*; *British Journal of Psychiatry*; *Clinical Medicine & Research*; *Contemporary OB/GYN*; *Diabetes Care*; *Diabetes, Obesity, and Metabolism*; *Endocrinology and Metabolism Clinics*; *European Eating Disorders Review*; *Health Affairs*; *Hormone Research in Pediatrics*; *Human Reproduction*; *International*

Journal of Behavioral Nutrition and Physical Activity; *International Journal of Obesity*; *Journal of Adolescent Health*; *Journal of the American Medical Association*; *Journal of Clinical Nursing*; *Journal of Genomics*; *Lancet*; *Lancet Oncology*; *Mediators of Inflammation*; *Medical Decision Making*; *Nature*; *Nature Communications*; *Nature Reviews Endocrinology*; *New England Journal of Medicine*; *Obesity Reviews*; *Obesity Surgery*; *PLoS Medicine*; *Stroke*; and *Trends in Pharmacological Sciences*.

Many excellent books and publications provided valuable insight into the obesity epidemic. Peter N. Stearns, in *Fat History: Bodies and Beauty in the Modern West* (1997), and Laura Fraser, in *Losing It: False Hopes and Fat Profits in the Diet Industry* (1998), offer detailed histories of magical cures and weight-loss fads. In *The Fattening of America: How the Economy Makes Us Fat, If It Matters, and What to Do about It* (2008), Eric A. Finkelstein and Laurie Zuckerman observe that Americans consumed 1,000 calories more per week in 2008 than they did in 1985. David A. Kessler, the former commissioner of the U.S. Food and Drug Administration, explains in *The End of Overeating: Taking Control of the Insatiable American Appetite* (2009) how the desire to eat and overeat originates in the brain and is triggered by a variety of combinations of salt, fat, and sugar in the American diet.

Medical and public health societies, along with advocacy organizations, professional associations, and foundations, offer a wealth of information about the relationship between weight, health, and disease. Sources cited in this edition include the Academy of Nutrition and Dietetics, the American Heart Association, the American Medical Association, the American Obesity Association, the Center for Consumer Freedom, the Center for Science in the Public Interest, the International Size Acceptance Association, the National Academy of Sciences, the National Association to Advance Fat Acceptance, the National Eating Disorders Association, the Pharmacy Benefit Management Institute, the Robert Wood Johnson Foundation, and the Trust for America's Health.

The Trust for America's Health/Robert Wood Johnson Foundation publication *The State of Obesity 2015: Better Policies for a Healthier America* (September 2015) provided data and insight into the obesity epidemic. The Gallup Organization makes available valuable poll and survey data about Americans' attitudes about overweight, obesity, physical activity, diet, and nutrition. Finally, many professional associations, voluntary medical organizations, and foundations dedicated to research, education, and advocacy about eating disorders, overweight, and obesity provided up-to-date information that was included in this edition.

INDEX

trying to lose weight, poll respondents, 177f

workplace sitting time, 169

worry about weight, 173, 176t

Genetics

attitudes toward obesity, 144

childhood overweight and obesity, 65–66

diet and weight-loss myths, 149

eating disorders, 48, 51–52, 54

and environmental influences, 33

metabolic syndrome, 45

and obesity, 31t, 32t

obesity causes, 31–33

research, 11–12

thinness, 33

Genomics. *See* Genetics

Gestational diabetes, 44

The G.I. Diet (Gallop), 89

Glucose, 19

Glycemic index, 89, 93–96

Gofman, John W., 86

Government agricultural subsidies, 132, 165

Group therapy, 53

Guaranteed success claims, 156

Gynoid obesity, 7

H

Hartwig, Dallas, 90

Hartwig, Melissa, 90

HDL cholesterol, 33–34, 45–46

Health care

behavioral counseling delivered by physicians, 113

employers' obesity-related costs, 124–125

obese patients, accommodating, 127

overweight and obesity expenditures, 117–120

preventive health services, 142

primary care physicians, 113

spending on, 1

weight bias among health professionals, 141–142

Health insurance

childhood and adolescent obesity treatment, 118–119

community prevention programs coverage, 170–171

obesity as a disease, 30

Obesity Society action plan, 137

weight-loss treatment coverage, 30

Health issues

added sugars, effects of, 133

android and gynoid obesity, 7

anorexia nervosa, medical complications of, 50

birth weight, effects of, 4

bulimia, 51

cancer, 42

cardiovascular disease, 33–36

classification of overweight and obesity by body mass index and waist circumference, 8t

consumer attitudes toward, 173, 175–176

eating disorders, health consequences of, 49t

fatty liver disease, 41

fruit and vegetable consumption, 165

gallbladder disease, 40–41

history of dieting, 86

metabolic syndrome, 44–46

morbidity and mortality related to overweight and obesity, 25

obesity during pregnancy, 43

osteoarthritis and joint injury, 39–40

overweight, obesity, and untreated dental carries, 34t–35t

overweight and obesity, 29t

overweight and obesity among children and adolescents, 76–77

physical activity benefits, 106, 107–108

risk factors for selected health conditions, by selected characteristics, 34t–35t

self-perceived well-being, 173, 175(t11.2)

sugar compared to tobacco, 131–132

type 2 diabetes, 36–39

very-low-calorie diets, 157–158

weight loss, harmfulness of, 115–116

weight-loss drug side effects, 109

women's reproductive health, 43–44

Health professionals, 113, 141–142

Health promotion programs, 55

Healthy, Hunger-Free Kids Act, 137

Healthy Communities initiative, 160

Healthy Eating Index, 167

Healthy Schools Program, 171–172

Healthy weight. *See* Ideal weight

Healthy Weight Commitment Foundation, 140–141

Heart defects, 44

Herbal products, 149

Heritability studies. *See* Genetics

High birth weight, 4, 5

High cholesterol, 33–34, 34t–35t, 86

High-density lipoprotein cholesterol, 33–34, 45–46

High-fat diets, 87–88

High-fructose corn syrup, 19, 20t–21t

High-protein diets, 87–88, 99

H.J. Heinz Company, 86

Hospitals, 127

Hot Topic (company), 127

Hydrostatic weighing, 7

Hyman, Mark, 114

Hyperandrogenism, 43

Hypercholesterolemia, 33–34, 34t–35t

Hyperlipidemias, 76

Hypertension, 34, 34t–35t, 36t–37t, 77

Hypnosis, 115

I

Ideal weight, 5–10, 64t

IFIC (International Food Information Council), 165, 171, 173

Impulsive behaviors, 52–53

Incentives for weight loss, 120, 151–152

Infants, 4, 5

Institute of Food Technologists, 167

Institute of Medicine, 75

Insurance. *See* Health insurance; Life insurance industry

Interagency Working Group on Food Marketed to Children, 71

Internal Revenue Service, 30

International Diabetes Federation, 45

International Food Information Council, 165, 171, 173

International issues

politics of obesity, 129–132

weight-based discrimination, 141

International Sugar Organization, 130

Interpersonal issues and eating disorders, 48

Interpersonal psychotherapy, 53

Ischemic strokes, 35

Israel, 58

Italy, 57–58

J

Jameson, Gardner, 87

Jay Z, 90

Jazzercise Inc., 143

Jenny Craig, 88, 114

Joint injury, 39–40, 40f

Juice fasts, 90

Junk food, 138

K

Khan, Mehmood, 140

Kind, Ron, 137

Knee pain, 40

L

Labels, nutrition, 134–135, 136f

Labor and delivery, 43

Lacto-ovo vegetarian menu, 98(t5.10)

Lancet, 7

Lane Bryant, 127

Lanzalotta, Stephen, 89

The Last Chance Diet—When Everything Else Has Failed (Linn), 88

Laws and regulations

New York City supersized soda ban, 179–180

penalizing obese people, 178–179

public opinion, 178

CPSIA information can be obtained
at www.ICGtesting.com
Printed in the USA
FFOW05n0905230916

9 781573 027069